RECENT ADVANCES IN HEMATOLOGY RESEARCH

THALASSEMIA

CAUSES, TREATMENT OPTIONS AND LONG-TERM HEALTH OUTCOMES

RECENT ADVANCES IN HEMATOLOGY RESEARCH

Additional books in this series can be found on Nova's website under the Series tab.

Additional e-books in this series can be found on Nova's website under the e-book tab.

RECENT ADVANCES IN HEMATOLOGY RESEARCH

THALASSEMIA

CAUSES, TREATMENT OPTIONS AND LONG-TERM HEALTH OUTCOMES

MAKENZIE GREENE
EDITOR

New York

For permission to use material from this book please contact us:
Telephone 631-231-7269; Fax 631-231-8175
Web Site: http://www.novapublishers.com

Library of Congress Cataloging-in-Publication Data

ISBN: 978-1-63117-954-9

Library of Congress Control Number: 2014938749

Published by Nova Science Publishers, Inc. † New York

Contents

Preface

Thalassemia is one of the most common genetic disorders worldwide and presents major public health and social challenges in areas of high incidence. The frequency of this disorder varies considerably with geographic locations and racial groups. Thalassemia refers to a group of inherited hemolytic anemia disorders that involve defects in the synthesis of hemoglobin α- or β-polypeptide chains. It leads to decreased hemoglobin production and hypochromic microcytic anemia associated with erythrocyte dysplasia and destruction. Homozygous β-thalassemia (also known as thalassemia major, Cooley's anemia, or Mediterranean anemia) is associated with the most severe signs and symptoms. Thalassemia major (TM) is a life-threatening condition that commonly manifests during early infancy, after which progressive pallor, severe anemia, and failure to thrive are common. Children with TM often develop feeding problems, recurrent fever, bleeding tendencies (especially epistaxis), susceptibility to infection, pathologic fractures of long bones and vertebrae, endocrine abnormalities, splenomegaly, lack of sexual maturation, and growth retardation. This book discusses cures and treatments available for thalassemia, as well as the causes and the type of long-term health outcomes it may cause.

Chapter 1 - Since the first cord blood transplantation performed by Gluckman and colleagues (1988), there have been many medical indications that have been proven for this stem cell therapy in the last two and half decades. Besides the standard hematological indications for bone marrow transplantation, such as leukemias, lymphomas, SCIDs, and aplastic anemia, cord blood transplantation has also been a proven curative therapy for non-hematological indications such as Krabbe's, osteopetrosis etc. As transplant related mortality, overall survival and disease-free survival for cord blood transplantation continue to improve with optimal conditioning regimens, better GvHD and infection prophylaxis and treatment, closer HLA matching and optimal cord blood product selection afforded by larger inventories, double cord blood transplantation and the availability of high cell dose cord blood products, the utility of this stem cell source will expand to certain indications which in the past, rarely used related or unrelated cord blood transplantation. For patients, families, referring and transplant physicians to accept allogeneic cord blood transplantation for indications such as thalassemia, sickle cell disease, severe autoimmune diseases or HIV, the benefit-risk ratio has to be significantly improved so that it is worthwhile for patients to take a chance on a risky procedure in order to prolong lifespan or improve quality of life. The authors review in this Chapter some of the efforts to improve clinical outcome of related and unrelated cord blood transplantation for thalassemia through increasing infused cord blood nucleated and CD34+ cell dosage using a combination of three strategies – (1) cord blood products manufactured using technologies that maximize cell dosage recoveries, (2) double cord blood transplantation whenever appropriate, and (3) the no-wash thaw and direct infusion method advocated by Chow et al.

Chapter 2 - Thalassemias are characterized by insufficient or absent synthesis of the globin chains. An imbalanced production of one of the globin chains leads to accumulation and precipitation of unpaired globin chains and consequently to ineffective erythropoiesis and hemolysis. Characteristically, patients affected with α or β-thalassemia show microcytic hemolytic anemia.

Although thalassemia is endemic to the Mediterranean basin and countries of the Far East, there is virtually no country in the world in which thalassemia does not affect some percentage of the inhabitants.

Thalassemia syndromes are among the most common genetic disorders worldwide, with 1.7% of the world's population carrying thalassemic genes in endemic countries represents a major public health problem. The β-thalassemias have an estimated annual incidence of symptomatic individuals of 1 in 100,000 throughout the world and 1 in 10,000 people in the European Union. Data from recent epidemiological surveys indicate that in Europe there are approximately 15,000 subjects with transfusion dependent thalassemia major.

While the majority of patients show significant microcytosis and some borderline anemia, the increase of HbA_2 mostly distinguishes β-thalassemia minor from other conditions like iron-deficiency.

The diagnosis of β thalassemia involves measuring $HgbA_2$ concentration of lysed red cells via high-performance liquid chromatography, with an ion-exchange column or electrophoresis methods. This measurement is considered the "gold standard".

Differentiation between thalassemic and non thalassemic microcytosis has important clinical implications, because each has entirely different cause, pathogenesis, prognosis and treatment.

As in all chronic diseases prevention is important in the overall management of the disease; the real danger of non-diagnosis or misdiagnosis of the carriers of thalassemia trait is the potential homozygous offspring: an appropriate screening, detection of patients and counselling of couples at risk are the most important procedures for the reduction of morbidity and mortality of the patients.

Iron-Deficiency Anemia (IDA) and thalassemia have different ethiologies, which renders typical profiles in the hemogram data, erythrocytosis and microcytosis in carriers, anisocytosis in iron deficiency; nevertheless, the results can be very similar and based on the individual parameters of the hemogram is difficult to recognise a carrier in daily practice.

A discriminant formula or index based on red cells parameters would be a useful tool in the investigation of microcytic anemia. The indices usefulness is to detect patients with a high probability to be β thalassemia carriers, so the best index must have as high sensitivity as possible, in order to detect almost all β thalassemia patients. Suspicious samples can be selected for HbA_2 analysis, to confirm the presumptive diagnosis of the disease.

β thalassemia can be diagnosed with confidence when raised HbA_2, erythrocytosis, microcytosis and normal serum ferritin are present.

The screening of hemoglobinopathies must rely on inexpensive methods, adding in the selection of highly suspicious samples for further analysis, more sophisticated and expensive.

Red Blood Cells (RBCs) indices are useful tools, can be calculated from data reported by the analyzers so every laboratory can apply this strategy, improving productivity, adding value and quality to the Laboratory reports.

Chapter 3 - The distribution of thalassaemias is global, with particular incidence in areas affected by malaria as the Mediterranean area (Italy, Greece, Turkey, Cyprus) and in southeast Asia (India, Vietnam, Cambodia). Screening of the heterozygous population is fundamental for keeping thalassaemic pathology diffusion under control.

Thalassaemia recognition is based on a first-level analysis performed with haemochromocytometric data and a second-level examination (HbA_2 quantification, globin chain synthesis, and genetic analysis). Many of the latter techniques are finalised to a secure diagnosis of the genetic defect and they are time-consuming and expensive, therefore it would be important to have a Computer Aided Diagnosis (CAD) support based mainly on the haemochromocytometric data and on the simple HbA_2 quantification. Such classification through CAD systems would contribute to the selection of cases that need further examination and could be helpful in laboratory quality control.

Several automated expert systems have been proposed to detect thalassaemias. There are different types of α-thalassaemia resulting from different gene mutations and their distribution is dissimilar in different geographic areas. The CAD systems are often optimized on the α-Thalassaemia and β-Thalassaemia types of the area where the software is built.

In this work an overview of some automated systems used for supporting the diagnosis of different Thalassaemia traits is presented.

Chapter 4 - Hemoglobinopathies, namely thalassemia and sickle cell disease, are the most frequent life-threatening non-infectious disease of children globally. In many countries, particularly in South Asia, where the majority of the pediatric population of our planet lives, a significant, and increasing, proportion of healthcare-related expenses is employed for the non-curative supportive care of patients with severe thalassemia.

Major advances in effective oral chelators have heralded a new thalassemia era in which patients are expected to have long and productive lives provided access to long-term appropriate care is available. Unfortunately, this is not always the case for most thalassemics, largely due to costs; appropriate life-long supportive therapy is estimated to cost a minimum of 7.000 USD/year, which is higher than the average income in many thalassemia-prone regions. Moreover, drug or transfusion intolerance, blood-borne infections, osteoporosis and pain, pulmonary hypertension and health-related quality of life (HRQoL) remain some open questions.

In parallel with improvements in supportive care also hematopoietic stem cell transplantation (blood and marrow transplantation or BMT) results have substantially improved over the last decade so that a low-risk patients with a compatible sibling is expected to enjoy over 90% cure probability with improved HRQoL. As opposed to supportive care, however, BMT costs have decreased to the point that it is possible to perform a bone marrow transplant for 15.000 USD, i.e. what is needed for 1-2 years of non-curative supportive care, thus making BMT highly cost-effective. Both the transplant community and international accreditation bodies are becoming increasingly aware that expensive and complex hospital infection control standards may not be required and that current reduced-intensity BMT strategies may be offered even on outpatient basis thus further cutting costs. The new thalassemia era has also provided the ability to induce negative iron balance, reverse some of the organ damage associated with chronic iron overload, downstage high-risk patients and further decrease transplant-related morbidity and mortality. Finally, it is become increasingly feasible to use partially matched related donors, e.g., mother of father, which are available for the great majority of patients. This latter option might be safer, more accessible, less expensive and as widely applicable as upcoming gene therapy.

Chapter 5 - Thalassemia comes from a greek word "*thalassa*" meaning the sea and "*amia*" for blood. The term thalassemia was first used in bordering countries of the Mediterranean Sea. Beta thalassemia is characterized by a quantitative deficiency of beta-globin chains and it is caused often for more than 200 punctual mutations than for deletions. The World Health Organization (WHO) has established that the hemoglobinopathies control, particularly the β-thalassemia, as a main priority in health care. In industrialized and in developing countries the strategies use to diagnose the illness are different, but there are three methods which are the most suitable to detect the anomaly: cellulose acetate membrane electrophoresis at alkaline pH, capillary electrophoresis, or high performance liquid chromatography. Screening programs are highly recommended for the identification of thalassemia carriers in countries where thalassemia prevalence is high. The prospective prevention includes identifying β-thalassemia trait carriers and counseling them about mate selection and prenatal diagnosis, to prevent the birth of a child with a major disease. Carrier diagnosis involves the accurate measurement of red blood count (RBC), mean corpuscular hemoglobin (MCH), mean corpuscular volume (MCV), HbA_2 and HbF values.

In developing countries a differential diagnosis of iron deficiency anemia is necessary. So, β-thalassemia trait carriers can be detected by screening tests like Naked Eye Single Tube Red Cell Osmotic Fragility Test (NESTROFT), and red cell indices, like Mentzer, Shine and Lal (SLI), Green and King, England and Fraser, RDWI (red blood distribution width index) and others. To increase NESTROFT sensitivity the authors proposed the spectrophotometer lecture, and for β-thalassemia trait detection, the use of Mentzer (MCV/RBC), SLI (MCV^2 x MCHb x 0.01) and RDWI (MCV x RDW/RBC) indexes. Ultimately, advances in molecular tests have facilitated the prenatal diagnosis of thalassemia and have allowed the genotyping of the β-thalassemia in different geographic areas. The majority of the common mutations tend to cluster within neighboring regions and its distribution depends of the ethnic group. The thalassemia mutations can be identified by PCR-based techniques. In northwestern of Argentina the authors have recognized the most prevalent mutations by real time PCR. They were a nonsense mutation, Cd39 (C→T), and a RNA processing mutation, IVS-I-1 (G→A).

Chapter 6 - Although in the original design for developing molecular therapies for monogenic diseases thalassemia was presented as the main candidate, yet genetic treatments were only available through two clinical trials only a few years ago with very few patients being enrolled in these studies. The reason for this inconsistency is mainly because molecular/genetic treatments must prove themselves to be safer than the current symptomatic therapies than include transfusion and iron chelation.

This review presents the current status of gene therapy for hemoglobin disorders, reviews the recent results and discusses how the knowledge gained from these trials can be used to develop a safe and effective gene therapy approach for the treatment of β-thalassemia. It also elaborates the next trend in molecular therapies for thalassemia that include manipulation of induced plupipotent stem cells (iPSCs) and gene editing.

Chapter 7 - Beta-thalassaemia (OMIM #613985) is the most common autosomal recessive disorder worldwide. In 2007, 42,409 global conceptions are affected by beta-thalassaemia and half of these occurred in Southeast Asia. To date, there are more than 800 variants in the beta-globin gene out of which more than 280 cause beta-thalassaemia with varying phenotypes (http://globin.bx.psu.edu/hbvar). Molecular diagnosis of these mutations are necessary for establishing proper treatment, disease prognosis and family planning. The development of molecular diagnostic methods to detect beta-thalassaemia is largely dependent on the prevalence and spectrum of mutations in the population. Direct sequencing is the gold standard to detect point mutations in or near the beta-globin gene which cause >90% of beta-thalassaemia defects. Multiplex ligation-dependent probe amplification (MLPA) detects deletions or duplications by quantitative amplification of multiple probe pairs hybridised across the beta-globin gene clusters. Other methods include amplification refractory mutation system (ARMS), reversed dot blot hybridisation (RDBH), and more recently, pyrosequencing in carrier screening and prenatal diagnosis will be described in this review. In prenatal diagnosis, invasive methods of obtaining fetal cells such as amniocentesis and chorionic villus sampling are necessary. These methods carry up to 1% risk of miscarriage and are unacceptable to some couples. Cell-free fetal DNA from maternal plasma offers an alternative source of fetal genetic material for noninvasive prenatal diagnosis. However, the presence of high levels of maternal DNA impedes the use of conventional methods in detecting mutations in the fetus. Developments including the use of next generation sequencing (NGS) to identify fetal alleles for the detection of beta-thalassaemia mutations amongst a high background maternal alleles will be discussed.

Chapter 8 - The cellular redox status in physiological condition is normally well-balanced between oxidant and antioxidant levels. Oxidative stress is defined as the disturbance state that the production of the oxidants is greater than the efficiency of the antioxidant system. In the pathogenesis of thalassemia, redox-active iron released from excess unpaired globin chains causes oxidative damage to the membrane of mature or immature red blood cells. This leads to increased premature removal of the affected red cells, ineffective erythropoiesis, chronic anemia, and finally, iron overload. Thus, patients with thalassemia have inevitably profound oxidative stress that triggers oxidation of intracellular biomolecules; causing tissue damage and then organ failure. Therefore, the antioxidant supplementation may be beneficial for the patients with thalassemia. This article briefly summarizes how oxidative stress raises and discusses several therapeutic strategies using antioxidant(s) to neutralize the oxidative burden in thalassemia; including direct scavenging of free radicals, detoxifying or removing oxidants, or boosting endogenous antioxidants. Several studies and clinical trials on the use of potential antioxidant agents such as pharmaceuticals, dietary compounds, and endogenous biomolecules in thalassemia have been reported. Some recent studies showed that various antioxidants when used in combination enhanced antioxidant capacity and decreased toxicity/side effects. Future research should address the optimization of combination strategies with the final goal to prevent hazardous complications and increase life expectancy of thalassemic patients. Moreover, it should focus on the investigation of the potential antioxidants for thalassemia which could be orally administered and readily absorbed, and highly bioavailable. Moreover, they should possess high antioxidative activities, have long half-life, do not interfere with other drugs, and are not toxic even at high concentrations.

Chapter 9 - Thalassemia is an important congenital hematological disorder. This congenital disorder result in hemoglobin defect and causes several signs and symptoms. This problem can be seen around the world and is still an important public health threat in several countries. There are many complications of thalassemia and those complications can be the causes of death. In the present short article, the authors will present and discuss on an important complication, calcification. The calcification is an important but usually forgotten complication. The calcified tissue can be seen in many organs and become the problem.

Chapter 10 - The primary defects in the β-hemoglobinopathies: β-thalassemia and sickle cell anemia (SCA), are quantitative and qualitative abnormalities in hemoglobin (Hb), respectively, leading to chronic anemia. To cure, these primary defects should be corrected. This can be accomplished by two therapeutic modalities: Hematopoietic stem cell transplantation and gene therapy. However neither is currently applicable to most patients with these diseases because of technical difficulties, the costs involved, and a lack of the highly sophisticated medical care necessary to provide these therapies in developing countries where the diseases are most prevalent. In addition to chronic anemia, which is treated by blood transfusion, other associated pathologies cause morbidity and mortality. Among these are: Ineffective erythropoiesis – the abortive attempt of the body to overcome the state of anemia; iron overload (IO) – the result of repeated blood transfusions and increased iron uptake, and oxidative stress – due to the instability of the Hb and iron-mediated generation of cytotoxic free radicals. Advances in the treatment of the chronic anemia and its accompanying IO significantly prolong the life-span of most patients, but with older age come additional pathologies associated with the underlying disease and its treatment modalities.

Treatment modalities are usually target-specific. Sometimes, such as in the case of malignancy, to achieve maximal efficacy a combination of drugs is used. For the β-hemoglobinopathies, each modality aims to treat one aspect of the disease: Blood transfusion for the chronic anemia, iron chelation for IO and anti-oxidants for oxidative stress. But usually drugs have more than one target. In most cases, their "side effects" on "secondary" targets are deleterious, causing therapy-associated symptoms. But sometimes the effects, either direct or indirect on "secondary" targets are beneficial, synergizing with the primary effect to optimize the therapeutic influence..

Many drugs used for treating β-hemoglobinopathies have a pleiotropic effect, and as such they are associated with a variety of effects, both beneficial and deleterious. Among the beneficial effects are: (A) Stimulation of erythropoiesis, aimed at ameliorating the state of anemia. (B) Specific stimulation of fetal Hb production, thereby decreasing the relative concentration of β^S-globin chains (leading to sickling in SCA), or the excess of α-globin chains – the main cause of the short life-span of RBC in β-thalassemia. (C) Reducing IO – by iron chelation, increasing iron utilization or decreasing iron uptake. (D) Amelioration of oxidative stress – by directly scavenging free radicals in erythroid and non-erythroid cells, as well as in the extracellular milieu, or by its indirect effect on iron. These effects may influence the proliferation and maturation of erythroid precursors in the bone marrow as well as the senescence and removal of RBC from the peripheral blood, and also reduce cytotoxicity to other cells in vital organs.

The following is a review of such modalities and a discussion of their potential application for treatment of β-hemoglobinopathies. author believe that on the basis of the data summarized in this review, the time has come to define, by studying *in vitro* and *in vivo* models, as well as by controlled clinical trials, the multi-target effects of drugs for the treatment of patients with various forms of these diseases.

Chapter 11 - The thalassaemias are a group of hereditary disorders caused by over 300 mutations on the beta globin loci and - over 160 affecting the alpha globin genes, responsible for the production of haemoglobin. They are regarded as the commonest of the clinically serious single gene disorders affecting humans. The thalassaemia genes were endemic in areas where falciparum malaria was common, suggesting an epistatic relationship between these genes and resistance of carriers to malaria. The endemic areas of the globe include the Mediterranean basin, the Middle East, central Asia, the Indian subcontinent, southern China and South East Asia. Population migrations have now introduced the conditions to non-endemic areas such as Northern Europe and the Americas. This geographical distribution was referred to as the thalassaemia belt. Sickle cell disease covers much of the Middle East but mainly Africa and the countries which over the centuries have received populations of African origin.

It is estimated that there are over 200 million carriers of the thalassaemia genes and that almost 60000 babies are born annually affected by clinically significant thalassaemia syndromes. It is noted that most countries in the thalassaemia belt are low or middle income countries, burdened with many acute health problems and chronic, hereditary disorders are not high in their health agenda. Despite this it has been proven, especially in Mediterranean countries that these conditions are both treatable and preventable. Optimum lifelong care has resulted in survival to an age where patients can fulfil their lives, and have a good quality existence. In addition prevention programmes have limited new births of affected individuals and have saved resources for the benefit of patients.

Priority of patient support organisations is the provision of services which can favour the good outcomes that have been demonstrated in the relatively few countries which have introduced comprehensive and effective programmes for the thalassaemias in their health systems. Such planning and service development is however impossible without epidemiological information. The World Health Organisation has recognised the global problem and has issued resolutions urging governments to adopt both prevention and patient care policies. Political will, budgetary allocation and health planning require knowledge of the disease, knowledge of the carrier prevalence and birth incidence and importantly the number of patients and their location.

Such data are difficult to collect especially in large non- homogeneous populations and even more in locations where the diseases are rare and imported through migrations.

In this chapter the authors discuss the development of epidemiological tools, such as carrier screening, patient registers, cost effectiveness studies, outcome measures which will provide the information for service development. In addition they provide such epidemiological and service information as they have available with some mapping of available services and examples of outcome. The objective is to develop a toolkit for gathering useful information on existing services in order to diagnose deficiencies especially where patient care is concerned.

Chapter 12 - Genetic blood diseases are frequent in Bahrain as in all Middle Eastern countries. Previous neonatal screening study 1984-1985 showed that the incidence of sickle cell disease (SCD) was 2.1%, of sickle cell trait (SCT) 11%, while the carrier rate for beta Thalassaemia was 3%.

The total number of Bahraini patients with thalassemia is 88 patients, Non Bahraini is 21, Age group between 2-35 years.

A ten years study on the prevalence of β thalassemia among the students in Bahrain was performed. The aim of the program was to raise awareness among the youth. A total of 88,000 students were screened from 1999 to 2013. The mean prevalence of ß thalessemia trait and major were 3.5% and 0.035% respectively. The frequency of β thalassemia in Bahrain was found to be low to moderate, in comparison with the situation in many other gulf countries.

In another study the authors measure the public awareness level about Beta thalassemia in Bahrain, Conducted in 2006 to 2007. A questionnaire was distributed among 2000 persons from the general public. It showed that (65.1%) knew about beta thalassemia. A majority of (77.8) strongly agreed that premarital checking can prevent it. Females showed better knowledge than males.

The molecular characterization of B-thalassemia mutations among Bahrainis was studied by using a variety of polymerase chain reaction (PCR)-based procedures including reverse dot blot (RDB), denaturing gradient gel electrophoresis (DGGE) and DNA sequencing. Thirteen different β-thal mutations were identified. It showed that four mutations (Intervening Sequence I (IVSI)-3' end (-25 base pairs (bp)) deletion; Codon (Cd) 39 (C→T) andIVSI-5 (G→C), account for ~80% of all β-thal alleles. and that IVSI-3' end (-25bp) deletion is the major β-thalassemic allele in Bahrain.

The authors have organized and directed the campaign to control genetic in the period between 1984-2013. The goals were to reduce the incidence, and to improve the standard of management for patients suffering from these diseases.

The prevention strategy depended on health education, screening and counseling. A comprehensive health education program has been launched, to increase public awareness of the diseases.

This program used the media, and targeted key opinion leaders in society and the community, in schools and other public places. Screening for haemoglobinopathies included sickle cell disease, thalassaemia, was undertaken on the following categories of the population: antenatal mothers, premarital couples, newborns, and school students, followed by counseling of families. The campaign was supported by both the policy makers and the community.

All these efforts continued for more than 25 years. It had tremendous effects in reducing the prevalence of Genetic Blood Diseases (GBD) among the newborns, in 1984 the incidence of SCD among newborn was 20 per thousand, now it is 4 per thousand with 75 % decline, while the number of affected newborn with beta thal is 0-2 per year.

During this campaign the Ethical legal and social issues were taken care of, such as: equity, informed consent, privacy, confidentiality and prevention of stigmatization and discrimination.

Treatment: available in Bahrain will be discussed, One of preventive measures is pnd prenatal diagnosis \ And pgd –preimplantation genetic diagnosis.

Chapter 13 - *Background.* Thalassemia is one of the most common genetic disorders worldwide and presents public health and social challenges in areas of high incidence. The manifestations of the condition are modulated by several genetic, racial, and environmental factors. The homozygous type of β-thalassemia (thalassemia major, TM) is associated with most severe signs and symptoms.

Subjects and methods. A total of 54 TM patients aged 5.5 to 18.3 years and healthy controls (when appropriate) were examined for dental caries, oral hygiene, periodontal status, orofacial features, tooth size and dental arch dimensions, dental development, and physical pattern.

Results. The caries prevalence in TM patients was significantly higher (P<0.001) than the control group. Among cases, 61.1% had poor oral hygiene. Supra- and subgingival calculus was found in 32.5% of TM patients versus 21.8% in the controls. Only 7.8% of TM patients showed no sign of gingivitis versus 25.2% in the controls. The mean periodontal pocket depth in the patients was 2.7 ±1.4 mm versus 2.3 ± 1.2 mm in the controls. Clinical orofacial features of TM were: frontal bossing (61.1%), saddle nose (59.2%), dental and jaw pain (40.7%), maxillary protrusion (24.1%), "chipmunk" like face (16.7%) and malocclusion. Radiographical examination showed the followings: thickened frontal bone (67%), thinned mandibular cortex (65%), and maxillary sinus hypoplasia (42%). More than one-third of the patients exhibited enlarged marrow spaces with course trabeculation producing "chicken-wire" appearance of the alveolar bone, thin lamina dura, faint inferior alveolar canal and widened dipolic spaces. All means of tooth size and dental arches dimensions were reduced relative to the controls, with 20 of the 24 and 14 of the 16 measurements, respectively were statistically significant ($P<0.05$ to $P<0.001$). Growth retardation was present in 75.9% of the thalassemic patients, worsened after the age of 10 years. Mean body mass index was 16.5 ± 2.2 kg/m^2.

Conclusion. TM produces a variety of signs, symptoms and complications including high risk dental caries, periodontal diseases and oral infection as well as dental and orofacial changes. These changes should be taken into account when planning treatment with emphasis to maintain preventive program.

In: Thalassemia
Editor: Makenzie Greene

ISBN: 978-1-63117-954-9

Chapter 1

Cure of Thalassemia Major Using Related and Unrelated Donor Cord Blood Stem Cell Transplantation

Lawrence D. Petz, M.D.[1], John Chow, M.D., Ph.D.[2], Tracie Dang[3], Andrew Song[4], Liang Liang[5], Michelle Chow[6], Christine Chow[6], Elizabeth Rao[6], Tang-Her Jaing, M.D.[7] and Robert Chow, M.D., A.M.[8*]

[1]StemCyte, Inc., Covina, California, US
[2]CyteTherapeutics Co. Ltd., Hong Kong;
[3]Pepperdine University, Malibu, California, US
[4]UC Irvine, Irvine, California, US
[5]UC San Diego, San Diego, California, US
[6]HMDC, LLC, Irvine, California, US
[7]Chang Gung Children's Hospital and Chang Gung University, Taoyuan, Taiwan
[8]CyteTherapeutics, Inc., Shanghai, People's Republic of China

Abstract

Since the first cord blood transplantation performed by Gluckman and colleagues (1988), there have been many medical indications that have been proven for this stem cell therapy in the last two and half decades. Besides the standard hematological indications for bone marrow transplantation, such as leukemias, lymphomas, SCIDs, and aplastic anemia, cord blood transplantation has also been a proven curative therapy for non-hematological indications such as Krabbe's, osteopetrosis etc... As transplant related mortality, overall survival and disease-free survival for cord blood transplantation continue to improve with optimal conditioning regimens, better GvHD and infection

* To whom correspondences should be addressed; Robert Chow, M.D., A.M. CyteTherapeutics, Inc. 6/F, 21st Century Tower, 210 Century Avenue, Pudong New Area, Shanghai, 200120, People's Republic of China; Email: rchow@cytetherapeutics.com, Telephone: +1-(818) 935 8588, +1-(818) 667 9860; Facsimile: +1-(626) 226 5988.

prophylaxis and treatment, closer HLA matching and optimal cord blood product selection afforded by larger inventories, double cord blood transplantation and the availability of high cell dose cord blood products, the utility of this stem cell source will expand to certain indications which in the past, rarely used related or unrelated cord blood transplantation. For patients, families, referring and transplant physicians to accept allogeneic cord blood transplantation for indications such as thalassemia, sickle cell disease, severe autoimmune diseases or HIV, the benefit-risk ratio has to be significantly improved so that it is worthwhile for patients to take a chance on a risky procedure in order to prolong lifespan or improve quality of life. We review in this Chapter some of the efforts to improve clinical outcome of related and unrelated cord blood transplantation for thalassemia through increasing infused cord blood nucleated and CD34+ cell dosage using a combination of three strategies – (1) cord blood products manufactured using technologies that maximize cell dosage recoveries, (2) double cord blood transplantation whenever appropriate, and (3) the no-wash thaw and direct infusion method advocated by Chow et al.

Introduction

Hemoglobinopathies such as thalassemia and sickle cell anemia are among the most common genetic disorders worldwide, with 4.83% of the world's population carrying some form of globin variants (Rund et al., 2005). Thalassemia is the most common single gene disorder and is widely distributed and prevalent in Southern Asia, South East Asia, Mediterranean and Middle East regions (Weatherall 1981). The worldwide birth rate of people who are homozygous or compound heterozygous for symptomatic globin disorders, including α-thalassemia and β-thalassemia, is no less than 2.4 per 1000 births, of which 1.96 have sickle cell disease and 0.44 have thalassemias (Rund et al., 2005).

Premature hemolysis and ineffective erythropoiesis cause the anemia in thalassemia, with the relative contributions between these two processes differ in variants of thalassemia. Ineffective erythropoiesis is associated with bone expansion and extramedullary hematopoiesis in the liver, spleen and other sites. Transfusion for the severe anemia and maintenance of hemoglobin levels of at least 9-10 g per deciliter allows for normal growth and development and serves to suppress the ineffective erythropoiesis, hepatosplenomegaly and bone deformities. In the past, the hemosiderosis as a result of frequent transfusion and enhanced gastrointestinal iron absorption causes severe iron overload and deposition in organs such as the heart, liver and endocrine glands, and eventually leads to multi-organ failure. Severe endocrinopathies often require hormone replacement; however, severe cardiac toxicity is life-threatening and the main cause of death in thalassemia patients. Since the advent of iron chelation therapy, many of these complications have been ameliorated and the life expectancy of thalassemia patients has doubled (Rund et al., 2005; Olivieri NF. 1999); however, without careful bone disease management, overly vigorous chelation can be associated with deferoxamine-induced bone dysplasia, which slow growth in children.

Deferoxamine was the first approved chelator; however, it was associated with several significant limitations, including the inconvenience, pain and associated reduced compliance of parenteral administration, side effects and prohibitive cost for most patients in developing countries (Olivieri NF. 1999). Deferiprone, an oral chelator, proved to be safe and effective, besides eliminating many of the problems associated with deferoxamine administration. It is still associated with several side effects; however, because of its ability to penetrate cell membrane, deferiprone can chelate intracellular iron and may be more effective in removing myocardial iron (Anderson et al., 2002; Piga et al., 2003; Hershko et al., 2005). Other new oral chelators such as Deferasirox appear to be effective but require longer follow up (Rund et al., 2005).

Hypertransfusion and iron chelation have been proven to improve life expectancy and quality of life. However, hypertransfusion can be associated with risks of alloimmunization and blood-transmitted infections, especially Hepatitis B and C, in areas where blood safety is poor. Moreover, iron chelation is prohibitively expensive to patients in most regions where thalassemia is prevalent and compliance in patients from developed countries is frequently poor. Despite modern supportive therapy of routine transfusion and chelation, only 68% of patients with beta-thalassemia are alive at the age of 35 (Cao at el. 2004). For sickle cell anemia, the median age of survival for females was 36.3 years and 38.7 years for male patients (Powars et al., 2005).

With all the improvements in transfusion management, infectious disease screening and innovations in oral iron chelation (Rund et al., 2005), hematopoietic cell transplantation is still the only curative therapy for hemoglobinopathies. For many patients, cure of their disease is their ultimate goal, sometimes because of failure of their medical support therapy or simply because of a desire for a normal life without chelation or transfusion. Since the first successful curative transplant in a child with thalassemia major by Thomas and colleagues at the Fred Hutchinson (Thomas et al., 1982) and the decades of optimization by the Italian groups (Lucarelli et al., 1998; 1990), over 1,000 patients with thalassemia and sickle cell disease have been cured, mostly using HLA-identical sibling donor bone marrow. For low-risk Pesaro class 1 or 2 patients, related bone marrow transplantation (BM transplantation) can achieve outstanding overall survival of 87 to 95% and thalassemia-free survival of 64 to 90%, depending on the disease severity (Lucarelli et al., 1998). Even with class 3 (with extensive liver damage from iron overload) patients, with certain new preparatory regimens, patients younger than 17 years old can achieve survival rates of 93% with only 8% autologous recovery rate (55 Sodani et al., 2004).

However, fewer than 30% of patients have unaffected HLA-matched siblings. Matched unrelated adult donors remain unavailable for most hemoglobinopathy patients, despite proving to be acceptable alternatives for patients with thalassemia who lack a compatible family donor (La Nasa et al., 2002). Related and unrelated umbilical cord blood may alleviate shortage of matched-unrelated donors, since less stringent HLA matching is acceptable. Moreover, due to the lower severity and incidence of GvHD after CB transplantation compared to BM transplantation (Gluckman et al., 1997; Rubinstein et al., 1998; Rocha et al., 2004; Laughlin et al., 2004), CB transplantation may be preferable to BM transplantation for thalassemia and other non-malignant diseases, as the potential long term elimination of GvHD prophylaxis greatly improves quality of life for transplant patients over medical therapy alone. For thalassemia and other transplant patients with non-malignant diseases, GvHD offers no advantage of relapse reduction as in the setting as for malignant diseases.

Recently, a number of studies have shown significant success using related and unrelated donor CB transplantation. Cell dose is the most critical factor for cord blood transplantation success, as revealed by almost every major study to date (Gluckman et al., 1997; Rubinstein et al., 1998; Rocha et al., 2004; Laughlin et al., 2004). Though theoretically cell dose may be less of a problem for hemoglobinopathies since transplantation are usually performed at an early age when patients have smaller body masses; however, due to the difficulties of eradicating the endogenous erythron, cell dose has been found to be just as critical for both related and unrelated CB transplantation (Locatelli et al., 2003, 2013; Lissini et al., 2008; Jaing et al., 2010, 2012).

As almost every major study has shown, the most critical factor for cord blood transplantation success is cell dose. Ruggeri et al. (2011) have shown superior outcome with a minimal TNC dose of 5 x 10^7/kg for related CB transplantation for thalassemia. For unrelated CB transplantation for thalassemia, Jaing et al. (2012) established institutional guidelines of 2.5 x 10^7/kg for single unit CB transplantation and >3.7 x 10^7/kg combined cell dose for double CB transplantation, with at least one unit exceeding 2 x 10^7/kg. Moreover, at Chang Gung, following the Minnesota recommendations of (Wagner et al., 2002), CD34+ cell dose of 1.5 x 10^5/kg is required for each unit, with the combined CD34+ cell dose exceeding 3.0 x 10^5/kg.

Due to the proven central importance of cell dose in cord blood transplantation, some groups have employed various strategies to optimize nucleated and CD34+ cell doses, such as the supplementation of bone marrow stem cells from the same donor to the cord blood graft (Goussetis et al., 2000; Fang et al., 2004; Walters et al., 2005), the use of double cord blood transplants when single cord blood units do not have sufficient cell doses (Jaing et al., 2007, 2008abc, 2010, 2012; Petz et al., 2012; Chow et al., 2012), avoidance of post-thaw wash (when indicated) which invariably results in loss of cells (Issaragrisil et al., 1995; Jaing et al., 2005, 2008abc, 2010, 2012; Chow et al., 2006, 2007acd, 2008abc, 2009, 2010, 2011ab, 2012; Rosenthal 2008; Petz et al., 2011, 2012), and usage of non-red cell reduced CB as red cell reduction results in decreased cell recovery (Jaing et al., 2005ab, 2006, 2007ab, 2008c, 2009, 2010, 2012; Petz et al., 2011, 2012; Chow et al., 2007a, 2008bc, 2009; 2010; 2011, 2012; Rosenthal et al., 2007; 2008; Graham et al., 2008).

Various other approaches have been tried, and some have been proven, to improve outcome of cord blood transplantation for thalassemia, ranging from usage of related HLA-identical donors (Locatelli et al., 2003, 2013; Lissini et al., 2008), preference for superior HLA matches (Jaing et al., 2005ab, 2006, 2007ab, 2008c, 2009, 2010, 2012), consideration of non-inherited maternal antigen (NIMA) matches (Rocha et al., 2012), directed sibling cord blood bank efforts (Walters et al., 2005; Smythe et al., 2007), preference for i.v. busulfan over oral formulations (Jaing et al., 2012), the addition of thiotepa to the conditioning regimen (Locatelli et al., 2013;Lissini et al., 2008), reduced intensity conditioning regimens (Ruggeri et al., 2011; Kharbanda et al., 2013; Soni et al., 2013), the avoidance of methotrexate in the prophylaxis regimen (Locatelli et al., 2003, 2013; Lissini et al., 2008), third party MSC co-infusion (Kharbanda et al., 2013), and intrabone direct injection of cord blood products (Brunstein et al., 2009; Rocha et al., 2013).

In this Chapter, we review the various clinical studies of CB transplantation for thalassemia and the approaches summarized above aimed at improving clinical outcome of related and unrelated CB transplantation for thalassemia major. By improving the benefit risk ratio of CB transplantation for a highly prevalent disease such as thalassemia, it is hoped that CB transplantation utilization for other non-malignant diseases that are curable with CB transplantation but rarely use HSCT today, might see greater usage of CB transplantation - for example, for HIV infections (Chow et al., U.S. patent 2003/0099621 AI; Chen et al., 2008; Hutter et al., 2009; 2011; Petz et al., 2013) and certain autoimmune diseases.

Related Donor Cord Blood Transplantation for Thalassemia

In 1995, the first cord blood transplantation for thalassemia was reported, using a HLA-identical sibling donor cord blood for a two and half year old (Issaragrisil et al.,). Busulfan/cyclophosphamide conditioning regimen and cyclosporine/methotrexate GvHD prophylaxis were used. The TNC dose was 3.9 x 10^7/kg and the thawed product was not washed and infused on June 12, 1993. Neutrophil and platelet engraftment were achieved by day +23 and d+27, respectively. The patient experienced no GvHD and the patient was alive and transfusion-independent 48 months after transplantation (Table 1).

Lau et al., (1998) followed up this effort with two patients (ages 2.2 and 3.8 years) with HLA-identical sibling donors, busulfan/cyclophosphamide conditioning regimen and cyclosporine +/- methotrexate GvHD prophylaxis (Table 1). TNC doses were 6.2 x 10^7/kg and 11.4 x 10^7/kg. Both patients engrafted, experienced grade III acute GvHD, resolved with steroid administration, and are alive and transfusion-independent, 11 to 24 months post-transplant.

Three patients (one Pesaro class 2 and two class 3) were transplanted by Goussetis et al., (2000) with the combination of HLA-identical sibling cord blood and bone marrow, because the cord blood nucleated cell doses were considered inadequate at 2, 1.2 and 2.5 x 10^7/kg. Neutrophil and platelet engraftments were achieved at days +17, +18, and +17, and days +19, 25, and +22, for the three patients respectively. All three patients are alive and transfusion-independent 23, 18, and 16 months post-transplant, respectively (Table 1).

The same group followed up in 2010 (Goussetis et al.,) with a total of three HLA-matched sibling cord blood transplantation and 5 cord blood transplantation combined with bone marrow from the same HLA-identical sibling donors (Table 1). The cord blood only group received nucleated cell dosage in excess of 5 x 10^7/kg, judged to be adequate – only one Pesaro class 1 patient engrafted. The other two experienced graft failure and were transplanted with bone marrow from the same sibling donor later. The five patients who received a combination of cord blood plus bone marrow grafts had cord blood nucleated cell doses below 4 x 10^7/kg. All five engrafted stably. Overall 7 of 8 are thalassemia-free and all patients survived.

Hongeng et al., reported their results of a 3-year child transplanted with a 4/6 HLA-matched related donor with a nucleated cell dose of 6.1 10^7/kg as detailed in Table 1. Though engraftment was achieved and the patient experienced only limited chronic GvHD, the patient eventually expired from severe infections at day +300.

Locatelli et al., (2003) studied related CB transplantation for 33 thalassemics and 11 patients with sickle cell disease (Table 1). No patients died; however, the 2–year event-free survival (EFS) was 79% for thalassemia, with 36 of 44 children remaining disease-free (81.8%) with a median follow up of 24 months. No grade III-IV acute GvHD and 2 of 36 experienced limited chronic GvHD. Univariate analysis of factors related to patients, disease and transplantation affecting EFS showed that the patients given methotrexate (MTX) as part of the GvHD prophylaxis had a significantly lower probability of EFS compared to those who did not (90% versus 55%; p=0.005). This finding of poorer EFS with MTX use was confirmed using a Cox regression model (hazard ratio = 6.6; 95% CI = 1.47 – 25.86; P=0.013).

Table 1. CB transplantation using Related Donors & Sibling Directed Donor CB Bank (SDCB) for patients with thalassemia

	Issaragrisil et al. 1995a,b	Lau et al. 1998	Goussetis et al. (1) 2000 (2) 2010	Hongeng et al. 2002	Locatelli et al. 2003	Fang et al. 2004	SDCB (1) Walters et al. 2005 (2) Smythe et al. 2007	Kabbara et al. 2008	Lisini et al. 2008	Locatelli et al. 2013
# Patients	1	2	(1) 3 CB+ BM (2) 3 CB 5 CB+BM	1	33 Thal 11 SCD	9; 2+baby donor's PB	(1) 14 Thal 4/14 +PB 4 SCD (2) 7 Thal	72 CB 48Thal 330 BM 184 Thal	27 Thal	CBT 66 Thal/30 SCD BMT Thal 259/ SCD130
Age (yrs) Median Range	2.5	2.2/3.8	(1)4,13,15	3	5 1-20	5.5 / 3.5-10	(1) NA 5.9 / 2-11	CB 5.5 BM 7.6	6 0.8-18	CB 5.9 / 2-20 BM 8.1 / 0.7-24
Pesaro Class 1 Class 2 Class 3	NA	NA	(1)0 (2)1 (1)1 (1)2 (2)7/8 class 2/3	NA	20 (61%) 13 (39%)	0 6 3	NA NA	CB 64%/36% 2/3 BM 36%/64% 2/3	16 (59%) 11 (41%)	CB 61% BM 33% CB 35% BM 31% CB 4% BM 13%
Conditioning Regimens	BU14 CY200	BU20 CY200 ATG	(1) BU16 CY200 ALG	BU20 CY200 ATG	BU/CY(16)+ ATG (10) or TT (9) or FLU (1) or FLU/TT (7)	BU14-20 CY160-200 MEL90 ATG/ALG	(1) NA	NA	Bu/Flu/T T 89% Bu/Cy/TT 11%	CB BU/CY 56% BU±CY+FL/TT4 2% BM BU/CY 89% BU±CY+FL/TT1 1%
GvHD Prophylaxis	CSA MTX	CSA+/- MTX	NA	CSA/MP	No MTX (32) + MTX (12)	Tacrolimus MP MTX	(1) NA	NA	CSA 100%	CB CSA +MTX 30% - MTX 70%
HLA A/B/DR 6/6 5/6 ≤ 4/6 Matches	1	2	(1)3 (2)8	0 0 1	41 3	6 1 2	(1)14 (2) 7	100% 0 0	100% 0 0	100% 0 / 0 0 / 0
TNC Dose Median Range	3.9	6.2 / 11.4	CB 2/1.2/2.5 Combined 3.2 /2.8 /3.7	6.1	5.1/1.2-13 PF 4.0/1.2-10 PT	6.6 / 3.4-12.7	(1) NA (2)4.7/0.8-7.6	NA	3.3 1.5-6	CB 3.9 (1.5-14)

	Issaragrisil et al. 1995a,b	Lau et al. 1998	Goussetis et al. (1) 2000 (2) 2010	Hongeng et al. 2002	Locatelli et al. 2003	Fang et al. 2004	SDCB (1) Walters et al. 2005 (2) Smythe et al. 2007	Kabbara et al. 2008	Lisini et al. 2008	Locatelli et al. 2013
CD34+ Cell Dose Median / Range	NA	NA	NA	NA	N/A	NA	NA (2)1.1/0.2-1.7	NA	N/A	NA
% CB Not Washed	1/1	NA	NA	NA	0%	N/A	(1) NA	Mostly washed	N/A	Mostly washed
% DCBT	None	None	None	None	None	None	None	None	None	None
Approaches to Maximize TNC	Non-Wash	NA	NA	NA	Related CB	NA	(1) None	Early Age	Early Age	Early Age
Engraftment Myeloiod (ANC500) Platelet 20K / 50K (Plt20K or 50K)	ANC 1/1 d+23 Plt 1/1 d+37	2 / 2	(1) 3/3 ANCD +17,18,17; Plt D+19, 25, 22 (2) 1/3CB 5/5 +BM	1 / 1	ANC 89% d+23 (12-60) Plt20K 90% D+39(19-92)	5/9	(1) Thal 12/14 SCD 4/4 (2) Thal 6/6 with engraftment data reporting	ANC CB 90±4% BM 94±2%	100% (27/27) 100% (27/27)	ANC CB 90±4%; D+23 BM 92±1%; D+19 Thal 91%;SCD 94% Plt CB 83±5%; D+38 BM 85±5%; D+25
Graft Failure; Primary (PGF); Secondary (SGF)	None	None	(1)None (2) 2/3 CB	None	7/33 (21%)	4/9; 2 PGF; 2 SGF	(1) 2 PGF+1 SGF (2) 1SGF		0 (0%)	CB 10.4% BM 7.4%
Acute GvHD	0	2/2 III SR	None	None	11% (4/38) II	3/9 I/II SR 1/9 IV	(1) NA	CB 9±4% BM 10±3%	0 (0%)	CB 11% II-IV BM 21% II-IV
Chronic GvHD	0	None	None	Limited	6% (2/36) Limited	1/9	(1) NA	CB 7±4% BM 5±2%	0 (0%)	CB 5±3%; 0 ext BM 12±2%; 12 ext
Severe Infections	None	None	None	Yes		None	(1) NA	NA	None	NA

Table 1. (Continued)

	Issaragrisil et al. 1995a,b	Lau et al. 1998	Goussetis et al. (1) 2000 (2) 2010	Hongeng et al. 2002	Locatelli et al. 2003	Fang et al. 2004	SDCB (1) Walters et al. 2005 (2) Smythe et al. 2007	Kabbara et al. 2008	Lisini et al. 2008	Locatelli et al. 2013
Survival	OS 1/1 DFS 1/1	2/2 Alive & TI	(1) 3/3 Alive & TI (2) OS 8/8 DFS 7/8	0/1 Died d+300	Thal OS 100% EFS 79%	OS 8/9; 1 death aGvHD IV 4 TI	(1) Thal OS 11/14; DFS 11/14 SCD OS ¾ (2) OS7/7 One used DLI for rejection episode.	CB 5YOS 95±3% DFS 86±5% BM 5YOS96±2% DFS 91±3% Thal 5YDFS CB 83% BM 88%	OS 27 (100%) DFS 27 (100%) TRM 0 (0%)	CB 6YOS 97±2% DFS 83±4% EFS 83±42 Thal DFS 80±5% SCD DFS 90±5% BM 6YOS 95±1% DFS 88±2% EFS 85±2% Thal DFS 86±2% SCD DFS 92±2%
Follow-up (M) Median/Range	48 (1995b)	11-24	(1) 18/ 16-23	10	24 / 4-76	49 / 38-64	12.4 / 0.5-77	32 / 2.1-116.6	40 / 15-89	CB 70 (12-151) BM 70 (12-165)

Thal = Thalassemia Major; SCD = Sickle Cell Disease; Other = Other Non-Malignant Indications; CB = Cord Blood; CBT = Cord Blood Transplant; PD = Non-Red Blood Cell Reduced Cord Blood; RCR = Red Cell Reduced Cord Blood; SCBT = Single Cord Blood Transplantation; DCBT = Double Cord Blood Transplantation; NW = Non-Wash Post-Thaw Processing; BU – Busulfan; CY = Cyclophosphamide; FLU = Fludarabine; TT = Thiotepa; ATG/ALG = Antithymocyte/lymphocyte globulins; N/A = Not Available; CSA = cyclosporin; MTX = Methotrexate; MP = Methylprednisolone; Tac = Tacrolimus; MMF = mycophenolate mofetil; LGF = Late Graft Failure; AR = Autologous Recovery; TI = Transfusion Independent; TNC = Total Nucleated Cells in X 10^7/kg patient weight; CD34+ = Total CD34+ Cells in X 10^5/kg patient weight; GvHD = Graft-versus-Host Disease; aGvHD = Acute Graft-versus-Host Disease; Ltd = Limited chronic GvHD; Ext = Extensive chronic GvHD; TRM=Transplant Related Mortality; M = Months; 3Y = 3 Year; 1Y=1 Year; D = Days post-transplant; OS = Overall Survival; DFS =Disease Free Survival; EFS = time interval from CBT to first event (death or autologous reconstitution or infusion of cryopreserved back up recipient hematopoietic stem cells); RR = Relative Risk; p = p value of PD versus RCR matched pair comparison; P = Paired Prentice-Wilcoxon Test p value; F/U = Follow Up; CI = Cumulative Incidence; KM = Kaplan Meier Estimator Survival; * = Modified Pesaro (no liver biopsy), which may underestimate the disease severity; @ = TC Data Audited by CIBMTR on site.

Table 2. Unrelated CB transplant for patients with thalassemia – Single Case Studies and Small Series

	Fang et al. 2003	Tan et al. 2004	Hall et al. 2004	Vanichsetakul et al. 2004	Jaing et al. 2005@	Jaing et al. 2007@	Soni et al. 2014	Kharbanda et al. 2014
# Patients	1	1	1 100% RCR CB	6 100% RCR CB	4 SCBT 1 DCBT 100% PD CB	5 DCBT 100% PD CB	2 1 Re-CBT	CBT/BMT+MSC 2 Thal 2 DCBT 4 SCD 1 SCBT 1 DCBT 2 BMT
Age (yrs) Median Range	5	5	0.2	5.5 2-15	3.7 2.3-11	11.1 10-13	5, 7	10 8-18
Pesaro Class	Class 3	Class 2	N/A	1 2 3	*5	N/A	2 Class 3	NA
Conditioning Regimens	BU20 CY200 ATG FLU150 TT6	BU18 CY120 ATG	BU CY200 ATG	BU16-20 CY200 +/-FLU200	BU14 CY200 ATG	BU14 CY200 ATG	RIC FLU30 TT10 MEL140 Alemtuzumab	RIC FLU150 MEL140 Alemtuzumab
GvHD Prophylaxis	Tacrolimus MP MTX	CSA MTX	CSA MP	CSA +/- MP	CSA MP	CSA MP	TAC MMF	CSA MMF
HLA A/B/DR 6/6 5/6 ≤ 4/6 Matches	1 0 0	0 0 1	0 0 1	3 1 2	0 3 2	1 0 4	1 / 1 1	Thal 0 SCD 0 Thal 1 SCD 0 Thal 3 SCD 3
TNC Dose Median Range	7.5	6	31.8 PF 19.1 PT	2.8 1.5-5.3	8.8 3.3-12	6.3 3.3-10	3.8 / 7.6 4.2	Thal 7.5 / 5.1 SCD 4.8 / 6.1
CD34+ Cell Dose Median / Range			6.1		2.48 2.31-3.75	4.53 4.1-8.44	NA / 2.0 2.5	Thal 6.7 / 4.4 SCD 5 / 3.3
% CB Not Washed	N/A	N/A	N/A	N/A	100%	100%	NA	
% DCBT	None	None	None	None	20%	100%	0	
Approaches to Maximize TNC	NA		NA	NA	100% PD CB/ NW/ ±DCBT	100% PD CB/ NW/ ±DCBT	NA	3rd Party MSC co-infusion to promote engraftment

Table 2. (Continued)

	Fang et al. 2003	Tan et al. 2004	Hall et al. 2004	Vanichsetakul et al. 2004	Jaing et al. 2005@	Jaing et al. 2007@	Soni et al. 2014	Kharbanda et al. 2014
Engraftment Myeloid(ANC500) Platelet 20K / 50K (Plt20K or 50K)	1/1	1/1	1/1 ANC d+13 Plt50K d+48	5/6	5/5	5/5	ANC 2/3 D+23 / 18 Plt20K D+34 / 32	ANC Thal 1/2 d+33 SCD 2/2 d+15/34 Plt Thal 0/2 SCD 2/2 d+37/56
Graft Failure	None	None	None	None	None	1/5 LGF	1/3 Re-CBT	3 / 6
Survival	1/1	1/1	1/1	5/6 1 death due to infection before ANC	5/5	4/5; 1 AR 1 Death (Evans' syndr., pulm. bleed)	OS 2/2 DFS 2/2	OS 2/6 Thal 0/2 SCD 2/4 DFS 0/6 Thal 0/2
F/U (M)Median/Range	20	24	60	7 / 2-30	10 / 4-12	18/11-32	7-8 years	
Acute GvHD	III SR	I	I	2/5 I	4/5 I/II 1/5 III	4/4 I/III	0	Thal 1/2 Grade 2 SCD 0/2
Chronic GvHD	None	None	None	None	None	4/4 Limited	0	
Severe Infections	None	None	E. coli	1	None	None	HHV-6	6/6

Thal = Thalassemia Major; SCD = Sickle Cell Disease; Other = Other Non-Malignant Indications; CB = Cord Blood; CBT = Cord Blood Transplant; PD = Non-Red Blood Cell Reduced Cord Blood; RCR = Red Cell Reduced Cord Blood; SCBT = Single Cord Blood Transplantation; DCBT = Double Cord Blood Transplantation; NW = Non-Wash Post-Thaw Processing; BU – Busulfan; CY = Cyclophosphamide; FLU = Fludarabine; TT = Thiotepa; ATG/ALG = Antithymocyte/lymphocyte globulins; N/A = Not Available; CSA = cyclosporin; MTX = Methotrexate; MP = Methylprednisolone; Tac = Tacrolimus; MMF = mycophenolate mofetil.

LGF = Late Graft Failure; AR = Autologous Recovery; TI = Transfusion Independent GvHD = Graft-versus-Host Disease; Ltd = Limited chronic GvHD; Ext = Extensive chronic GvHD.

TNC = Total Nucleated Cells in X 10^7/kg patient weight; CD34+ = Total CD34+ Cells in X 10^5/kg patient weight; OS = Overall Survival; DFS =Disease Free Survival; EFS = time interval from HSCT to first event (death or autologous reconstitution or infusion of cryopreserved back up recipient hematopoietic stem cells); TRM=Transplant Related Mortality; M = Months; 3Y = 3 Year; 1Y=1 Year; D = Days post-transplant.

RR = Relative Risk; p = p value of PD versus RCR matched pair comparison; P = Paired Prentice-Wilcoxon Test p value; F/U = Follow Up; CI = Cumulative Incidence; KM = Kaplan Meier Estimator Survival.

* = Modified Pesaro (no liver biopsy), which may underestimate the disease severity; @ = TC Data Audited by CIBMTR on site.

Table 3. Unrelated CB transplantation for patients with thalassemia – Large Series

	Jaing et al., 2008abc PD CB @	Jaing et al. 2008abc RCR CB @	Jaing et al. 2010 @	Ruggeri et al. 2011	Jaing et al. 2012 @	Petz et al. 2012 @	Chow et al. 2012 @
# Patients Type of CB	58 Thal patients 48 PD patients MP performed on 30 PD patients vs. 10 RCR patients	58 Thal patients 10 RCR patients MP performed on 10 RCR patients vs. 30 PD patients	45 total; 32 Thal 13 Other 13 DCBT 100% PD CB	35 Thal 100% RCR CB	35 Thal patients 5 Re-CBT 40 CBT 13 DCBT 100% PD CB	120 total; 46 Thal. 3 SCD 71 Other 100% PD CB	91 Thal. 79 PD CBT; 12 RCR CBT
Age (yrs) Median Range	5.0 / 0.3-20 MP 4.0 / 0.3-12	2.8 / 1-12 MP 2.8 / 1-12	4.5	4	5.5 1.2-14	3.5 / 0.1-14	PD 5.3 / 0.3-20 RCR 4.0 / 0.8-12
Pesaro Class 1 Class 2 Class 3 N/A	* 1-46% /2-17% /3-0% MP* 1-57%/2-23% /3-0%	1-50%/2-20% /3-10% MP 1-50%/2-30% 3-20%	21 9 0 2	9 2 4 20	N/A	N/A	31 (*PD 27 RCR 6) 19 (*PD 17 RCR 2) 2 (*PD 0 RCR 2) 39 (*PD 35 RCR 2)
Conditioning Regimens	Multi-inst. series Mostly BU/CY/ATG	Multi-inst. series Mostly BU/CY/ATG	Thal BU14 CY200 ATG	30/35 myelo-ablative	BU14 CY200 ATG	Multi-inst. series Mostly BU/CY/ATG	Multi-inst. series Mostly BU/CY/ATG
GvHD Prophylaxis	CSA MP	CSA MP	CSA MP	CSA 80% Tac 20%	CSA MP	Multi-institution series	Multi-institution series
HLA A/B/DR 6/6 5/6 ≤ 4/6 Matches	Median 4.8 Range 3-6 MP Median 4.5 Range 3-6	Median 4.4 Range 4-6 MP Median 4.4 Range 3-6	11 25 27	5 14 16	8 16 28	26 48 53	PD 21 RCR 1 PD 38 RCR 3 PD 45 RCR 8
TNC Dose Median Range	9.1 / 2.5-47 MP 9.1 / 3.4-20	8.9 / 2.3-19 MP 8.9 / 2.3-19	7.6 /2.8-15.0	6 / 2-32	7.8 / 2.8-14.7	10.5 Pre-Freeze 7.7 Infused	PD 9.8 / 2-23.7 RCR 8.7 / 2-18.6
CD34+ Cell Dose Median / Range	N/A		4.0 / 1.3-19.9	N/A	4.0 / 1.7-19.9	3.7	PD 3.6 / 0.4-10.3 RCR1.5/0.4-13.5
% CB Not Washed	N/A		10)%	NA	100%	70 (58%)	PD 89%; RCR 77%
% DCBT	11 (23%) MP 5 (17%)	1 (10%) MP 1 (10%)	0	0	10/35 (27%)	15 (12%)	PD 20% RCR 8%

Table 3. (Continued)

	Jaing et al., 2008abc PD CB @	Jaing et al. 2008abc RCR CB @	Jaing et al. 2010 @	Ruggeri et al. 2011	Jaing et al. 2012 @	Petz et al. 2012 @	Chow et al. 2012 @
Approaches to Maximize Cell Dose	100% PD CB/ NW/ ±DCBT/	±NW/ ±DCBT/	100% PD CB/ NW/ ±DCBT/ CD34+ Priority	NA	100% PD CB/ NW/ ±DCBT/ CD34+ Priority	100% PD CB/ NW/ ±DCBT	PD 89% NW RCR 77% NW NW/ ±DCBT
Engraftment Myeloiod (ANC500) Platelet 20K / 50K (Plt20K or 50K)	ANC PD 96±4% vs. RCR 75±15% RR=1.31; p=0.56 Plt50K PD 95±5% vs. RCR 75±15% RR=1.24; p=0.64 MPANC PD 88±12% vs. RCR80±14% RR=1.05; p=0.90; P=0.92 Plt50K PD 88±12% vs. RCR 70±17% RR=1.01; p=0.98; P=0.73		ANC500 88% D+16 / 10-46 Plt20K 82% D+	ANC500 15/35 42.8%	ANC 88 % (35/40 CBT with 5 re-CBT engraftments) Plt20K 78%	ANC 87±6% D+21 Plt20K 81±6% D+49	ANC 83.2% Plt20/50K 79%/76%
Graft Failure	MP 1Y PD 7±5%; RCR 22±14% RR=0.31; p=0.24; P=0.04		4 Primary	20 / 35 57.2%	5 Primary 1 Secondary	3±2%	N/A
Survival	OS PD 89±6% vs. 53±20% RR=0.32; p=0.17 P DFS PD 89±6% vs RCR 38±17% RR=0.17; p =0.01 Matched Pair Comparisons (MP) 3Y OS PD 96±4% vs RCR 53±18% RR=0.09; p=0.03; P=0.001 3Y DFS PD 89±6% vs RCR 40±15% RR=0.17; p=0.01;P=0.0001 3Y TRM PD 4±4% vs RCR 47±18% RR=0.09; p=0.03; P=0.001		5-Year OS 88.1% 5-Year DFS 77.1% 40/45 alive and disease free 2-Year TRM 12%	OS 23/35 (66%) KM 62±9% DFS 8/35 (23%) KM 21±7%	5-Year OS 88.3±6.7% 5-Year DFS 73.9±7.4% (1st CBT only) 85.7% or 30/35 (1st & 2nd CBT) 2-Year TRM 11.7±6.7%	1Y OS 79±4% DFS 72±5% 3Y OS 79±4% DFS 70±6% 100 Day TRM 10±3% 3Y TRM 20±4%	OS 72.8% DFS 61.4% PD OS 73.3% DFS 61.4% RCR OS 75.0% DFS 50.0%
F/U (M)Median/Range	9.5	6	26 / 3-66	21 / 3-138	36 / 6-76	6.5	23.7
Acute GvHD	N/A		II-IV 76% III-IV 42±%	23±2%	6 I; 12 II 15 III; 1 IV	0-II 7 38±5% III-IV 19±4%	0-II76% / III-IV24% PD 75% / 25% RCR 80% / 20%

	Jaing et al., 2008abc PD CB @	Jaing et al. 2008abc RCR CB @	Jaing et al. 2010 @	Ruggeri et al. 2011	Jaing et al. 2012 @	Petz et al. 2012 @	Chow et al. 2012 @
Chronic GvHD	N/A		35% 1/14 extensive	8/35 Ltd 2/35 Ext.	13/35 Limited 1/35 Limited	36±6% Ltd. 12±4% Ext.	60% Ltd. 5% Ext. PD 60% / 5% RCR 100% / 0%
Severe Infections	N/A		1	4/35	2/35		N/A

Thal = Thalassemia Major; SCD = Sickle Cell Disease; Other = Other Non-Malignant Indications; CB = Cord Blood; CBT = Cord Blood Transplant; PD = Non-Red Blood Cell Reduced Cord Blood; RCR = Red Cell Reduced Cord Blood; SCBT = Single Cord Blood Transplantation; DCBT = Double Cord Blood Transplantation; NW = Non-Wash Post-Thaw Processing; BU – Busulfan; CY = Cyclophosphamide; FLU = Fludarabine; TT = Thiotepa; ATG/ALG = Antithymocyte/lymphocyte globulins; N/A = Not Available; CSA = cyclosporin; MTX = Methotrexate; MP = Methylprednisolone; Tac = Tacrolimus; MMF = mycophenolate mofetil.

LGF = Late Graft Failure; AR = Autologous Recovery; TI = Transfusion Independent GvHD = Graft-versus-Host Disease; Ltd = Limited chronic GvHD; Ext = Extensive chronic GvHD.

TNC = Total Nucleated Cells in X 10^7/kg patient weight; CD34+ = Total CD34+ Cells in X 10^5/kg patient weight; OS = Overall Survival; DFS =Disease Free Survival; EFS = time interval from CBT to first event (death or autologous reconstitution or infusion of cryopreserved back up recipient hematopoietic stem cells); TRM=Transplant Related Mortality; M = Months; 3Y = 3 Year; 1Y=1 Year; D = Days post-transplant.

RR = Relative Risk; p = p value of PD versus RCR matched pair comparison; P = Paired Prentice-Wilcoxon Test p value; F/U = Follow Up; CI = Cumulative Incidence; KM = Kaplan Meier Estimator Survival.

* = Modified Pesaro (no liver biopsy), which may underestimate the disease severity; @ = TC Data Audited by CIBMTR on site.

MP = PD versus RCR CBT Matched pair analysis used a logistic regression model to find patients with similar characteristics to form 30 pairs, with 3 PD patients matched to each RCR patient (30 PD patients to 10 RCR patients). Factors matched for were Age, Weight, #HLA Matches, TNC Dose, Transplant Center Experience. Univariate comparisons and Paired-Prentice-Wilcoxon Test were performed for the matched pairs.

Among thalassemia patients, the use of BU/TT/CY or BU/TT/FLU preparative regimens was associated with a significantly higher probability of EFS compared with the BU/CY alone (94% versus 62%; p=0.03). EFS of Pesaro class 1 and 2 thalassemia patients were 89% and 62%, respectively.

Nine more related donor cord blood transplantation with two supplemented by the baby donor's own peripheral blood were reported by Fang et al., (2004). Median age was 5.5 with a range of 3.5 to 10 years in this cohort, with 5 Pesaro class 2 and 3 class 3 patients. Six donor-recipient pairs were HLA-identical, one was 5/6 and two were 4/6 HLA-matched (Table 1). Busulfan/Cyclophosphamide/Melphelan/ATG conditioning regimen and Tacrolimus/ Methotrexate/ Methylprednisolone were used for GvHD prophylaxis. Median TNC dose was 6.6 x 10^7/kg with a range of 3.4-12.7 x 10^7/kg. Only 5 patients engrafted; two experienced primary graft failure and two suffered secondary graft failures. Three patients had grade 1/II acute GvHD, resolved with steroids. One died from Grade IV acute GvHD. Of the eight patients who survived, only four were transfusion-independent, with a median follow up period of 49 months (range 38-64 months).

Related cord blood transplantation using products cryopreserved at sibling directed donation cord blood banks were reported by Walters et al., (2005) and Smythe et al., (2007). The authors reported low usage rates for cord blood products stored. Fourteen of 96 related CB products (32 HLA identical) stored were released for transplantation by the Oakland group (Walters et al., 2005), with 11 patients surviving and transfusion-independent (Table 1). Four of the fourteen received a combination of cord blood and bone marrow or peripheral blood progenitor cells. One patient experienced graft failure, one with late graft failure and autologous recovery and one patient died of pulmonary toxicity. The National Blood Service of U.K. reported 7 CB transplantation for thalassemia, all HLA-identical at 10/10 and with a median nucleated cell dose of 4.7 x 10^7/kg with a range of 0.8-7.6 x 10^7/kg (Smythe et al., 2007). Median CD34+ cell dose of 1.1 x 10^5/kg with a range of 0.2-1.7 x 10^5/kg. Six of six patients with data engrafted. One patient suffered late graft loss followed by transplantation using bone marrow from the same related donor. Donor lymphocyte infusion was used on one patient to rescue rejection. All patients survived.

To study causes of graft failure allogeneic hematopoietic cell transplantation for thalassemia, Lisini et al., (2008) compared 27 consecutive related donor CB transplant recipients against 42 related donor bone marrow transplant patients and 37 unrelated donor bone marrow transplant patients (Table 1). There were statistically significant differences (p <0.05) in overall cumulative incidences of acute GvHD, chronic GvHD, graft rejection, and overall probability of survival and thalassemia-free survival in favor of related CB transplantation. Overall cumulative incidence of transplant-related mortality was not significantly different between related CB transplantation (0%), related BM transplantation (5%) and unrelated BM transplantation (9%).

Using univariate analysis for graft rejection in this study, patients' gender, donors' gender, donor->recipient gender, patients' age, Pesaro class, related versus unrelated donor, conditioning regimen, bone marrow or cord blood cell dose infused were all insignificant variables; however, CB as a stem cell source (p<0.05), related donor CB versus related or unrelated bone marrow (p<0.05), avoidance of methotrexate in GvHD prophylaxis (p<0.05), and not having worsening mixed chimerism (p<0.001) were all significant factors in avoiding graft rejection. Use of ATG trended towards higher cumulative incidence of rejection at 18% versus 9% for conditioning regimens without ATG (p=0.09).

This study, along with the previous Eurocord study (Locatelli et al., 2003), confirmed that related donor cord blood transplantation is a safe and highly efficacious procedure. The results of Lisini et al., (2008) appear to be superior in terms of survival and disease-free survival (both 100%), whereas significant number of patients in the Locatelli et al., (2003) series experienced primary and secondary graft failure (Table 1). Lisini et al., speculated that none of their patients were given methotrexate as part of the GvHD prophyalaxis after CB transplantation and all received thiopeta in the conditioning regimen, both factors found to be strongly correlated with sustained donor engraftment in the Locatelli et al., study (2003).

In 2013, Locatelli et al., published a landmark study (2013) on the comparison of related HLA-identical CB transplantation (66 thalassemia and 30 sickle cell disease) against bone marrow transplantation (259 thalassemia and 130 sickle cell disease) for hemoglobinopathies (Table 1). This was a follow-up study to an earlier abstract with a smaller cohort and shorter follow-up as reported by Kabbara et al., (2008; Table 1) with 72 CB (48 thalassemia) and 330 BM (184 thalassemia). The CB transplant cohort was younger (median age of 6 years versus 8 years; p=0.02), transplanted more recently (median year 2001 versus 1999; p < 0.01), and had higher disease severity for the thalassemia patients (Pesaro II-III 39% versus 44%; p<0.01). Patients receiving CB products were more likely to receive fludarabine or thiotepa-based regimens than BM transplant recipients. Moreover, a significantly higher percentage of BM transplant patients received methotrexate GvHD prophylaxis than CB product recipients. Transplantation were performed at 28 participating centers, with no patients excluded except for patients who received both CB and BM products. Most thawed CB products were thawed and washed per procedure described by Rubinstein et al., (1995; 1998)

The 96 patients given CB transplant had slower neutrophil engraftment, less acute GvHD and no extensive cGvHD, compared to the 389 BM transplant recipients. Graft failure occurred in 10/96 (10.4%) of the CB transplanted patients (2 received methotrexate and were re-transplanted and engrafted stably with BM from the same donor) and 29/389 (7.4%) of the recipients of BM grafts (p=0.33). Eight of the thalassemia patients who received CB graft experienced graft failure versus two for sickle cell disease. Cumulative incidence of primary graft failure was 9±4% and 6±4% after CB and BM transplantation, respectively. Six patients experienced secondary graft failure after CB transplantation at a median of day +151 (range day +51 - 202). Table 1 shows that cumulative incidence of neutrophil engraftment was 90±4% and 92±1% (p=0.01) after CB and BM transplantation, respectively, and 83±5% and 85±5% for platelet engraftment. For patients who engrafted, the median time to neutrophil recovery was day +23 and +19 for CB (range day +9 - 60) and BM (range day +8 - 56) transplant, and day +38 (range day +13 – 125) and +25 for CB and BM transplant, respectively (p=0.004). The proportion of long-term sustained mixed chimerism was 37% after CB transplant, significantly higher than 22% for BM transplant (p = 0.01).

Only 11% (11/96) of CB transplant recipients experienced grade II-IV acute GvHD (no grade IV), versus 21% (83/389) of BM transplant recipients (with 2% or 8 patients with grade IV acute GvHD), which resulted in a significant difference (p=0.04) in cumulative incidence 10±3% and 21±2% (Table 1). Only 6 of 84 evaluable CB recipients experienced chronic GvHD with no extensive grade versus 42 of 355 (12 extensive) patients of BM transplant who survived past 100 days, with the cumulative incidence of chronic GvHD at 5±3% and 12±2% (p=0.12) and with cumulative incidence of extensive chronic GvHD at 0% and 5±9%, respectively (Table 1). Twenty-one patients expired from transplant-related causes - three after CB and 18 after BM transplants.

Most importantly, with a median follow up of 70 months, 93 of 96 CB transplant patients survived – 79 disease-free. This compares with 342 disease-free out of the 371 who survived after BM procedure (Table 1). The 6-year Kaplan-Meier estimates of overall survival, disease-free survival and event-free survival after CB and BM transplants were and 97±2% and 95±1% (p=0.92), 83±4% and 88±2% (p=0.18), and 83±2% and 85±2% (p=0.36), respectively. For thalassemia, the 6-year disease-free survival was 80% and 86% for CB and BM transplanted patients, respectively (Table 1), whereas the 6-year disease-free survival was 90% and 92% for CB and BM transplanted sickle cell disease patients, respectively, with no difference in DFS between CB transplant and BM transplant in multivariate analysis. This study proved definitively that CB transplant using related donor for thalassemia and sickle cell disease is as efficacious and safe as bone marrow transplantation, with potentially better long-term quality of life due to low chronic GvHD with minimal extensive grades. The authors point out that the quality of life for bone marrow transplant patients with extensive GvHD are worse than patients on medical therapy.

For CB transplant, methotrexate was again shown in multivatate analysis negatively influencing disease-free survival (HR 3.81, CI 1.40 – 10.87; p = 0.004), with 6-year DFS at 90±4% if methotrexate was avoided versus 60±11% (p<0.001). Similar to previous studies, thiotepa-containing preparative regimen and Pesaro classification 1 were shown to correlate with better outcome after CB transplantation. The author speculated that due to the higher nucleated cell dosage for most of the CB recipients, nucleated cell dosage was not shown to influence engraftment or disease-free survival.

Given that low percentages of donor mixed chimerism is sufficient to provide transfusion independence, it may be tempting to use reduced-intensity preparative regimen in patients with thalassemia to reduce early toxicity and many of the long term complications associated with conventional myeloablative hematopoietic cell transplantation (Buchbinder et al., 2012); however, available evidence so far indicate that barrier to stable partial donor engraftment after non-myeloablative transplantation in patients with thalassemia may be more difficult to overcome than adults with hematological malignancies (Ruggeri et al., 2011; Kharbanda et al., 2013; Soni et al., 2013).

Taken together, these large series using related CB transplantation, demonstrate the clinical utility and high margin of safety of related cord blood stem cells for hematopoietic cell transplantation for thalassemia. Re-transplant using bone marrow stem cells from the same donor was able to achieve sustained donor engraftment. All the studies confirmed that despite persistent mixed chimerism, patients are still transfusion-independent. Methotrexate GvHD prophylaxis was proven to be detrimental to favorable outcome and the addition of thiopeta to busulfan and cyclophosphamide conditioning regimen favored sustained donor engraftment.

Unrelated Donor Cord Blood Transplantation for Thalassemia

A number of single case studies employing unrelated CB transplantation successfully for thalassemia were reported between 2003-04, with all three patients achieving neutrophil engraftment and transfusion-independence (Fang et al., 2003; Tan et al., 2004; Hall et al.,

2004). Busulfan/Cyclophosphamide/ATG-containing regimen were used in these three patients; however, Fang et al., and Tan et al., used methotrexate containing GvHD prophylaxis. Nucleated cell dose was high, with the minimum of 6 x 10^7/kg. One patient received 6/6 HLA-matched CB and two others were transplanted with 4/6 HLA-matched CB. None of the patients experienced chronic GvHD or Grade IV acute GvHD.

Vanichsetakul et al., (2004) reported on 6 patients transplanted with three 6/6, one 5/6 and two 4/6 HLA-matched cord blood from unrelated donors. Patients ranged from 2 to 15 years old with a median of 5.5 years. Busulfan, cyclophosphamide and fludarabine conditioning was used with cyclosporine and methypredisolone GvHD prophylaxis. Median TNC dose was 2.8 (range 1.5 to 5.3). Five patients engrafted and survived, while one expired due to infection prior to engraftment.

Soni et al., (2014) reported on unrelated CB transplantation of two Pesaro class III patients with reduced intensity conditioning, with one recipient requiring re-transplantation with CB. After re-transplant, both patient engrafted and were thalassemia-free, with a follow-up of 7 and 8 years. Lastly, Kharbanda et al., (2014) reported on the use of unrelated cord blood supplemented with co-infusion of third party mesenchymal stromal cells (MSC) in two thalassemia. Reduced intensity condition was employed. Only one of two thalassemia patients engrafted, with neither surviving.

In 2004, Jaing et al., embarked on a long-term study using unrelated CB transplantation for thalassemia patients in Taiwan with the hypothesis that if conditions were optimized, perhaps HLA mismatched unrelated CB transplantation may produce results as favorable as unrelated BM transplantation as well as approach that of related BM and CB transplantation. One strategy was to transplant patients as early as possible when disease stage is least severe. As Chang Gung does not perform liver biopsy on thalassemia patients for scoring purposes, true Pesaro scores are not available. Because of the dearth of unrelated CB products from Asian donors, up to 3 HLA mismatches were allowed at high resolution levels. Several approaches to optimize cell dose were employed: (1) Utilization of CB products that were not reduced in red blood cells (PD CB) whenever possible. Such non-red blood cell (PD) CB products have been shown to have significantly higher recovery for nucleated cell, CD34+ cells, and colony forming unit (CFU) following processing (Chow et al., 2007, 2011ab, 2012; Petz et al., 2011, 2012). (2) Avoidance of post-thaw washing unless contraindicated, which have been shown by several groups to be safe and offer enhance infused cell dose due to zero cell loss from washing (Hahn et al., 2003, Nagamura-Inoue et al., 2003, Laroche et al., 2005; Stiff et al., 2005; Issaragrisil et al., 1995; Jaing et al., 2005, 2008abc, 2010, 2012; Chow et al., 2006, 2007acd, 2008abc, 2009, 2010, 2011ab, 2012; Rosenthal 2008; Petz et al., 2011, 2012). (3) Double CB transplantation whenever cell dosage for single CB units was insufficient to meet the study thresholds for nucleated and CD34+ cell doses (Barker et al., 2005). In practice, the study complied with the first two conditions completely for all patients from Chang Gung that have been reported by sourcing all of its CB products from a single multi-national CB bank that manufactured non-red cell reduced CB products. As a result, the median and mean cell dosages achieved in Chang Gung patients were higher than every other large unrelated CB transplantation series for thalassemia. A fairly standard myeloablative conditioning regimen consisting of busulfan, cyclophosphamide and ATG and GvHD prophylaxis of cyclosporine and methylprednisolone were used on all Chang Gung patients. Initially, oral formulations of busulfan was used; however, after a cluster of several autologous recoveries within a short span, IV busulfan accompanied by drug level monitoring and adjustment is now used at Chang Gung. Initially, pre-freeze nucleated and CD34+ cell dose criteria were set at 2 x 10^7/kg and 1.7 x 10^5/kg, respectively; however, these criteria was raised later to 2.5 x 10^7/kg (for single CB transplantation) and 2.0 x 10^5/kg, respectively (Table 5). Importantly, the outcome data for Chang Gung transplant recipients were audited by CIBMTR on site using actual patient records, and verified to be 98.5% accurate.

From 2005 onwards, Jaing and collaborators published and reported their experience of a number studies using unrelated CB transplantation for thalassemia (Tables 2, 3 and 6) – both single institution experiences at Chang Gung Children Hospital (Jaing et al., 2005a,b, 2007a, 2008c, 2009, 2010, 2012) and multi-institutional studies (Jaing et al., 2006, 2007b, 2008ab; Chow et al., 2007b, Chow et al., 2008c; Chow et al., 2012; Rosenthal et al., 2007, 2008). The first thalassemia patient transplanted by Jaing et al., on October 2003 also had the distinction of being the first disease-free surviving cord blood transplant recipient in Taiwan (2005a). The patient was a three and a half year-old girl, who received a one-antigen HLA mismatched CB product that had 2.48 x 10^5/kg CD34+ cell and 8.78 x 10^7/kg nucleated cell dose. Neutrophil and platelet engraftment and RBC transfusion independence occurred at day +17, 49, and 34 respectively.

The next Chang Gung study contained their experience with their first five consecutive patients, incorporating the first patient cited above (2005b). Median nucleated cell dose was kept high at 8.8 x 10^7/kg with 1 or 2 or 6 HLA antigen mismatched CB. All patients engrafted, attained transfusion independence, and survived (Table 2). Median time to neutrophil engraftment, RBC transfusion independence, and platelet engraftment occurred at days+ 12, 34 and 46 – considered early for unrelated CB transplantation – at least partially enabled by the high cell dose undoubtedly. At the time of cut-off for the study, with a range of follow up of 120-360 days, all patients had grade II-III acute GvHD, but none experienced grade IV or extensive chronic GvHD.

In 2007, Jaing et al., published their experience with their first five consecutive patients transplanted for thalassemia major using double cord blood transplantation (2007a). Median age was 11.1 years and CB units were 4/6 HLA-matched or better with the recipients with a minimum combined CD34+ cell dose of 3.0 x 10^5/kg (Table 2). All patients engrafted at a median of 15 days (range 12-19); however, one suffered secondary graft failure at day +52. Four experiencing grade I-III acute GvHD and none developing extensive chronic GvHD. Median days to platelet engraftment and RBC transfusion independence were attained at days +49 and 32 post-transplant. One patient suffered Evans' syndrome and expired from pulmonary hemorrhage.

The Chang Gung group also studied the utility of double CB re-transplantation in cases where the first cord blood transplantation resulted in early graft failure (2009a). One of the initial transplant employed double CB transplantation. This involved using a Busulfan/Cyclophosmide/ATG conditioning regimen that is modified from that employed for the first transplant, while maintaining the same GvHD prophylaxis. From subsequent reports (Jaing et al., 2012), it appeared that the first transplant employed oral formulation of busulfan, whereas the second transplants employed i.v. busulfan. Neutrophil and platelet engraftment were attained for all three patients on days +15, +23 and +26 and days +33, +61, +53, respectively. Without experiencing grade III-IV acute and extensive chronic GvHD, all patients are alive and transfusion-independent. This study demonstrated that re-transplant using double CB transplantation for thalassemia was feasible and effective, even when total cell dosage and the number of HLA mismatches for the first and re-transplant were similar.

A single institution series of unrelated CB transplantation of 45 patients with non-malignant disease, including 32 thalassemia cases, were reported by Jaing et al., in 2010 (Table 3). Eighty-two patients received an HLA-mismatched CB graft, with median infused nucleated and CD34+ cell doses at 7.6 x 10^7/kg and 4.0 x 10^5/kg, respectively. With cumulative incidence of neutrophil and platelet engraftment at 88% and 82%, four patients experienced primary graft failure. Three patients experienced grade IV acute GvHD and only one patient suffered extensive chronic GvHD, which appear to be higher than the related CB transplantation experience of Locatelli et al., (2013) With a median follow up of 25 months, five year overall survival and disease-free survival were 88.1% and 77.1%, respectively and transplanted related mortality was 12% at 2 years.

To study the effect of non-red blood cell reduced (PD) CB, in a series of 58 thalassemia patients performed in 14 transplant centers (9 U.S. and 5 non-U.S.), Jaing et al. (2008ab) compared 48 patients who received PD CB against 10 patients who received red cell reduced (RCR) CB (Table 3). Though not rigorously matched, patients were similar among two groups in age, weight, disease severity, TNC dose, #HLA matches, conditioning regimen, no post-thaw wash, and transplant center experience. There were more double CB transplantation in the PD group (23% versus 10%). The result of the raw comparisons between the two groups (Table 3) showed no significant differences the speed or cumulative incidence in neutrophil (PD 96±4% vs. RCR 75±15%; RR=1.31; p=0.56) or platelet 50K engraftment (PD 95±5% vs. RCR 75±15%; RR=1.24; p=0.64). Moreover, overall patient survival at 1-year was similar (PD 89±6% vs. RCR 53±20%; RR=0.32; p=0.17); however, thalassemia-free survival was significantly different at 89±6% for PD CB compared to 38±17% (RR=0.17; p=0.01).

To further minimize patient population differences and selection bias, Jaing et al. (2008a, b) next performed the comparison with a matched pair analysis using a logistic regression model to find patients with similar characteristics to form 30 pairs (Table 3), with 3 PD patients matched to each of the available RCR patient (30 PD patients to 10 RCR patients). Since all RCR patients available to the study were used, and the best-matched PD patients were used in the matched pair, differences in the matched factors were minimized and certain selection biases were avoided. Factors matched were age, weight, #HLA matches, TNC Dose, and transplant center experience. Univariate comparisons and Paired-Prentice-Wilcoxon Test (PPW) were both performed for the matched pairs. After matched pairing, age, disease severity, # HLA matches, TNC dose and usage of double cord blood transplants were quite similar for the two groups, with no significant differences. The results of the matched pair (Table 3) showed that though neutrophil and platelet engraftment did not appear to improve significantly, autologous recovery rates was significantly lower in the PD group (RR=0.31; p=0.04) at 7±5% versus 22±14%. Moreover, 3-year overall survival (96±4% vs 53±18%; RR=0.09; p=0.03 univariate and p=0.001 PPW), thalassemia-free survival (89±6% vs 40±15%; RR=0.17; p=0.01 univariate and p=0.0001 PPW), and transplant-related mortality (4±4% vs 47±18%; RR=0.09; p=0.03 univariate and p=0.001 PPW) were significantly improved for the PD group. It should be noted again that the RCR and PD overall and thalassemia-free survival rates in this study were similar to that of previously reported series using unrelated CB (Ruggeri et al., 2011, Jaing et al., 2012, 2007, 2005). Lastly, the outcome data for PD CB transplant recipients was audited by CIBMTR on site at transplant centers using actual patient records, and verified to be 97.3% accurate, with no errors for major variables, such as engraftment, survival, mortality, autologous recovery, etc...

Petz et al., (2012a) extended this observation of the utility of non-red cell reduced CB to other diseases, with a series of transplantation of 120 non-malignant patients, 46 for thalassemia (38.3%), 3 for sickle cell disease and 71 other non-malignant indications. Besides using exclusively PD CB, double cord blood transplantation was used in 15 (12%) and non-wash thaw procedure was used in 70 (58%) of the patients, as strategies to maximize cell dose. Median TNC dose at collection was 10.5 x 10^7 per kilogram patient weight and 7.7 x 10^7 per kilogram on infusion, and median CD34+ cell dose at collection was 3.7 x 10^5 per kilogram patient weight. Twenty-six, forty-eight and fifty-three patients were matched at zero, one and two or more HLA mismatches at A/B/DR loci. Myeloid and platelet 20K engraftment occurred at a median of days +21 and +49, respectively. The cumulative incidence to myeloid and platelet 20K engraftment were 87±6% and 81±6%, respectively, whereas platelet 50K engraftment occurred in 79±6% of patients at a median of day +62. Autologous recovery occurred in only 3±2% of the patients in this population made up of 38.3% thalassemics and 40.8% hemoglobinopathy patients. Importantly, overall survival at 1-year and 3-year were both 79±4%, whereas 1-year and 3-year disease free survivals were 72±5% and 70±6%, respectively. Transplant-related mortality at 100 days and 3-year were 10±3% and 20±4%, respectively.

The authors performed a univariate analysis of the risk factors (including TNC, CD34+ cell dose, HLA and ABO matches, age, myeloablative preparation regimen, CMV sero-positivity, and use of double CB transplantation) that impact engraftment, acute GvHD, overall and disease-free survival. Within the statistical power of this series, the analysis showed that ABO match, recipient sex, age, myeloablative conditioning regimen, and CMV sero-positivity were not significant predictors of particular outcome. Double CB transplantation was associated with a significantly higher incidence of acute GvHD grades II to IV (relative risk 2.23; p=0.05). Higher pre-freeze CD34+ dose improved myeloid (RR=1.55; p=0.05) and platelet (RR=2.73; p=0.05) engraftment, overall survival (RR of death=0.30; p=0.05) and disease-free survival (RR of death or relapse=0.27; p=0.02). In this study, TNC was not a significant factor, unlike previous reports (Ruggeri et al., 2011); however, that was probably because the usage of typical TNC dose thresholds of 2.5 or 4.0 x 10^7 per kilogram for analysis was not possible in this series, due to the low numbers of patients with such low TNC doses, making statistical comparisons not possible. This anomaly is likely due to the higher median and average TNC doses afforded by the usage of PD CB products. Tissue match at 5 or 6 out of 6 HLA matches trended towards improved neutrophil engraftment (RR=1.44; p=0.09), but inexplicably, were also associated with worse overall (RR=2.83; p=0.04) and disease-free survival (RR=2.38; p=0.05).

It should be noted that in this multi-institutional series with 46 U.S. and international centers, with divergent conditioning and GvHD prophylaxis, by using these three simple strategies to improve infused cell dose - PD CB exclusively, not washing cord blood upon thawing (58%) and double cord blood transplantation (12%), results that are apparently superior to other reported series using unrelated RCR CB are obtained (Vanichsetakul et al., 2004; Ruggeri et al., 2011). In fact, these results approached that of Jaing et al., (2012) in 35 thalassemia patients from a single institution controlled environment (also transplanted exclusively with unrelated donor PD CB that were unwashed upon thawing), showing that adoption of this combination approach to improve cell dose may be of utility in diverse settings.

Table 4. Advantages and disadvantages of CB transplantation for thalassemia

HLA-identical Related CB transplantation	Advantages	Disadvantages
Related CBT	High overall and thalassemia-free survival	Limited HSC, TNC and CD34+ progenitor cell dose
	Low transplant related mortality and morbidity	Somewhat higher incidence of graft failure
	Lower incidence and less severe aGvHD Negligible extensive cGvHD – improved quality of life	Delayed and lower cumulative incidence of neutrophil & platelet engraftment than related BMT
	Even low mixed chimerism (as low as 10-20%) may confer transfusion independence	Delayed immune reconstitution
	Low incidence of severe infection due to low GvHD	No second graft in some cases - graft failure/autologous recovery
	Directed sibling donation makes earlier transplant possible	Undetected underlying donor genetic disorder
	No donor morbidity, especially important for pediatric sibling donors	
	Possible second DLI (Smythe et al. 2007) or MSC or backup BM from same sibling donor in some cases	
Unrelated CBT	Advantages	Disadvantages
	Improved overall and thalassemia-free survival for patients who cannot afford lifelong medical therapy	Limited HSC, TNC and CD34+ progenitor cell dose – Need higher cell dose than related donor CBT
	Low transplant related mortality and morbidity with higher cell dose	Higher incidence of graft failure and autologous recovery
	Acceptable incidence of aGvHD and cGvHD, with decreased severity compared to unrelated BMT – possible improved long term survival and quality-of-life	Delayed and lower cumulative incidence of neutrophil & platelet engraftment than related CBT/BMT and unrelated BMT.
	Mixed chimerism may confer transfusion independence	Delayed immune reconstitution
	Lower financial burden for family versus life-long costs of expensive transfusion/chelation	No second graft from same donor in cases of graft failure/autologous recovery
	Earlier transplant possible than BM grafts	No backup BM, DLI or MSC from same donor
	No donor morbidity	Undetected underlying donor genetic disorder
	Negligible transfusion transmitted infections	Rare donor cell derived hematologic malignancies (Frazer et al. 2005) & new autoimmune disease (Daikeler et al. 2013)

CBT = Cord Blood Transplant; BMT = Bone Marrow Transplantation; HSCT = Hematopoietic Stem Cell Transplantation; NC = nucleated cell; TNC = total nucleated cell; MSC = mesenchymal stromal cells; DLI = Donor leukocyte/lymphocyte infusion; GvHD = Graft-versus-host disease; aGvHD = Acute Graft-versus-host disease; cGvHD = Chronic Graft-versus-host disease.

Chow et al., (2012) reported a multi-center series of 91 thalassemia patients transplanted between 1999 and 2011 with unrelated CB, 79 with PD CB and 12 with RCR CB (Table 3 and 6), the largest series to date of unrelated CB transplantation for thalassemia. The authors also reported on 10 sickle cell disease patients for a total of 101 hemoglobinopathy patients transplanted using unrelated CB (Table 6). Patient median age was 5.6 years (range 0.3-20) and median patient weight was 18.8 kg (range 4-80), with 45% male recipients. HLA matches between patients and donors were 23 at 6/6, 45 at 5/6, 54 at 4/6 and 3 at 3/6 HLA matches. Median pre-freeze TNC dose was 9.4 $x10^7$/kg and median pre-freeze CD34+ dose was at 3.2 $x10^5$/kg – quite high due to the combination of patients' young age and the usage of PD CB products exclusively. Three-quarter of the patients were Asian. Eighty-four percent of the CB was infused directly without post-thaw wash/reconstitution. Most centers reported the usage of preparative regimens without the usage of total body irradiation (TBI) or ones that included Busulfan/Cytoxan/ATG. Seven patients received a second CB transplant due to graft failure. Acute GvHD grade II-IV and III-IV occurred in 76% and 24% of the patients, respectively, in this patient population; whereas 60% and 5% of the patients exhibited limited and extensive chronic GvHD, respectively. Overall, cumulative incidence of myeloid, platelet 20K and 50K engraftment of 83%, 79% and 76% were achieved, respectively. Median times to myeloid and platelet 20K engraftment were 17 days and 47 days, respectively. Moreover, 180-day overall survival, 1-year overall survival and thalassemia-free survival of 79.2%, 74.3 % and 61.4 % of the patients were reported, respectively, with a median follow up of 711 days. The disease-free survival of this multi-center study of unrelated CB transplantation appears to be inferior to the 80±5% 6-year thalassemia-free survival for HLA-identical related CB transplantation reported by Locatelli et al., (2013). Moreover, as the comparison of PD versus RCR CB transplants has not been published yet, the break down of outcome by CB product type is not yet available. However, it should be noted that 10 of the 12 RCR patients and 48 of the 79 PD patients overlapped with this group's earlier series and the matched pair comparisons cited above (Jaing et al., 2008a,b), which showed significant improvement in autologous recovery, transplant-related mortality, overall and thalassemia-free survival for recipients of PD CB versus RCR CB. Again, it is important to emphasize that the outcome data for PD CB transplant recipients were audited by CIBMTR on site at transplant centers using actual patient records, and verified to be 97.3% accurate, without errors in engraftment and patient survival.

Ruggeri et al., (2011) reported their multi-institutional study (combined data of Eurocord, New York Blood Center, and Center for International Blood and Marrow Transplant Registry) on 35 thalassemia and 16 sickle cell disease patients (Table 3). With median age of 4 years old, and mostly Pesaro class 1 and 2 patients (11 out of 15), this study used a variety of conditioning regimens (30/35 myeloablative regimens) and mostly calcinuerin inhibitor containing GvHD prophylaxis (65% cyclosporine). As outcome for most PD CB products transplanted for thalassemia were only reported to the PD CB bank and not reported to New York Blood Center, Eurocord or CIBMTR, this series is believed to have used exclusively RCR CB products. Myeloid engraftment was reported only for 15 of the 35 patients (42.8%), with primary graft failure occurring in 20 patients (57.2%). As shown in Table 3, twenty-three of thirty-five patients (66%) were alive and only eight were alive and thalassemia-free (23%).

Table 5. Recommendations, suggestions and considerations for cord blood transplantation for thalassemia

Factors	Recommendations
Conditioning	Myeloablative conditioning regimens still preferred, with most TCs experienced in using BU/CY/ATG. Results with TT or FLU additions have been encouraging (Lisini et al. 2008; Locatelli et al. 2013). IV busulfan with pharmacokinetic monitoring of levels and careful dosage adjustment may be recommended over uneven bioavailability of oral formulations (Jaing et al. 2012)
GvHD Prophylaxis	Avoidance of MTX (Locatelli et al. 2003, 2013; Lisini et al. 2008)
Transplant Age	As early as possible while some centers advocate waiting for the HLA-identical sibling donor is at least 2 years old so that "back up cells" are available in case of graft failure (Pinto et al. 2008)
Pesaro Class	Transplant prior to multiple transfusions and increased disease severity. Transplant patients with lower Pesaro classifications associated with more favorable outcome.
CB Selection – CB Bank	Reputation of the CB Bank, availability of attached segments for CT and comprehensive infectious disease screening and sterility are important considerations, especially for unrelated CB transplants (McCullough et al., 2005, 2009; Spellman et al., 2011)
CB Selection - Source	Related sibling donor HLA-identical matched CB preferred (Lisini et al., 2008; Locatelli et al., 2013), with potential supplementation of additional donor's peripheral blood or bone marrow stem cells (Goussetis et al. 2000; Fang et al. 2004; Walters et al., 2005; Kanathezhath et al., 2010)
CB Selection - HLA Match	Highest HLA matches, with NIMA match considerations for unrelated CBT (Rocha et al. 2012)
CB Selection - Cell Dose	Balance of highest nucleated and CD34 +cell doses, with minimal thresholds of 2.5-5.0 x 10^7/kg and 1.5 x 10^5/kg, respectively (Wagner et al. 2002; Eapen et al. 2010; Jaing et al. 2012; Ruggeri et al. 2011; Locatelli et al. 2013; Petz et al. 2012; Chow et al. 2007a, 2008c, 2009; 2010; 2011, 2012)
CB Selection - Type	Non-red blood cell (PD) CB products have been shown to have significantly higher recovery for nucleated cell, CD34+ cells, and colony forming unit (CFU) following processing (Chow et al. 2007, 2011ab, 2012; Petz et al. 2011, 2012). The use of PD CB appears to achieve acceptable outcome in unrelated CBT for thalassemia (Jaing et al. 2005ab, 2006, 2007ab, 2008c, 2009, 2010, 2012; Petz et al. 2011, 2012; Chow et al. 2007a, 2008c, 2009; 2010; 2011, 2012; Rosenthal et al. 2007; 2008), and appear to improve outcome for unrelated CBT as shown in matched pair analysis versus red cell reduced CB units (Jaing et al. 2008ab; Chow et al. 2008b; Graham et al., 2008).
CB Selection - Double	In cases of insufficient cell dose for unrelated single CBT, double cord extends access (Jaing et al. 2007, 2008abc, 2010, 2012; Petz et al. 2012; Chow et al. 2012).
CB Post-Thaw Processing	Strict adherence to CB banks' manufacturer instructions is paramount to avoid SAEs, especially with respect to minimizing time from thawing to infusion, or to dilution in cases of washing or reconstitution. Except in related CBT or when high cell dosage is assured due to low recipient weight, avoidance of post-thaw wash may be considered in most cases of unrelated CBT, especially if TC has relatively little experience with thaw handling of CB products (Hahn et al. 2003, Nagamura-Inoue et al. 2003, Stiff et al. 2005; Issaragrisil et al. 1995; Jaing et al. 2005, 2008abc, 2010, 2012; Chow et al. 2006, 2007acd, 2008abc, 2009, 2010,2011ab, 2012; Rosenthal 2008; Petz et al. 2011, 2012). Contraindications to direct infusion – known sensitivity to DMSO or RBC, significant co-morbidities, kidney function impairment, DMSO dose > 0.5g/kg recipient weight (Laroche et al. 2005, Chow et al. 2006, 2007acd, 2008abc, 2009, 2010, 2011ab, 2012; Petz et al. 2011, 2012;).
Intravenous versus Intrabone Injection	Unequivocal results; however, larger series appear to show faster engraftment and lower aGvHD (Brunstein et al., 2009 and Rocha et al., 2013).

Table 5. (Continued)

Factors	Recommendations
MSC Co-Infusion	No success so far in thalassemia (Kharbanda et al. 2014)
Mixed donor chimerism	Mixed chimerism (as low as 10% donor) may still confer transfusion independence (Locatelli et al. 2003,2013; Jaing et al. 2007, 2012; Lisini et al. 2008). State of donor-recipient reciprocal tolerance?
Autologous Recovery	Back up graft using BM/PBSC from autologous or same related donor are recommended.
Post-Transplant Chelation	Until serum ferritin has decreased to the level mandated by individual TC (Jaing et al. 2012)
DLI for late graft failure	DLI from same related donor has been used rarely to overcome rejection and prevent late graft failure (Smythe et al. 2007; Pinto et al. 2008)

TC = Transplant centers; HSC = hematopoietic stem cell; CB = Cord Blood; BM = Bone Marrow; PBSC = Peripheral Blood Stem Cells; HSCY = Hematopoietic Stem Cell Transplantation; CBT = Cord Blood Transplantation; BMT = Bone Marrow Transplantation; PD = Non-Red Blood Cell Reduced Cord Blood; RCR = Red Cell Reduced Cord Blood; NC = nucleated cell; MSC = mesenchymal stromal cells; DLI = Donor leukocyte/lymphocyte infusion; aGvHD= Acute Graft-versus-host disease; SAE = Severe Adverse Events; CT = confirmatory typing; BU – Busulfan; CY = Cyclophosphamide; FLU = Fludarabine; TT = Thiotepa; ATG/ALG = Antithymocyte/lymphocyte globulins; MTX = Methotrexate.

Table 6. Summary of Patient, Disease, CB, and Transplant Characteristics of Chow et al., series (2012)

Patient Characteristics	All Patients 101 CBT	Thalassemia 79 PD CBT	Thalassemia 12 RCR CBT	SCD 9 PD CBT	SCD 1 RCR CBT
Age (yrs) Median/ Range	5.6 / 0.3 – 20	5.3 / 0.3 – 20	4.0 / 0.8 – 12	12.4 / 4 – 20	NA
Weight (kg) Median/ Range	18.8 / 4 – 80	18.5 / 8 - 45	15.1 / 4 – 36	34.0 / 17–80	NA
Male Sex (%)	46%	43%	58%	44%	NA
Race, number (%)					
Asian/API/Indian	75 (%)	71 (%)	4 (%)	-	-
Caucasian/Middle Eastern	9 (%)	4 (%)	5 (%)	-	-
African American	8 (%)	-	-	8 (%)	-
Unknown	9 (%)	4 (%)	3 (%)	1 (%)	1 (%)
CB Graft Characteristics	129 CB Products	105 PD CB	13 RCR CB	9 PD CB	2 RCR CB
≤3/6 HLA Matches	3	3	0	0	-
4/6 HLA Matches	54	42	8	4	-
5/6 HLA Matches	45	38	3	4	-
6/6 HLA Matches	23	21	1	1	-
Not Available	4	1	1	0	2
TNC Median/ Range	9.4 / 2.3-23.7	9.8 / 2.5-23.7	8.7 / 2.3-18.6	4.4 / 2.6-10.0	NA
CD34+ Median/ Range	3.2 / 0.4-13.5	3.6 / 0.4-10.3	1.5 / 0.4-13.5	1.8 / 0.8-3.1	NA
% infused without wash	84%	89%	77%	56%	0%
% of Double CBT	21/108 (19%)	19/86 (20%)	1/12 (8%)	0/9 (0%)	1/1 100%

CBT = Cord Blood Transplant; PD = Non-Red Blood Cell Reduced; RCR = Red Cell Reduced.

Overall and thalassemia-free survival at 2-year post-transplant as estimated by Kaplan-Meier method was 62±9% and 21±7%, respectively (Table 3). Referring to the Jaing et al., series (2010), the authors concluded that "For UCB, only 1 group has reported 80% DFS at 2 years specifically in recipients of busulfan, cyclophosphamide, and ATG limited to patients with thalassemia. Although most patients in the current analysis received a myeloablative transplant-conditioning regimen with ATG or alemtuzumab, DFS was not as good as previously reported by Jaing and colleagues." Besides the single center versus multi-institutional aspects of the two groups, the most obvious differences were the higher TNC dosage in the Jaing et al., series (2005, 2007, 2008a,b, 2010, 2012) and exclusive utilization of RCR CB units in the Ruggeri et al. series (2011) versus 100% PD CB products used in the Jaing et al., series (2005, 2007, 2008a,b, 2010, 2012). In a similar multi-institutional setting, using exclusively PD CB products with 38.3% thalassemia patients, Petz et al., (2012) published 3-year OS at 79±4% and DFS at 70±6% (Table 3). As discussed above, Chow et al., (2012) showed in 91 thalassemia patients, employing PD CB in 86.8% of the recipients, higher patient survival at 72.8% and DFS at 61.4% were achieved than patients from the Ruggeri et al., series who received RCR CB units exclusively (Table 3).

In further comparison, Jaing et al., (2012), using exclusively unrelated PD CB, transplanted 35 thalassemia patients, with 12 patients receiving double cord blood transplantation (Table 3). The authors explained that their initial approach of using oral busulfan resulted in 5 primary and 1 secondary graft failures due to high pharmacokinetic variability exhibited with oral busulfan, necessitating 6 re-transplants. In this series, 88% of the transplants (35 first and 5 second transplants combined) achieved neutrophil engraftment. Five-year overall survival was 88.3±6.7%, whereas 5-year disease-free survival was 73.9±7.4% after first CB transplants and 85.7% (30 of 35 patients) disease-free survival if re-transplants were taken into consideration, in this exclusive PD CB single institution series. The thalassemia-free survival of this single center experience compares very favorably with 80±5% 6-year thalassemia-free survival for HLA-identical related CB transplantation reported for the multi-institution study by Locatelli et al., (2013).

Discussion

Hematopoietic stem cell transplantation is currently the only known curative therapy for thalassemia major currently, despite advances in gene therapy and medical management (Gaziev et al., 2005). For years, allogeneic bone marrow transplantation using HLA-identical sibling donors for thalassemia major as pioneered by Thomas et al., (1998) was the standard of care. However, BM transplantation is limited by the high cost in developed countries and scarcity of HLA-matched, related donors, especially among minority patients who comprise the majority of hemoglobinopathy patients. Despite 14 million potential unrelated adult donors registered in various international registries, only 20% Asians who may benefit from unrelated donor transplantation are able to find a suitably HLA-matched unrelated adult donor (Eapen et al., 2010). Though costs are quite high for HCT, allogeneic transplantation costs vary greatly between developed countries and developing countries. For example, the transplantation medical cost was reported to be approximately US $ 40,000 for unrelated CB transplantation in Taiwan (Jaing et al., 2005b) – considered far less than that of the U.S. Moreover, this one-time cost is offset by the elimination of lifelong transfusion support and chelation therapy; therefore the cumulative lifetime cost of supportive therapy may often be lower than that of HCT.

Scarcity of HLA-matched related donors can be alleviated by the expansion of unrelated hematopoietic cell donor registries and the development of alternative sources of hematopoietic cell stem cells, such as cord blood transplants (CB transplantation). Since the establishment of large adult donor registries, unrelated donor bone marrow or peripheral blood transplantation have achieved outcomes similar to those of matched, related donors (La Nasa et al., 2002). However, only a small proportion of the donors in the world's adult donor registries are of non-Caucasian background; therefore, except for certain Mediterranean regions, most of the world's thalassemic population in China, India, southeast Asia and other areas, do not have suitable matched unrelated adult donors.

Due to far less stringent HLA matching requirements and the less severe graft-versus-host disease, related and unrelated CB transplantation represent an ideal hematopoietic cell source for most thalassemia patients who cannot access suitable matches in adult stem cell donor registries. In the past, due to the large number of hematopoietic stem cells needed to sustain hematopoiesis and prevent graft rejection and autologous bone marrow reconstitution in thalassemics, several initial cord blood transplantation studies have shown low and slow engraftment rates, frequent primary and secondary graft failures, autologous reconstitution and suboptimal thalassemia-free or event-free survival (Hongeng et al., 2002; Locatelli et al., 2003; Fang et al., 2004; Walters et al., 2005; Ruggeri et al., 2011). Recently, usage of HLA-identical sibling donor CB, transplanting at a younger age with lower Pesaro risk classification, optimization with conditioning regimen, GvHD prophylaxis, and for unrelated CB transplantation, employment of various strategies to maximize cell dose through choice of higher cell dose products including non-red cell reduced CB, double cord blood transplantation when single units do not suffice, and avoidance of post-thaw wash in certain situations, have all contributed to significant outcome improvements in both related and unrelated cord blood transplantation for thalassemia (Kabbara et al., 2008; Lisini et al., 2008; Locatelli et al., 2013; Jaing et al., 2005, 2007, 2008abc, 2010, 2012; Petz et al., 2012; Chow et al., 2012). Currently, HLA-identical sibling CB transplantation is considered to be the "gold standard", as safe as related BM transplantation, with significantly less long term complications from cGvHD and prophylaxis than BM transplantation, resulting in better quality of life and probably lower financial burdens than life-long hypertransfusion and chelation (Lisini et al., 2008; Locatelli et al., 2013).

Unrelated CB transplantation, with judicious CB graft selection and consideration of the factors detailed in table 5, has also achieved significantly improved overall, thalassemia-free survival and transplant-related mortality than past efforts. Certain single institution efforts have achieved thalassemia-free survival approaching that of related CB transplants (Jaing et al., 2012); however, several investigators still advocate that unrelated CB transplantation be reserved for carefully controlled clinical trials (Locatelli et al., 2013). In fact, without significant experience managing thalassemia transplant patients, carefully optimizing cell dosage and employing the various strategies outlined in Table 5, unrelated CB transplantation for thalassemia patients may be a risky proposition, as have been shown by many investigators. Transplant cener experience (even performing as few as just 5 HSCT for thalassemia) was shown to be a significant positive variable for outcome in univariate analysis (Jaing et al., 2008ab data not shown). TC experience with thalassemia HSCT management is likely to be important and most of the centers in Chow et al. (2012) and Petz et al. (2012) have performed few HSCT for thalassemia, and this importance appears to be reflected in the results of these two multi-institutional studies (Petz et al.and Chow et al.

2012) versus the Chang Gung single center experience. With the largest single center experience of unrelated donor CB transplantation for thalassemia (35 patients), Chang Gung has achieved 5-year DFS (85.7% including re-transplant with CB and 73.9±7.4% after first CB transplants) comparable to the impressive 6-year 80±5% thalassemia-free survival of related CB transplantation results of Locatelli et al. (2013) - likely showing the combined effects of their center experience and their various optimization strategies. Therefore, in order to properly address the widespread utility of unrelated CB transplantation for thalassemia, most centers have to gain additional experience. It appears that without doing more transplants for thalassemia, it may not be easy for transplant centers to improve their outcome for thalassemia - a chicken and egg scenario.

Survival and thalassemia-free survival for unrelated CB transplantation, even with industry's best practice today, is still not considered optimal at most institutions. However, as patients in many developing countries where thalassemia is most prevalent, cannot access or afford the latest advances in hypertransfusion and oral chelation regimens, unrelated CB transplantation may be a viable and reasonable option. It should be noted that benefit-risk ratio may be relatively different for patients who can access proper medical therapy versus people with no such access. For the vast number of thalassemia patients from developing countries, even current best practices of unrelated CB transplantation may offer them significant benefits - better quality of life, improved long-term survival, the reduced long-term financial burdens.

Moreover, it is highly likely that even centers with the best clinical outcomes in performing unrelated CB transplantation for thalassemia patients, can further improve on their results. For example, the use of thiotepa and fludarabine as advocated and shown by the European groups to improve outcome in related CB transplantation (Lisini et al., 2008; Locatelli et al., 2013), may be attempted. In another example, the Chang Gung group credited improved control of graft failure with the switch from oral busulfan to i.v. busulfan when a cluster of several autologous recoveries and graft failures were observed in their initial thalassemia cord blood transplantation patients (Jaing et al., 2012). It should be noted that the valuable transplantation experience with thalassemia patients of the Italian groups took decades and hundreds of patients to acquire, culminating in the impressive survival and event-free survival with related CB transplantation (Lisini et al., 2008; Locatelli et al., 2013); however, related CB transplantation elsewhere, have not matched the European experiences (Table 1). With further experience at management of patients undergoing unrelated CB transplantation, improvements in clinical outcome may be similarly anticipated.

Over the years, investigators have tried many theoretically promising measures, such as reduced intensity conditioning regimens and co-infusion of third-party mesenchymal stromal cells to enhance engraftment, so far these strategies have failed to improve engraftment and survival (Soni et al., 2014; Kharbanda et al., 2014). Because of the difficulty of eradicating the endogenous bone marrow in thalassemics, it has long been considered essential to administer the myeloablative conditioning regimens for HCT. However, other measures such as those that enhanced nucleated and CD34+ cell dose, optimal conditioning and GvHD prophylaxis, and transplant at an early age, have yielded tangible improvements and it is believed that a combination of these strategies will result in further improvements in unrelated CB transplantation for thalassemia.

References

Anderson LJ, Wonke B, Prescott E, Holden S, Walker JM, Pennell DJ. Comparisons of effects of oral deferiprone and subcutaneous desferrioxamine on myocardial iron concentrations and ventricular function in beta-thalassemia. *Lancet* 2002;360:51-20.

Barker JN, Weisdorf DJ, DeFor TE, Blazar BR, McGlave PB, Miller JS, Verfaillie CM, Wagner JE. Transplantation of 2 partially HLA-matched umbilical cord blood units to enhance engraftment in adults with hematologic malignancy. *Blood.* 2005 Feb 1;105(3):1343-7. Epub 2004 Oct 5.

Boncimino A, Bertaina A, Locatelli F. Cord blood transplantation in patients with hemoglobinopathies. *Transfus Apheresis Sci* 2010;42:277-281.

Brunstein CG, Barker JN, Weisdorf DJ, Defor TE, McKenna D, Chong SY, Miller JS, McGlave PB, Wagner JE. Intra-BM injection to enhance engraftment after myeloablative umbilical cord blood transplantation with two partially HLA-matched units. *Bone Marrow Transplant.* 2009 Jun;43(12):935-40. doi: 10.1038/bmt.2008.417. Epub 2009 Jan 12.

Buchbinder D, Nugent DJ, Brazauskas R, Wang Z, Aljurf MD, Cairo MS, Chow R, Duncan C, Eldjerou LK, Gupta V, Hale GA, Halter J, Hayes-Lattin BM, Hsu JW, Jacobsohn DA, Kamble RT, Kasow KA, Lazarus HM, Mehta P, Myers KC, Parsons SK, Passweg JR, Pidala J, Reddy V, Sales-Bonfim CM, Savani BN, Seber A, Sorror ML, Steinberg A, Wood WA, Wall DA, Winiarski JH, Yu LC, Majhail NS. Late Effects in Hematopoietic Cell Transplant Recipients with Acquired Severe Aplastic Anemia: A Report from the Late Effects Working Committee of the Center for International Blood and Marrow Transplant Research. *Biol. Blood Marrow Transplant.* 2012; 18(12):1776-84. doi: 10.1016/j.bbmt.2012.06.018. Epub 2012 Aug 1.

Cao A. Quality of life and survival of patients with beta-thalassemia major. *Haematologica.* 2004;89: 1157-1159.

Chen TK, Moore TB, Territo M, Chow R, Tonai R, Petz L, Rossi F, Mitsuyasu R, Rosenthal F, Forman S, Zaia FA, Bryson YF, The Feasibility of Using CCR532Δ/32Δ Hamatopoietic Stem Cell Transplants for Immune Reconstitution in HIV-Infected Children. *Biol. Blood & Marrow Transplantation* 2008;14 (2S):119.

Chow R, Nademanee A, Rosenthal J, Karanes C, Jaing T, Tan P, Graham M, Gjertson D, and Petz L. Hematopoietic Stem Cell Transplantation (HSCT) using Plasma Depleted Umbilical Cord Blood Units (UCB) and the Effect of Post-Thaw Washing. IN Wagner, J, Champlin, R, Petz, L. Proceedings of the 4th Annual International Cord Blood Transplantation Symposium. *Biol. Blood & Marrow Transplantation* 2006; 12:1206-1217.

Chow R. Gindy L. "Plasma Depletion Technology & Post-Thaw Direct Infusion" ISCT Telegraft (Spring 2006/2007) 14:6-9.

Chow R, Nademanee A, Rosenthal J, Karanes C, Jaing TH, Graham ML, Tsukahara E, Wang B, Gjertson D, Tan P, Forman S, Petz LD. Analysis of hematopoietic cell transplants using plasma-depleted cord blood products that are not red blood cell reduced. *Biol Blood Marrow Transplant.* 2007a;13:1346-1357. Epub 2007 Sep 21.

Chow, R. Bhat R, Petz L, Tan P, Rosenthal J, Wang B, Hsieh H, Chow T, Chase S, and Jaing T. Unrelated HLA-mismatched cord blood transplantation for transfusion-dependent thalassemia and sickle cell disease – Is the benefit risk ratio there yet? *VAK* 2007b; 2:57-66.

Chow R, Wang B, McCarter M, Brown R, Gjertson D, Petz L. Selection of Post-Thaw Manipulations Prior to Transplantation of Plasma Depleted Umbilical Cord Blood (PD CB) *Products. Transfusion* 2007c; 47(3S):28A.

Chow R, Wang B, Rosenthal J, Nademanee A, Karanes C, Jaing TH, Graham M, Delaney C, Gjertson D, Petz L, Forman S, Kurtzberg J. Avoidance of Post-Thaw Wash Prior to Transplantation of Plasma Depleted Cord Blood (PD CB) is Associated With Improved Engraftment & Decreased Severity of Chronic GVHD (cGvHD) Without Increased Relapse. *Blood* 2007d; 110:494a.

Chow R, Graham M, Rosenthal J, Nademanee A, Karanes C, Jaing T, Fiederlein R, Wang B, Chow T, Gjertson D, Petz L. Matched Pair Comparisons of Unrelated Cord Blood Transplantation (CBT) using Plasma Depleted Cord Blood (PD CB) products Versus Red Cell Reduced (RCR) CB in 92 Pair of Patients with Pediatric Malignancies. *Cytotherapy* 2008a;10 (supple 1):178.

Chow R, Wang B, Rosenthal J, Nademanee A, Karanes C, Jaing TH, Graham M, Delanye C, Gjertson D, Petz L, Forman S, Kurtzberg J. A Novel Method to Reduce Rates of Extensive Chronic GVHD (cGvHD) without Increased Relapse for Cord Blood Transplant. *Biol. Blood & Marrow Transplantation* 2008b; 14 (2S):11.

Chow R, Tan P, Jaing TH, Rosenthal J, Nademanee A, Karnes C, Graham M, Eames G, Ballen K, Wang B, Tan AM, Tan PL, Lin HP, Gjertson D, Petz L. Avoidance of Post-Thaw Washing Prior to Transplantation of Plasma Depleted Umbilical Cord Blood (PD CB) Improves Outcome in a Matched Pair Audited Analysis of 258 Patients. *Transfusion* 2008c; 48:(2S:17A) S43-020F.

Chow R, Law P, Wang B, Rosenthal J, Nademanee A, Karanes C, Jaing TH, Graham M, Delaney C, Gjertson D, Petz L, Kurtzberg J. Negative Impact of Post-Thaw Washing on the Overall Survival (OS) and Disease Free Survival (DFS) of Patients Receiving Plasma Depleted (PD) Cord Blood (CB) Transplantation. Biol. *Blood & Marrow Transplantation* 2009;15:2-2.

Chow R, Cord Blood Unit Selection: Engraftment, GVHD and Overall Survival Using Cord Blood Units Processed using Plasma Depletion" in "Symposium Summary of the 7th Annual International Cord Blood Transplantation Symposium. eds. Wagner, J. Laughlin M. and Petz L. *Biol. Blood & Marrow Transplantation*. 2010;16:12-27.

Chow R, Tonai R, Klich I., Wang B, Chow M, Ratajczak J, Petz L, Ratajczak MZ. Optimal Recovery of SSEA-4+/Oct-4+/CD133+/CXCR4+/Lin-/CD45- Very Small Embryonic-Like (VSEL) stem Cells from Umbilical Cord Blood (CB) Using Plasma Depletion/Reduction (PDR) Compared to Red Cell Reduction (RCR). *Biol. Blood & Marrow Transplantation*. 2011a;17:2-2.

Chow R, Lin A, Tonai R, Bolanos R, Connor C, Mendoza A, Heminger R, Chow M, Ho E, Kang J, Gindy L, Fu C, Rao A, Gau JF, Wang BC, Klich I, Ratajczak J, Ratajczak M, Petz LD. Cell Recovery Comparison between Plasma Depletion/Reduction & Red Cell Reduction Processing of Umbilical Cord Blood. *Cytotherapy* 2011b;13:1105-1119. doi: 10.3109/14653249.2011.592524. Epub 2011 Aug 26.

Chow, R., Jaing T., Chan L., Tan P., Lin H., Graham M., Rosenthal J., Karanes, C., Nademanee A., Wang B., Yen L., Chow, M., Dang T., Kurtzberg J. and Petz L. Unrelated

Cord Blood Transplantation (CBT) of 101 Hemoglobinopathy (HGB) Patients. *Biol. Blood & Marrow Transplantation* 2012; 18:2-2; S268.

Daikeler T, Labopin M, Ruggeri A, Crotta A, Abinun M, Hussein AA, Carlson K, Cornillon J, Diez-Martin JL, Gandemer V, Faraci M, Lindemans C, O'Meara A, Mialou V, Renard M, Sedlacek P, Sirvent A, Socié G, Sora F, Varotto S, Sanz J, Voswinkel J, Vora A, Yesilipek MA, Herr AL, Gluckman E, Farge D, Rocha V. New autoimmune diseases after cord blood transplantation: a retrospective study of EUROCORD and the Autoimmune Disease Working Party of the European Group for Blood and Marrow Transplantation. *Blood.* 2013 Feb 7;121(6):1059-64. doi: 10.1182/blood-2012-07-445965. Epub 2012 Dec 17.

Eapen M, Rocha V, Sanz G, Scaradavou A, Zhang MJ, Arcese W, Sirvent A, Champlin RE, Chao N, Gee AP, Isola L, Laughlin MJ, Marks DI, Nabhan S, Ruggeri A, Soiffer R, Horowitz MM, Gluckman E, Wagner JE. Effect of graft source on unrelated donor haematopoietic stem-cell transplantation in adults with acute leukaemia: a retrospective analysis. *Lancet Oncol.* 2010;11:653-660.

Fang J, Huang S, Chen C and Zhou D. Umbilical cord blood transplantation for beta-thalassemia. *Journal of Tropical Pediatrics*. 2003; 49:71-73.

Fang J, Huang S, Chen C, Zhou D, Li CK, Li Y, Huang K. Umbilical cord blood transplantation in Chinese children with beta-thalassemia. *J. Pediatr. Hematol. Oncol.* 2004;26:185-9.

Fraser CJ, Hirsch BA, Dayton V, Creer MH, Neglia JP, Wagner JE, Baker KS. First report of donor cell-derived acute leukemia as a complication of umbilical cord blood transplantation. *Blood.* 2005 Dec 15;106(13):4377-80. Epub 2005 Aug 23.

Gaziev J, Lucarelli G. Stem cell transplantation and gene therapy for hemoglobinopathies. *Curr. Hematol. Rep*. 2005;4:126-131.

Gluckman E, Broxmeyer HA, Auerbach AD, Friedman HS, Douglas GW, Devergie A, Esperou H, Thierry D, Socie G, Lehn P, et al., Hematopoietic reconstitution in a patient with Fanconi's anemia by means of umbilical-cord blood from an HLA-identical sibling. *N. Engl. J. Med.* 1989;321:1174-1178.

Gluckman E, Rocha V, Boyer-Chammard A, Locatelli F, Arcese W, Pasquini R, Ortega J, Souillet G, Ferreira E, Laporte JP, Fernandez M, Chastang C. Outcome of cord-blood transplantation from related and unrelated donors. Eurocord Transplant Group and the European Blood and Marrow Transplantation Group. *N. Engl. J. Med.* 1997; 337:373-381.

Goussetis E, Peristeri J, Kitra V, Kattamis A, Petropoulos D, Papassotiriou I, Graphakos S. Combined umbilical cord blood and bone marrow transplantation in the treatment of beta-thalassemia major. *Pediatric Hematology and Oncology*. 2000; 17:307-314.

Goussetis E, Petrakou E, Theodosaki M, Kitra V, Peristeri I, Vessalas G, Dimopoulou MN, Spiropoulos A, Papassavas AC, Stavropoulos-Giokas C, Graphakos S. Directed sibling donor cord blood banking for children with beta-thalassemia major in Greece: usage rate and outcome of transplantation for HLA-matched units. *Blood Cells Mol. Dis.* 2010 Mar-Apr;44(2):107-10. doi: 10.1016/j.bcmd.2009.10.011.

Graham M., Fiederlein R., Wang B., Rosenthal J., Karanes C., Nademanee A., Jaing TH, Chan LL, Tan PL, Gjertson D, Petz L, Chow R. A Retrospective Study and Matched Pair Analysis of 240 pediatric Patients with Malignancies Transplanted with Plasma Depleted

(PD) or Red Cell Reduced (RCR) Cord Blood (CB) Products. *Biol. Blood & Marrow Transplantation* 2008; 14 (2S):133.

Hahn T, Bunworasate U, George MC, Bir AS, Chinratanalab W, Alam AR, Bambach B, Baer MR, Slack JL, Wetzler M, Becker JL, McCarthy PL Jr. Use of nonvolume-reduced (unmanipulated after thawing) umbilical cord blood stem cells for allogeneic transplantation results in safe engraftment. *Bone Marrow Transplant.* 2003;32:145-150.

Hall JG, Martin PL, Wood S, Kurtzberg J. Unrelated umbilical cord blood transplantation for an infant with beta-thalassemia major. *J. Pediatr. Hematol. Oncol.* 2004;26:382-5.

Hershko C, Link GM, Kohnjin AM, Cabantchik ZI. Iron chelation therapy. *Curr. Hematol. Rep* 2005; 4:110-6

Hongeng S, Chuansumrit A, Hathirat P, Rerkamnuaychoke B, Chaisiripoomkere W, Jootar S. Full chimerism in nonmyeloablative stem cell transplantation in a beta-thalassemia major patient (class 3 Lucarelli). *Bone Marrow Transplant* 2002; 30:409-10.

Hutter G, Nowak D, Mossner M, Ganepola S, Mussig A, Allers Z, Schneider T, Hofmann J, Kucherer c, Blau 0, Blau IW, Hofmann WK, and Thiel E. Long-term control of HIV by CCR5 Delta32/Delta32 stem-cell transplantation. *N. Engl. J. Med. 2009;* 360:692-698.

Hutter G, Ganepola S. Eradication of HIV by transplantation of CCR5-deficient hematopoietic stem cells. *The Scientific World Journal 2011;* 11:1068-1076.

Issaragrisil S, Visuthisakchai S, Suvatte V, Tanphaichitr VS, Chandanayingyong D, Schreiner T, Kanokpongsakdi S, Siritanaratkul N, Piankijagum A. Brief report: transplantation of cord blood stem cells into a patient with severe thalassemia. *N. Engl. J. Med.* 1995;332:367-369.

Jaing T, Hung I, Yang C, Lin T, Chow R, Hsieh S. Successful unrelated cord blood transplantation in a child with beta-thalassemia major. *J. Trop. Ped.* 2005a; 51:122-124.

Jaing TH, Hung IJ, Yang CP, Chen SH, Sun CF, Chow R. Rapid and complete donor chimerism after unrelated mismatched cord blood transplantation in five children with beta-thalassemia major. *Biol. Blood & Marrow Transplantation* 2005b; 11:349-353.

Jaing T, Tan P, Rosenthal J, and Chow R. Rapid and durable engraftment after unrelated cord blood transplantation (CBT) for children with transfusion-dependent thalassemia. In Wagner, J, Champlin, R, Petz, L. Proceedings of the 4th Annual International Cord Blood Transplantation Symposium Biol. *Blood & Marrow Transplantation* 2006; 12:1206-1217.

Jaing TH, Yang CP, Hung IJ, Chen SH, Sun CF, Chow R. Transplantation of unrelated donor umbilical cord blood utilizing double-unit grafts for five teenagers with transfusion-dependent thalassemia. *Bone Marrow Transplantation* 2007a; 40:307-311.

Jaing T, Tan P, Rosenthal J, Chan L, Lin H, Tan P, Nademanee A, Karanes C, Gjertson D, Wang B, Petz L and Chow R. Unrelated Cord Blood Transplantation (UCBT) for Transfusion-Dependent Thalassemia - A Retrospective Audited Analysis of 41 Consecutive Patients. *Biol. Blood & Marrow Transplantation*. 2007b; 13: suppl. 2: 62.

Jaing TH, Tan P, Rosenthal J, Chan LL, Lin HP, Tan PL, Nademanee A, Karanes C, Gjertson D, Wang B, Petz L, Chow R. Unrelated Cord Blood Transplantation (UCBT) for Transfusion-Dependent Thalassemia-A CIBMTR Audited Retrospective Analysis of 51 Consecutive Patients. *Biol. Blood & Marrow Transplantation* 2008a;14(2S):6.

Jaing J, Tan T, Graham M, Rosenthal J, Wang B, Chow T, Gjertson D, Petz L, Chow R. Matched Pair Comparisons of Unrelated Cord Blood Transplantation (CBT) using

Plasma Depleted Cord Blood Products (PD CB) Versus Red Cell Reduced (RCR) CB in 30 Pair of Patients with Thalassemia. *Cytotherapy* 2008b;10, supple 1.

Jaing T, Wang B, Gjertson D, Law P, Petz L, and Chow R. Unrelated Cord Blood Transplantation (UCBT) for Transfusion-Dependent Thalassemia - A CIBMTR Audited Retrospective Analysis of 30 Consecutive Patients from a Single Center. *Blood* 2008c;112:11.

Jaing TH, Wang B, Gjertson D, Petz L, Chow R. Unrelated Cord Blood Transplantation (UCBT) of 30 Consecutive Patients with Transfusion-Dependent ß-Thalassemia from a Single Center. *Biol. Blood & Marrow Transplantation* 2009; 15:2-2.

Jaing TH, Hung IJ, Yang CP, Tsai MH, Lee WI, Sun CF. Second transplant with two unrelated cord blood units for early graft failure after cord blood transplantation for thalassemia. *Ped. Transplant.* 2009a; 13:766-768.

Jaing TH, Chen SH, Tsai MH, Yang CP, Hung IJ, Tsay PK. Transplantation of unrelated donor umbilical cord blood for nonmalignant diseases: a single institution's experience with 45 patients. *Biol. Blood Marrow Transplant* 2010;16(1):102-107.

Jaing TH, Hung IJ, Yang CP et al., Unrelated cord blood transplantation for thalassaemia: a single-institution experience of 35 patients. *Bone Marrow Transplant* 2012;47:33-39.

Kabbara N, Locatelli F, Rocha V, Ghavamzadeh A, Bernaudin F, Li CK, Vermylen C, Stein J, Beruchel A, Cordonnier C, Roberts I, Socie G, Gluckman E, Walters M. A multicentric comparative analysis of outcomes of HLA-identical related cord blood and bone marrow transplantation in patients with beta-thalassemia or sickle cell disease. *Biol. Blood Marrow Transplant* 2008;14:3-4.

Kanathezhath B, Walters MC. Umbilical cord blood transplantation for thalassemia major. *Hematol. Oncol. Clin. N. Am.* 2010; 24:1165-1177.

Kharbanda S, Smith AR, Hutchinson SK, McKenna DH, Ball JB, Lamb LS Jr, Agarwal R, Weinberg KI, Wagner JE Jr., et al., Unrelated donor allogeneic hematopoietic stem cell transplantation for patients with hemoglobinopathies using a reduced-intensity conditioning regimen and third-party mesenchymal stromal cells. *Biol. Blood Marrow Transplant* 2014; 2013 Dec 24. pii: S1083-8791(13)01161-0. doi: 10.1016/j.bbmt.2013.12.564. [Epub ahead of print]

La Nasa G1, Giardini C, Argiolu F, Locatelli F, Arras M, De Stefano P, Ledda A, Pizzati A, Sanna MA, Vacca A, Lucarelli G, Contu L. Unrelated donor bone marrow transplantation for thalassemia: the effect of extended haplotypes. *Blood* 2002; 99:4350-6.

Laroche V1, McKenna DH, Moroff G, Schierman T, Kadidlo D, McCullough J. Cell loss and recovery in umbilical cord blood processing: a comparison of postthaw and postwash samples. *Transfusion.* 2005;45:1909-1916.

Lau YL, Ma ES, Ha SY, Chan GC, Chiu D, Tang M, Hawkins BR, Chan V, Liang RH. Sibling HLA-matched cord blood transplant for beta-thalassemia: report of two cases, expression of fetal hemoglobin, and review of the literature. *J. Pediatr Hematol. Oncol.* 1998;20:477-481.

Lisini D, Zecca M, Giorgiani G, Montagna D, Cristantielli R, Labirio M, Grignani P, Previderè C, Di Cesare-Merlone A, Amendola G, Bergami E, Mastronuzzi A, Maccario R, Locatelli F. Donor/recipient mixed chimerism does not predict graft failure in children with b-thalassemia given an allogeneic cord blood transplant from an HLA-identical sibling. *Haematologica* 2008; 93:1859-1867. doi: 10.3324/haematol.13248. Epub 2008 Oct 22.

Locatelli F, Rocha V, Reed W, Bernaudin F, Ertem M, Grafakos S, Brichard B, Li X, Nagler A, Giorgiani G, Haut PR, Brochstein JA, Nugent DJ, Blatt J, Woodard P, Kurtzberg J, Rubin CM, Miniero R, Lutz P, Raja T, Roberts I, Will AM, Yaniv I, Vermylen C, Tannoia N, Garnier F, Ionescu I, Walters MC, Lubin BH, Gluckman E; Eurocord Transplant Group. Related umbilical cord blood transplantation in patients with thalassemia and sickle cell disease. *Blood.* 2003;101:2137-2143.

Locatelli F, Kabbara N, Ruggeri A, Ghavamzadeh A, Roberts I, Li CK, Bernaudin F, Vermylen C, Dalle JH, Stein J, Wynn R, Cordonnier C, Pinto F, Angelucci E, Socié G, Gluckman E, Walters MC, Rocha V; Eurocord and European Blood and Marrow Transplantation (EBMT) group.. Outcome of patients with hemoglobinopathies given either cord blood or bone marrow transplantation from an HLA-identical sibling. *Blood* 2013;122:1072-1078. doi: 10.1182/blood-2013-03-489112. Epub 2013 May 21.

Lucarelli G, Galimberti M, Giardini C, Polchi P, Angelucci E, Baronciani D, Erer B, Gaziev D. Bone marrow transplantation in thalassemia. The experience of Pesaro. *Ann. N Y Acad. Sci.* 1998. 850:270-275.

Lucarelli G, Galimberti M, Polchi P, Angelucci E, Baronciani D, Giardini C, Politi P, Durazzi SM, Muretto P, Albertini F. Bone marrow transplantation in patients with thalassemia. *N. Engl. J. Med..* 1990;322:417-421.

McCullough J, McKenna D, Kadidlo D, Schierman T, Wagner J. Issues in the quality of umbilical cord blood stem cells for transplantation. *Transfusion.* 2005 Jun;45(6):832-41.

McCullough J, McKenna D, Kadidlo D, Maurer D, Noreen HJ, French K, Brunstein C, Wagner JE. Mislabeled units of umbilical cord blood detected by a quality assurance program at the transplantation center. *Blood.* 2009 Aug 20;114(8):1684-8. doi: 10.1182/blood-2009-02-205047. Epub 2009 Jun 1.

Laughlin MJ, Eapen M, Rubinstein P, Wagner JE, Zhang MJ, Champlin RE, Stevens C, Barker JN, Gale RP, Lazarus HM, Marks DI, van Rood JJ, Scaradavou A, Horowitz MM. Outcomes after transplantation of cord blood or bone marrow from unrelated donors in adults with leukemia. *N. Engl. J. Med.* 2004; 351:2265-2275.

Miniero R, Rocha V, Saracco P, Locatelli F, Brichard B, Nagler A, Roberts I, Yaniv I, Beksac M, Bernaudin F, Gluckman E. Cord blood transplantation in hemoglobinopathies. *Bone Marrow Transplant.* 1998; 22:S78-S79.

Nagamura-Inoue T, Shioya M, Sugo M, Cui Y, Takahashi A, Tomita S, Zheng Y, Takada K, Kodo H, Asano S, Takahashi TA. Wash-out of DMSO does not improve the speed of engraftment of cord blood transplantation: follow-up of 46 adult patients with units shipped from a single cord blood bank. *Transfusion.* 2003;43:1285-1295.

Olivieri NF. The β-thalassemias. *N. Engl. J. Med.* 1999; 341:99-109.

Petz L & Chow R. Correspondence: selection of unrelated cord blood grafts. *Blood (*2011) 118:478-479. doi: 10.1182/blood-2011-01-331389.

Petz L, Jaing TH, Rosenthal J, Karanes C, Nademanee A, Chan LL, Graham M, Lin HP, Tan P, Wang BC, Chen F, Chow M, Forman S, and Chow R. Analysis of 120 pediatric patients with non-malignant disorders transplanted using unrelated plasma depleted/reduced cord blood. *Transfusion* 2012; 52:1311-1320. doi: 10.1111/j.1537-2995.2011.03452.x. Epub 2011 Nov 21.

Petz LD, Redei I, Bryson Y, Regan D, Kurtzberg J, Shpall E, Gutman J, Querol S, Clark P, Tonai R, Santos S, Bravo A, Spellman S, Gragert L, Rossi J, Li S, Li H, Senitzer D, Zaia J, Rosenthal J, Forman S, Chow R. Hematopoietic cell transplantation with cord blood for cure of HIV infections. *Biol. Blood Marrow Transplant*. 2013 Mar;19(3):393-7. doi: 10.1016/j.bbmt.2012.10.017. Epub 2012 Oct 23.

Piga A, Gaglioti C, Fogliacco E, Tricta F. Comparative effects of deferiprone and deferoxamine on survival and cardiac disease in patients with thalassemia major: a retrospective analysis. *Haematolotica* 2003;88:489-96.

Pinto FO and Roberts I. Cord blood stem cell transplantation for haemoglobinopathies. *Brit. J. Haematol.* 2008; 141:309-324.

Powars DR; Chan LS; Hiti A; Ramicone E; Johnson C. Outcome of sickle cell anemia: a 4-decade observational study of 1056 patients. *Medicine* (Baltimore). 2005; 84(6):363-76.

Rocha V, Labopin M, Sanz G, Arcese W, Schwerdtfeger R, Bosi A, Jacobsen N, Ruutu T, de Lima M, Finke J, Frassoni F, Gluckman E. Transplants of umbilical-cord blood or bone marrow from unrelated donors in adults with acute leukemia. *N. Engl. J. Med.* 2004; 351:2276-2285.

Rocha V, Spellman S, Zhang MJ, Ruggeri A, Purtill D, Brady C, Baxter-Lowe LA, Baudoux E, Bergamaschi P, Chow R, Freed B, Koegler G, Kurtzberg J, Larghero J, Lecchi L, Nagler A, Navarrette C, Prasad V, Pouthier F, Price T, Ratanatharathorn V, van Rood JJ, Horowitz MM, Gluckman E, Eapen M; Eurocord-European Blood and Marrow Transplant Group and the Center for International Blood and Marrow Transplant Research. Effect of HLA-matching recipients to donor noninherited maternal antigens on outcomes after mismatched umbilical cord blood transplantation for hematologic malignancy. *Biol. Blood Marrow Transplant.* 2012 Dec;18(12):1890-6. doi: 10.1016/j.bbmt.2012.07.010. Epub 2012 Jul 17.

Rocha V, Labopin M, Ruggeri A, Podestà M, Gallamini A, Bonifazi F, Sanchez-Guijo FM, Rovira M, Socie G, Baltadakis I, Michallet M, Deconinck E, Bacigalupo A, Mohty M, Gluckman E, Frassoni F. Unrelated cord blood transplantation: outcomes after single-unit intrabone injection compared with double-unit intravenous injection in patients with hematological malignancies. *Transplantation.* 2013 May 27;95(10):1284-91. doi: 10.1097/TP.0b013e318288ca4d.

Rosenthal J, Jaing T, Chan L, Eames G, Graham M, Tan A, Lin H, Nademanee A, Karanes C, Wang B, Chow T, Wu T, Tan P, Gjertson D, Petz L, Chow R and Forman S. Unrelated Cord Blood Transplantation (UCBT) for 59 Pediatric Patients with Benign Indications Using Plasma Depleted Cord Blood (PD CB) An Audited Retrospective Analysis. *Biol. Blood & Marrow Transplantation* (2007) 13: suppl. 2: 7.

Rosenthal J, Jaing TH, Chan LL, Eames G, Graham M, Tan AM, Lin HP, Nademanee A, Karanes C, Wang B, Chow T, Tan P, Gjertson D, Petz L, Chow R, Forman S. Improved Outcome for Transplantation of Pediatric patients with Non-Maligant Disorders with Unwashed Plasma Depleted Cord Blood (PD CB) *Biol. Blood & Marrow Transplantation.* 2008; 14 (2S):28.

Rubinstein P1, Dobrila L, Rosenfield RE, Adamson JW, Migliaccio G, Migliaccio AR, Taylor PE, Stevens CE. Processing and cryopreservation of placental/umbilical cord blood for unrelated bone marrow reconstitution. *Proc. Natl. Acad. Sci. USA.* 1995; 92:10119-10122.

Rubinstein P, Carrier C, Scaradavou A, Kurtzberg J, Adamson J, Migliaccio AR, Berkowitz RL, Cabbad M, Dobrila NL, Taylor PE, Rosenfield RE, Stevens CE. Outcomes among 562 recipients of placental-blood transplants from unrelated donors. *N. Engl. J. Med.*. 1998; 339:1565-1577.

Ruggeri A1, Eapen M, Scaravadou A, Cairo MS, Bhatia M, Kurtzberg J, Wingard JR, Fasth A, Lo Nigro L, Ayas M, Purtill D, Boudjedir K, Chaves W, Walters MC, Wagner J, Gluckman E, Rocha V; Eurocord Registry; Center for International Blood and Marrow Transplant Research; New York Blood Center. Umbilical cord blood transplantation for children with thalassemia and sickle cell disease. *Biol. Blood Marrow Transplant* 2011; 17:1375-1382.

Rund D, and Rachmilewitz E. β-Thalassemia. *N. Engl. J. Med.* 2005; 353:1135-1146. REVIEW.

Smythe J, Armitage S, McDonald D, Pamphilon D, Guttridge M, Brown J, Green A, Brown C, Warwick RM, Lankester A, Fehily D, Contreras M, Navarrete C, Watt SM. Directed sibling cord blood banking for transplantation: the ten year experience in the National Blood Service in England. *Stem Cells* 2007; 25:2087-2093.

Sodani P, Gaziev D, Polchi P, Erer B, Giardini C, Angelucci E, Baronciani D, Andreani M, Manna M, Nesci S, Lucarelli B, Clift RA, Lucarelli G. New approach for bone marrow transplantation in patients with class 3 thalassemia aged younger than 17 years old. *Blood* 2004; 104:1201-1203.

Soni S., Breslin N, and Cheerva A. Successful unrelated umbilical cord blood transplantation for class 3 β-thalassemia major using a reduced-toxicity regimen. *Pediatric Transplantation* 2014; 18:E41-E43.

Spellman S, Hurley CK, Brady C, Phillips-Johnson L, Chow R, Laughlin M, McMannis J, Reems JA, Regan D, Rubinstein P, Kurtzberg J; National Marrow Donor Program Cord Blood Advisory Group. Guidelines for the development and validation of new potency assays for the evaluation of umbilical cord blood. *Cytotherapy*. 2011 Aug;13(7):848-55. doi: 10.3109/14653249.2011.571249. Epub 2011 Mar 30.

Stiff P, Shane M, and Rodriguez T. Successful umbilical cord blood transplants in adults who received a nucleated cell dose = 1×10(7) cells/kg processed by a post-thaw non-wash procedure. *Blood.* 2005;106.

Tan PH, Hwang WY, Goh YT, Tan PL, Koh LP, Tan CH, Quah TC. Unrelated peripheral blood and cord blood hematopoietic stem cell transplants for thalassemia major. *Am. J. Hematol.* 2004;75:209-212.

Thomas ED, Buckner CD, Sanders JE, Papayannopoulou T, Borgna-Pignatti C, De Stefano P, Sullivan KM, Clift RA, Storb R. Marrow transplantation for thalassemia. *Lancet.* 1982;2:227-229.

Vanichsetakul P, Wacharaprechanont T, O-Charoen R, Seksarn P, Kupatawintu P. Umbilical cord blood transplantation in children with beta-thalassemia diseases. *Journal of the Medical Association of Thailand.* 2004;87 (suppl. 2): S62-67.

Wagner JE, Barker JN, DeFor TE, Baker KS, Blazar BR, Eide C, Goldman A, Kersey J, Krivit W, MacMillan ML, Orchard PJ, Peters C, Weisdorf DJ, Ramsay NK, Davies SM. Transplantation of unrelated donor umbilical cord blood in 102 patients with malignant and nonmalignant diseases: influence of CD34 cell dose and HLA disparity on treatment-related mortality and survival. *Blood.* 2002;100:1611-1618.

Walters MC, Patience M, Leisenring W, Eckman JR, Scott JP, Mentzer WC, Davies SC, Ohene-Frempong K, Bernaudin F, Matthews DC, Storb R, Sullivan KM. Bone marrow transplantation for sickle cell disease. *N. Engl. J. Med.*. 1996;335:369-376.

Walters MC1, Quirolo L, Trachtenberg ET, Edwards S, Hale L, Lee J, Morton-Wiley J, Quirolo K, Robertson S, Saba J, Lubin B. Sibling donor cord blood transplantation for thalassemia major: experience of the sibling donor cord blood program. *Ann. N Y Acad. Sci.* 2005; 1054:206-13.

Weatherall DJ, Clegg JB. The thalassemia syndromes. Oxford: Blackwell Scientific. 1981:1-875.

In: Thalassemia
Editor: Makenzie Greene

ISBN: 978-1-63117-954-9

Chapter 2

The Differential Diagnosis of Microcytosis

Eloísa Urrechaga Igartua[1,*], Silvia Izquierdo Álvarez[2,†] and Jesús Fernando Escanero Marcén[3,‡]

[1]Laboratory. Hospital Galdakao – Usansolo. Galdakao, Vizcaya, Spain
[2]Biochemical Chemistry Service. University Hospital Miguel Servet, Zaragoza, Spain
[3]Department of Pharmacology and Physiology. Faculty of Medicine, University of Zaragoza, Spain

Abstract

Thalassemias are characterized by insufficient or absent synthesis of the globin chains. An imbalanced production of one of the globin chains leads to accumulation and precipitation of unpaired globin chains and consequently to ineffective erythropoiesis and hemolysis. Characteristically, patients affected with α or β-thalassemia show microcytic hemolytic anemia.

Although thalassemia is endemic to the Mediterranean basin and countries of the Far East, there is virtually no country in the world in which thalassemia does not affect some percentage of the inhabitants.

Thalassemia syndromes are among the most common genetic disorders worldwide, with 1,7% of the world's population carrying thalassemic genes in endemic countries represents a major public health problem. The β-thalassemias have an estimated annual incidence of symptomatic individuals of 1 in 100,000 throughout the world and 1 in 10,000 people in the European Union. Data from recent epidemiological surveys indicate that in Europe there are approximately 15,000 subjects with transfusion dependent thalassemia major.

* Eloisa Urrechaga Igartua: Laboratory. Hospital Galdakao – Usansolo. Galdakao, Vizcaya. Spain. E-mail: eloisa.urrechagaigartua@osakidetza.net

† Silvia Izquierdo Álvarez: Biochemical Chemistry Service. University Hospital Miguel Servet, Zaragoza, Spain. E-mail: sizquierdoa@hotmail.com.

‡ Jesús Fernando Escanero Marcén: Department of Pharmacology and Physiology. Faculty of Medicine. University of Zaragoza. Spain. E-mail: escanero@unizar.es.

While the majority of patients show significant microcytosis and some borderline anemia, the increase of HbA_2 mostly distinguishes β-thalassemia minor from other conditions like iron-deficiency.

The diagnosis of β thalassemia involves measuring $HgbA_2$ concentration of lysed red cells via high-performance liquid chromatography, with an ion-exchange column or electrophoresis methods. This measurement is considered the "gold standard".

Differentiation between thalassemic and non thalassemic microcytosis has important clinical implications, because each has entirely different cause, pathogenesis, prognosis and treatment.

As in all chronic diseases prevention is important in the overall management of the disease; the real danger of non-diagnosis or misdiagnosis of the carriers of thalassemia trait is the potential homozygous offspring: an appropriate screening, detection of patients and counselling of couples at risk are the most important procedures for the reduction of morbidity and mortality of the patients.

Iron-Deficiency Anemia (IDA) and thalassemia have different ethiologies, which renders typical profiles in the hemogram data, erythrocytosis and microcytosis in carriers, anisocytosis in iron deficiency; nevertheless, the results can be very similar and based on the individual parameters of the hemogram is difficult to recognise a carrier in daily practice.

A discriminant formula or index based on red cells parameters would be a useful tool in the investigation of microcytic anemia. The indices usefulness is to detect patients with a high probability to be β thalassemia carriers, so the best index must have as high sensitivity as possible, in order to detect almost all β thalassemia patients. Suspicious samples can be selected for HbA_2 analysis, to confirm the presumptive diagnosis of the disease.

β thalassemia can be diagnosed with confidence when raised HbA_2, erythrocytosis, microcytosis and normal serum ferritin are present.

The screening of hemoglobinopathies must rely on inexpensive methods, adding in the selection of highly suspicious samples for further analysis, more sophisticated and expensive.

Red Blood Cells (RBCs) indices are useful tools, can be calculated from data reported by the analyzers so every laboratory can apply this strategy, improving productivity, adding value and quality to the Laboratory reports.

1. Disease Characteristics

Beta-thalassemia (β-thalassemia) syndromes are a group of hereditary blood disorders characterized by reduced synthesis of the hemoglobin beta chain that results in microcytic hypochromic anemia.

Most thalassemias are inherited as recessive traits. Table 1 summarizes the different types of beta-thalassemia.

Apart from the rare dominant forms, subjects with thalassemia major are homozygotes or compound heterozygotes for $beta^0$ or $beta^+$ genes, subjects with thalassemia intermedia are mostly homozygotes or compound heterozygotes and subjects with thalassemia minor are mostly heterozygotes.

2. Clinical Description

The phenotypes of the homozygous β-thalassemias include thalassemia major and thalassemia intermedia. The clinical severity of the β-thalassemia syndromes depends on the extent of alpha globin chain/non-alpha globin chain (i.e., $\beta^+ \gamma$) imbalance.

Table 1. Classification of Beta-thalassemia

Type of Beta-thalassemia	Subclassification
Beta-thalassemia	Thalassemia major (referred to as "Cooley´s Anemia" and "Mediterranean Anemia")
	Thalassemia intermedia
	Thalassemia minor ("beta-thalassemia carrier", "beta-thalassemia trait" or "heterozygous beta-thalassemia")
Beta-thalassemia with associated Hb* anormalies	HbC/Beta-thalassemia
	HbE/Beta-thalassemia
	HbS/Beta-thalassemia (clinical condition more similar to sickle cell disease than to thalassemia major or intermedia)
Hereditary persistence of fetal Hb and beta-thalassemia	
Autosomal dominant forms	
Beta-thalassemia associated with other manifestations	Beta-thalassemia-tricothiodystrophy
	X-linked thrombocytopenia with thalassemia

*Hemoglobin (Hb).

The non-assembled alpha globin chains that result from unbalanced alpha globin chain/ non-alpha globin chain synthesis precipitate in the form of inclusions. These alpha globin chain inclusions damage the erythroid precursors in the bone marrow and in the spleen, causing ineffective erythropoiesis. Individuals with thalassemia major usually come to medical attention within the first two years of life; they subsequently require regular red blood cell transfusions to survive. Those who present later and rarely require transfusion are said to have thalassemia intermedia [1].

β-thalassemia major. Clinical presentation of thalassemia major occurs between ages six to 24 months. Affected infants fail to thrive and become progressively pale. Feeding problems, diarrhea, irritability, recurrent bouts of fever, and progressive enlargement of the abdomen caused by splenomegaly may occur. If the diagnosis of thalassemia major is established at this stage and if a regular transfusion program that maintains a minimum Hb concentration of 95 to 105 g/L is initiated, growth and development are normal until ten to 11 years of age.

After age ten to 11 years, affected individuals are at risk of developing severe complications related to iron overload, depending on their compliance with chelation therapy. Complications of iron overload in children include growth retardation and failure of sexual maturation and in adults include involvement of the heart (dilated cardiomyopathy), liver (fibrosis and cirrhosis), and endocrine glands (resulting in diabetes mellitus and insufficiency of the parathyroid, thyroid, pituitary, and, less commonly, adrenal glands). In individuals who have been regularly transfused, iron overload results mainly from transfusions. Other complications are hypersplenism, chronic hepatitis (resulting from infection with the viruses that cause hepatitis B and/or hepatitis C), cirrhosis (from iron overload and chronic hepatitis), HIV infection, venous thrombosis, and osteoporosis. The risk for hepatocellular carcinoma is increased secondary to liver viral infection, iron overload, and longer survival [2].

At present, prognosis for individuals who have been well transfused and treated with appropriate chelation is open-ended. Myocardial disease caused by transfusional siderosis is the most important life-limiting complication of iron overload in β-thalassemia.

In fact, cardiac complications are reported to cause 71% of the deaths in individuals with β-thalassemia major [2].

The classic clinical picture of thalassemia major is presently only seen in some developing countries, in which the resources for carrying out long-term transfusion programs are not available. The most relevant features of untreated or poorly transfused individuals are growth retardation, pallor, jaundice, brown pigmentation of the skin, poor musculature, genu valgum, hepatosplenomegaly, leg ulcers, development of masses from extramedullary hematopoiesis, and skeletal changes that result from expansion of the bone marrow. These skeletal changes include deformities of the long bones of the legs and typical craniofacial changes (bossing of the skull, prominent malar eminence, depression of the bridge of the nose, tendency to a mongoloid slant of the eye, and hypertrophy of the maxillae, which tends to expose the upper teeth), and osteoporosis. Individuals who have not been regularly transfused usually die before the third decade. Individuals who have been poorly transfused are also at risk for complications of iron overload.

β-thalassemia intermedia. Clinical features are pallor, jaundice, cholelithiasis, liver and spleen enlargement, moderate to severe skeletal changes, leg ulcers, extramedullary masses of hyperplastic erythroid marrow, a tendency to develop osteopenia and osteoporosis, and thrombotic complications resulting from iron accumulation and hypercoagulable state secondary to the lipid membrane composition of the abnormal red blood cells [3, 4]. By definition, transfusions are not required or only occasionally required. Iron overload occurs mainly from increased intestinal absorption of iron caused by deficiency of hepcidin, a 25-amino acid peptide produced by hepatocytes that plays a central role in the regulation of iron homeostasis [5, 6]. The associated complications of iron overload present later, but may be as severe as those seen in individuals with thalassemia major who depend on transfusions.

3. From Genotype to Phenotype: Clinical Diversity of β Thalassemia

Carriers for β-thalassemia are typically clinically asymptomatic; they may have a mild anemia with characteristic hypochromic microcytic red blood cells, elevated levels of HbA_2 and variable levels of Hb F. However, even the heterozygous states for β-thalassemia show a phenotypic diversity comparable with that of thalassemia major.

In some cases, the β-thalassemia allele can be phenotypically ‘silent’, with no anemia or any hematological abnormalities.

In others, the heterozygous state causes a phenotype almost as severe as the major forms, that is, the β-thalassemia allele is dominantly inherited.

Although definition of the two extremes of the clinical spectrum of β-thalassemia is easy, assigning the severity of the intermediate form can be problematical. Criteria such as age and level of hemoglobin at presentation, transfusion history and the requirements for intermittent blood transfusion have been used, but these have their inherent limitations and are highly subjective and clinician dependent.

The underlying pathophysiology of β-thalassemia relates to a quantifiable deficiency of functional β globin chains, which leads to an imbalanced globin chain production and an excess of α globin chains [7, 8].

The latter aggregates in red cell precursors, forming inclusion bodies that cause mechanical damage and their premature destruction in the bone marrow, i.e. ineffective erythropoiesis. Red cells that survive to reach the peripheral circulation are prematurely destroyed in the spleen. Anemia in β-thalassemia thus results from a combination of ineffective erythropoiesis, peripheral hemolysis and an overall reduction in hemoglobin synthesis. Factors which reduce the degree of chain imbalance and the magnitude of α chain excess in the red cell precursors, have an ameliorating effect on the β-thalassemia phenotype.

A direct effect of the anemia is the increased production of erythropoietin, which leads to intense proliferation and expansion of the bone marrow with the resulting skeletal deformities. These secondary complications of bone disease, splenomegaly, endocrine and cardiac damage can be related to the severity of anemia and the iron loading that results from the increased gastrointestinal absorption and the blood transfusions. Recently, it has become apparent that these complications of β-thalassemia may also be genetically modified by variability at other loci (tertiary modifiers) [9].

The clinical manifestations of β-thalassemia are extremely diverse, spanning a broad spectrum from the transfusion-dependent state of thalassemia major to the asymptomatic state of thalassemia trait. The most severe end of the spectrum is characterized by the complete absence of β globin production and results from the inheritance of two β° thalassemia alleles, homozygous or compound heterozygous states. This combination of genotype usually results in β-thalassemia major and, at their worst; the patients present within 6 months of life, and if not treated with regular blood transfusions, die within their first 2 years. Conversely, many patients who have inherited two β-thalassemia alleles may have a milder disease, ranging from a condition that is only slightly less severe than transfusion dependence, through a spectrum of decreasing severity to one that is asymptomatic and often mistaken as β-thalassemia trait. This diverse collection of phenotypes between the two extremes of thalassemia major and thalassemia trait constitute the clinical syndrome of thalassemia intermedia [10, 11].

In a large number of patients with thalassemia intermedia, the reduced disease severity can be explained by the inheritance of the milder β-thalassemia alleles (β^{++} and 'silent') that allow the production of a significant proportion of β globin chains. A substantial number, however, have β° thalassemia, and in such cases, the absence of β globin chains is compensated by an inherent ability to produce fetal hemoglobin (Hb F $\alpha^2\gamma^2$). Yet other thalassemia patients have inherited only one β-thalassemia allele. Most cases of unusually severe heterozygous β-thalassemia are due to the co-inheritance of extra α globin genes while others are due to the nature of the underlying β-thalassemia mutation itself. Hence, the underlying genotypes of β-thalassemia intermedia are extremely heterogeneous; the genetic basis can be the inheritance of one or two β thalassemia alleles interacting with other genetic variables [12, 13].

In some instances, heterozygous β-thalassemia may lead to the phenotype of thalassemia intermedia instead of the asymptomatic carrier state. Heterozygosity for mutations in the gene encoding β chain (HBB), that result in hyper-unstable hemoglobins (dominant β-thalassemia), which precipitate in the red cell membrane together with unassembled alpha globin chains, resulting in markedly ineffective erythropoiesis.

Most of these HBB mutations lie in the third exon and lead to the production of a markedly unstable Hb variant often not detectable in peripheral blood [14].

Compound heterozygosity for typical β-thalassemia mutations and the triple or (less frequently) quadruple alpha gene arrangement (αα/αα or ααα/ααα or αααα/αα) may increase the imbalance in the ratio of alpha/non- alpha globin chains. Duplications of the entire alpha globin gene cluster have been reported as causing thalassemia intermedia in association with the β-thalassemia carrier state [15].

4. Pathophysiology of Thalassemia

Despite discoveries concerning the molecular abnormalities that led to the thalassemic syndromes, it still is not fully understood how accumulation of excess globin leads to red blood cell hemolysis in the peripheral blood, and premature destruction of erythroid precursors in marrow (ineffective erythropoiesis).

During erythroid differentiation and maturation, it is critical that the components of hemoglobin are made in stoichiometric amounts. In thalassemia, ineffective erythropoiesis is characterized by apoptosis of the maturing nucleated erythroid cells; limited differentiation plays a role in the development of ineffective erythropoiesis. This would further exacerbate anemia and increase iron absorption [16].

Iron absorption is increased in conditions of ineffective erythropoiesis. The poor elimination of reactive oxygen species, which are increased under conditions of iron overload, may also hamper erythropoiesis and the oxidant injury may cause hemolysis [17].

4.1. Ineffective Erythropoiesis

Ineffective erythropoiesis could develop under conditions in which erythroid progenitor precursors either fail to mature, die in the process of becoming erythrocytes, or develop into erythrocytes that are abnormal and die prematurely. Although the erythron is expanded in ineffective erythropoiesis, this results in only a limited number of erythrocytes being produced, far fewer than the same number of erythroid progenitor cells could generate under normal circumstances.

The notion of ineffective erythropoiesis in thalassemia was first described using ferrokinetic parameters by Huff et al. [18] and further elaborated on by Finch and colleagues [19-22]. Ineffective erythropoiesis was further characterized showing that apoptosis of the erythroid precursors, due to chain imbalances, leads to medullary as well as intravascular hemolysis [23, 24]. However, the apoptotic patterns in thalassemic patients as well as in mouse models of thalassemia point to additional mechanisms that may contribute to this process. Ineffective erythropoiesis leads to erythroid marrow expansion.

Extramedullary erythropoietic tissues, primarily in the thorax and the paraspinal regions, can lead to characteristic deformities of the skull and face, osteopenia, and demineralization of the bones, which are then prone to fractures. The excessive erythropoietic activity exacerbates the anemia by progressive splenomegaly. Splenic sequestration of red cells may develop, accelerating destruction of abnormal as well as transfused normal red blood cells (RBCs).

Splenectomy may help decrease transfusion requirements for patients with splenomegaly.

Unfortunately, after the spleen is removed, patients may be at a greater risk for stroke and infections [25]. Patients affected by the most severe forms of thalassemia require chronic blood transfusions to sustain life and chelation therapy to prevent iron overload. Those affected by beta-thalassemia intermedia do not require chronic blood transfusions but eventually develop elevated body iron loads also due to increased gastrointestinal iron absorption [26].

As loading continues, the capacity of transferrin, the main transport protein of iron, to bind and detoxify this essential metal may be exceeded. The resulting nontransferrin-bound iron (NTBI) fraction within plasma may promote the generation of reactive oxygen species (ROS), propagators of oxygen-related damage [27-29].

Iron overload is responsible for the most damaging effects of the thalassemias, making iron chelation a major focus of the management of these diseases. In addition, as iron accumulates in the organs, dysfunction of the liver, endocrine glands, and heart become the main factors in limiting the survival of patients with betathalassemia [30, 31].

Iron absorption is increased in conditions of ineffective erythropoiesis. Iron absorption studies in patients affected by betathalassemia intermedia show that the rate of iron loading from the gastrointestinal tract is approximately three to four times greater than normal [26, 32-34]. In nontransfused patients with severe thalassemia, abnormal dietary iron absorption results in an increased body iron burden between 2 and 5 g per year depending on the severity of erythroid expansion [35]. Analysis of nontransfused adult patients with HbH disease also indicates that iron overload is common in this disorder [36].

If regular transfusions are required, as in beta-thalassemia major patients, this doubles the rate of iron accumulation. In addition to the transfusion-related iron overload, increased iron absorption also plays a role in beta-thalassemia major, in which its importance is inversely related to Hb levels [37, 38].

Erythropoiesis and iron metabolism are extremely intertwined in that alteration of one of the two may have a major impact on the second. In thalassemia, the mechanisms that control iron homeostasis are likely mediated by the relative levels of ineffective erythropoiesis, hypoxia, and iron overload [39]. Hepcidin, a circulating peptide hormone [40], responds to iron overload, limiting or preventing the activity of ferroportin, the iron export molecule, which is expressed in enterocytes and macrophages [41]. However, hepcidin expression can be greatly reduced in conditions of high erythroid demand, apoptosis, hypoxia, and if levels of erythropoietin (Epo) are increased [42-46]. Therefore, though very low levels of hepcidin are extremely helpful in resolving acute or transient blood loss, its continued downregulation will result in iron overload due to the inadequacy of ineffective erythropoiesis in addressing anemia.

4.2. Role of Oxidant Injury

Evaluating the possible role of oxidant injury caused by the presence of reactive oxygen species (ROS) is potentially important because anti-oxidant therapy could be clinically useful while improvements from genetic-based therapies are awaited. ROSs include superoxide anion radical, hydrogen peroxide, singlet molecular oxygen, and hydroxyl radical; recently, the role of nitric oxide radicals as been appreciated [47].

These ROSs are generated in increased amounts in thalassemic red blood cells (RBCs) because the depositions of excess unmatched globin chains contain free iron, nonheme iron, and hemichromes.

These compounds can generate ROS by several mechanisms, including action as a Fenton reagent. The failure of therapeutic trials with agents like vitamin E is not surprising given newer information on the highly specific actions of the different free radicals, which in turn produce equally specific alterations in membrane lipids, intracellular hemoglobin, and membrane proteins like band 3 [47, 48]. The evidence supporting the role of oxidant injury in thalassemic RBCs can be reviewed briefly.

Previous studies showed that in thalassemia intermedia, band 4.1 had undergone partial oxidation and, accordingly, was only 50% effective in generating the important spectrin-actin-band 4.1 membrane skeleton ternary complex [49, 50].

Furthermore, globin-associated hemichromes induced oxidant injury that led to clustering of band 3, which in turn produced a neoantigen that bound IgG and complement [51].

Membrane-associated IgG and complement provided signals for macrophages to remove such affected RBCs. The excess globin chains bound to the membrane skeleton had lost thiols, presumably because of oxidative attack [50].

More recent data showed that in comparison with children with iron deficiency anemia, children with thalassemia had elevated plasma levels of conjugated dienes and thiobarbituric acid-reactive substances.

These are markers of lipid oxidation. The levels of RBC protective antioxidant enzymes, superoxide dismutase, and glutathione peroxidase were increased [52], implying that ongoing intraerythrocytic oxidant injury led to induction of antioxidant mechanisms. Iron compounds that could generate reactive oxygen species have been identified on thalassemia intermedia RBC membranes. Thus, membrane bound free iron, nonheme iron, and heme compounds (mainly hemichromes and methemoglobin) are very much increased, particularly in the RBCs of splenectomized subjects [53]. This finding suggests that the spleen normally removes the most heavily iron-loaded and thus severely damaged RBCs.

The level of the RBC antioxidant glutathione is reduced by almost 70% [53, 54]. To summarize: there is evidence of oxidant injury to RBC hemoglobin, membrane proteins, and lipids; the possible sources of generation of ROS in thalassemic RBC have been identified; antioxidant RBC enzyme activity is increased; and the RBC level of the anti-oxidant glutathione is much reduced.

Investigators are beginning to consider the role of nitric oxide in the hemoglobinopathies. Nitric oxide from the blood or endothelial cells diffuses into RBCs but cannot diffuse out to perform its vasodilatory function. Nitric oxide entering RBCs binds first to the heme of hemoglobin and then is transferred to the chain cysteine 93, forming hemoglobin-derived S-nitrosothiol.

S-nitrosothiol is associated with the RBC membrane, binding to the cytosol face of band 3 (also known as anion exchanger AE1), forming AE1–S-nitrosothiol. Upon deoxygenation, normally nitric oxide is released from this membrane site, entering the circulation and performing its vasodilatory function.

In thalassemia, hemoglobin may be oxidatively altered at the 93 cysteine site [50], and it is known that band 3 has undergone oxidative clustering [51]. These alterations could impair nitric oxide release, and the lack of vasodilator activity could contribute to the pulmonary hypertension now being reported in beta thalassemia intermedia [55].

5. Microcytic Anemia in the Laboratory

5.1. Diagnosis/Testing of Beta-Thlassemia

The diagnosis of β-thalassemia relies on measuring red blood cell indices that reveal microcytic hypochromic anemia, nucleated red blood cells on peripheral blood smear, hemoglobin analysis that reveals decreased amounts of HbA_2 and increased amounts of hemoglobin F (HbF) after age 12 months, and the clinical severity of anemia. Molecular genetic testing of *HBB*, the gene encoding the hemoglobin subunit beta, may be useful for predicting the clinical phenotype in some cases as well as presymptomatic diagnosis of at-risk family members and prenatal diagnosis. Table 2 shows red blood cell indices.

Affected individuals demonstrate morphologic changes of erythrocytes: microcytosis, hypochromia, anisocytosis, poikilocytosis (spiculated tear-drop and elongated cells), and nucleated red blood cells (i.e., erythroblasts). The number of erythroblasts is related to the degree of anemia and is markedly increased following splenectomy.

Carriers demonstrate reduced mean cell volume (MCV), mean cell hemoglobin (MCH) (see Table 2) and RBC morphologic changes that are less severe than in affected individuals. Erythroblasts are normally not seen.

In Table 3 shows the results of qualitative and quantitative analysis of hemoglobin [56].

5.2. Differential Diagnosis of Microcytic Anemia

Microcytic anemia is frequently due to iron deficiency (IDA) or thalassemia. The differentiation between thalassemic and non thalassemic microcytosis has important clinical implications.

Table 2. Red blood cell indices in Beta-Thalassemia

Red Blood Cell Index	Normal		Affected	Carrier
	Male	Female	β-Thal Major	β-Thal Minor
Mean cell volume (MCV fL)	89.1±5.01	87.6±5.5	50.0-70.0	<79.0
Mean cell hemoglobin (MCH pg)	30.9±1.9	30.2±2.1	12.0-20.0	<27.0
Hemoglobin (Hb g/dL)	15.9±1,0	14.0±0.9	<7.0	Males: 11.5-15.3 Females: 9.1-14.0

Table 3. Hemoglobin Patterns in Beta-Thalassemia (Age > 12 Months)

Hemoglobin Type	Normal	Affected		Carrier
		β^o-Thal Homozygotes	β^+-Thal Homozygotes or β^+/β^o Compound Heterozygotes	β-Thal Minor
HbA_0	96.0-98.0	0	10.0-30.0	92.0-95.0
HbF	<1.0	95.0-98.0	70.0-90.0	0.5-4.0
HbA_2	2.0-3.0	2.0-5.0	2.0-5.0	>3.5

(Hb values in %)

Differentiation between thalassemic and non thalassemic microcytosis has important clinical implications, because each has entirely different cause, pathogenesis, prognosis and treatment [57].

β-thalassemia is prevalent in populations in the Mediterranean, Middle East, Transcaucasus, Central Asia, Indian subcontinent, and Far East.

It is also common in populations of African heritage. The highest incidences are reported in Cyprus (14%), Sardinia (12%), and Southeast Asia.

The high frequency of β-thalassemias in these regions is most likely related to selective pressure from malaria. This distribution is quite similar to that of endemic *Plasmodium falciparum* malaria. However, because of population migration and, in a limited part, the slave trade, β-thalassemia is now also common in northern Europe, North and South America, the Caribbean, and Australia [58].

As in all chronic diseases prevention is important in the overall management of the disease; the real danger of non-diagnosis or misdiagnosis of the carriers of thalassemia trait is the potential homozygous offspring: an appropriate screening, detection of patients and counselling of couples at risk are the most important procedures for the reduction of morbidity and mortality of the patients [59].

The diagnosis of β-thalassemia involves measuring $HgbA_2$ concentration of lysed red cells via high-performance liquid chromatography, with an ion-exchange column or electrophoresis methods [60, 61]. This measurement is considered the "gold standard" and is useful for assessing sensitivity and specificity of other testing methods.

On the basis of classical hematological parameters subjects with IDA are inappropriately discriminated from subjects with anemia due to thalassemia or chronic disease [62]. As a state of iron deficiency proceeds MCV, MCH and RBC tend to decline, but results in both microcytic anemias overlap.

The combination of two or more individual parameters in the form of discriminant indices and ratios leads to a great improvement in discriminant efficiency, therefore several mathematical indices have been proposed for the differential diagnosis of β-thalassemia trait and iron deficiency (Table 4).

In order to be useful in selecting microcytic samples for β-thalassemia testing, the index must detect the maximum number of thalassemic patients (high sensitivity), while eliminating as many non thalassemic as possible (high specificity): 100% sensitivity is required for screening purposes.

A number of formulae and indexes have been proposed to differentiate iron deficiency from heterozygous β-thalassemia using formulas that incorporate at least 2 of the red cell parameters provided by the modern automated hematological analyzers (MCV; MCH; RBC count; red cell distribution width, RDW) and Hb, in various combinations [63-69]. These indices, defined to quickly discriminate IDA and β thalassemia, can be effective for use as a preliminary screening tool to allow the reflex HbA_2 analysis, when a proper cut off is chosen.

For a certain degree of anemia MCV and MCH tend to be lower in β-thalassemia than in IDA. Thus, most indices use MCV, MCH, and RBC count to amplify these differences. Another significant difference between these two types of anemia is the level of anisocytosis [70, 71]. In iron deficiency states, RBCs are continuously produced in the bone marrow as the iron stores progressively decrease. As a result, they tend to be more and more microcytic. Because of their long life span of approximately 4 months, several cohorts of normocytic and increasingly microcytic RBCs coexist in the peripheral blood, leading to anisocytosis.

Table 4. Indices for differential diagnosis of microcytic anemia

Indices	Year	IDA	Thalassemia
Mentzer = MCV / RBC	1973	>13	<13
Srivastava = MCH / RBC	1973	>3.8	<3.8
England & Fraser = MCV - RBC - 5*Hb - 3.4	1976	>0	<0
Ricerca = RDW / RBC	1987	>4.4	<4.4
Green & King = MCV^2 * RDW / 100* Hb	1989	>65	<65
MH ratio (Technicon) = %micro / %hypo	1992	<1	>1
Sirdah = MCV - RBC - 3*Hb	2008	>27	<27
MH ratio (Siemens)	2008	<3.4	>3.4
Ehsani = MCV - (10* RBC)	2009	>15	<15
%MicroR - %Hypo He	2010	<11.5	>11.5
%MicroR - %Hypo He - RDW	2011	<-7.6	>-7.6
MH ratio (Abbott)	2013	<6.4	>6.4

Hb: hemoglobin concentration; IDA Iron deficiency anemia; MCH: mean cell hemoglobin; MCHC: mean cell hemoglobin concentration; MCV: mean corpuscular volume; RBC red blood cells; RDW red cell distribution width; %Hypo percentage of hypochromic erythrocytes (Technicon, Siemens, Abbott); %HypoHe percentage of hypochromic erythrocytes (Sysmex); %MicroR: percentage of microcytic erythrocytes (Sysmex); %Micro percentage of microcytic erythrocytes (Technicon, Siemens, Abbott).

On the contrary, the underlying pathological anomaly in β-thalassemia has no fluctuations, and as a result, the bone marrow produces a constantly uniform population of microcytic erithrocytes.

Consequently, RDW, which is an index of anisocytosis, tends, theoretically, to be increased in IDA and normal in β-thalassemia, therefore some indices defined in the 80s include RDW in the formulae. All those indices have been evaluated applied to different populations around the world [72-80].

Automated blood cell counters have changed substantially during the last 30 years. Technological progress has meant that in recent years modern analyzers report new parameters that provide further information from the traditional count. Flow Cytometry expand information at a cellular level, provides information on red cells individual characteristics and the percentages of erythrocyte subsets can be reported (RBC extended parameters).

The measurement of microcytic and hypochromic red cells, as reported by the Technicon analyzers, was soon recognized as a useful tool in differentiating the ethiology of microcytic anemia [81].

The [% microcytic / % hypochromic] or [% hypochromic / % microcytic] ratios were studied over recent decades and their usefulness in the differential diagnosis of β thalassemia was assessed [81-83]; the ratio between % microcytic and % hypochromic RBCs has proved to be very useful in distinguishing these two common types of microcytic anemias.

Although IDA and thalassemia are microcytic anemias, hypochromia and microcytosis exhibit opposite trends in both diseases; the percentage of microcytic and hypochromic give insights into the pathology of both entities.

In 1992 Onofrio et al. [81] using a Technicon H*1 analyzer found that there was an inverse relationship between the percentages of the microcytes (MCV < 60 fl) and the hypochromic cells (MCHC 280 g/L) in IDA and carriers. Percentile of microcytes (mean 33,1%) was higher than the hypochromic cells (mean 13,9%) in thalassemia. On the contrary, in IDA, the percentage of hypochromic cells (mean 34,6%) was higher than the percentage of microcytes (mean 12,8%).

Iron deficient erythropoiesis is characterized by the production of RBCs with a decreased Hb concentration, so a high hypochromic cells percentage is present, the number of microcyte increases with the degree of anemia, while microcytes of β thalassemia are generally smaller, with more preserved Hb concentration [84].

As exposed on section 4.1, β-thalassemia is characterized by an increase in RBCs, as a result of the chronic increase of erythropoiesis, and a high rate of microcytosis.

Microcytes of β-thalassemia have a small volume due to severely impaired globin synthesis, but almost normal Hb concentration. It is only when these patients also have an iron deficiency that the percentage of hypochromic cells increases [85]. The threshold value for this index MH ratio was set on 1.

Based on these data published in the 90s, in 2007 we evaluated the performances of MH ratio as generated by the Advia 2120 analyzer (Siemens), which represent the next generation of the old Technicon H*1.

The results verified that measurement of microcytic and hypochromic red cells shows opposite results in patients with uncomplicated and untreated β-thalassemia, and IDA. The new cut off was set in 3,7 [86, 87].

Recently, a new software version was made available for the Abbott CELL-DYN Sapphire hematology analyzer (Abbott Diagnostics, Santa Clara, CA, US), including a set of extended RBC parameters. They correlate highly with the ones measured in Advia analyzers, but also show systematic differences, which make analyzer-specific reference ranges and clinical decision values necessary [88]. The MH ratio, as measured on CELL-DYN Sapphire, is a reliable discriminant index for the differential diagnosis of microcytic anemia. A microcytic to hypochromic ratio > 6,4 was found to be strongly indicative of thalassemia [89].

The measurement of the red cell subsets was restricted to the analysers of a single manufacturer, ADVIA series Siemens (Siemens Medical Solutions Diagnostics, Tarrytown NY), until Sysmex XE 5000 (Sysmex Corporation, Kobe, Japan) was available in the market in 2008.

The analyzer incorporates four new RBC extended parameters including: %Micro R, (percentage of microcytic red cells with a volume lower than 60 fL) and %Hypo He, which indicates the percentage of hypochromic red cells with an Hb content lower than 17 pg.

The results differ from those obtained in Advia analyzers [81, 86, 87], the reason is the definition of hypochromia, low Hb concentration (Advia, Siemens) or Hb content (XE 5000, Sysmex).

The former, as thalassemic microcytes are more microcytic, Hb concentration despite low Hb content seems to be more preserved, so the percentages of hypochomic cells (defined as those with MCHC < 28,0 g/dL), tend to be low. In the latter, the state of ineffective erythropoiesis, due to the lack of iron or to lack of globin, renders similar high percentages of hypochromic cells (defined as those with MCH < 17pg), and shows the impairment of hemoglobin synthesis in both clinical conditions [90].

The relative values of %MicroR and %Hypo He in IDA and thalassemia trait have consequences when trying to define a new index with discriminant purposes. Derived from the Sysmex parameters new formulae have been proposed for differential diagnosis of microcytic anemia and the screening of thalassemia: MicroR - %Hypo-He (M-H) and %MicroR - %Hypo-He - RDW (M-H-RDW) [91, 92].

In summary, a discriminant formula or index based on red cells parameters, derived from automated blood cell analysers, with a high level of specificity and sensitivity for detecting thalassemia trait, would be a useful tool in the investigation of microcytic anemia, a matter of great interest in geographic areas where nutritional deficiencies and thalassemia are present with high prevalence.

These indices are based on RBC parameters obtained from automated analyzers and have been defined to quickly discriminate IDA and β-thalassemia trait; these formulae can be effective for use as a preliminary screening tool for selecting suspicious samples for further analysis to confirm the disease.

Nevertheless none of the formulae provides 100% sensitivity and 100% specificity for discrimination purposes, so further confirmatory test must be performed before the patient can be correctly diagnosed.

The screening of hemoglobinopathies must rely on inexpensive methods, aiding in the selection of highly suspicious samples for further analysis, more sophisticated and expensive. Screening by cell counter–based indices and formulae is rapid, automated, and inexpensive and can be done without additional costs to medical systems.

RBC indices are useful tools, can be calculated from data reported by the analyzers so every laboratory can apply this strategy, improving productivity, adding value and quality to the Laboratory reports.

By enabling the clinician to reach a prompt accurate diagnosis, the applications of the formulae reduces unnecessary diagnostic testing and avoid inappropriate treatment, which would result in a considerable reduction of health care costs.

References

[1] Origa, R. and Galanello, R. (2011) Pathophysiology of β-thalassemia. *Pediatric Endocrinology Reviews* 8(2),263-270.

[2] Borgna-Pignatti, C., Vergine, G., Lombardo, T., et al. (2004) Hepatocellular carcinoma in the thalassaemia syndromes. *British Journal of Haematology* 124,114-117.

[3] Eldor, A. and Rachmilewitz, E. A. (2002) The hypercoagulable state in thalassemia. *Blood* 99, 36-43.

[4] Cappellini, M. D., Musallam, K. M., Poggiali, E., et al. (2012) Hypercoagulability in non-transfusion-dependent thalassemia. *Blood Reviews* 26 Suppl. 1, S20-23.

[5] Nemeth, E. and Ganz, T. (2006) Hepcidin and iron-loading anemias. *Haematologica* 91,727-732.

[6] Origa, R., Galanello, R., Ganz, T., et al. (2007) Liver iron concentrations and urinary hepcidin in beta-thalassemia. *Haematologica* 92,583-588.

[7] Weatherall, D. J. and Clegg, J. B. (2001) *The Thalassaemia Syndromes*. 4th edn. Blackwell Science, Oxford.

[8] Schrier, S. L. (2002) Pathophysiology of thalassemia. *Current Opinion in Hematology* 9, 123-126.

[9] Thein, S. L. (2004) Genetic insights into the clinical diversity of b thalassaemia. *British Journal of Haematology* 124, 264-274.

[10] Uda, M., Galanello, R., Sanna, S., et al. (2008) Genome-wide association study shows BCL11A associated with persistent fetal hemoglobin and amelioration of the phenotype of beta-thalassemia. *Proceedings of the National Academy of Sciences US*. 105, 1620-1625.

[11] Thein, S. L., Menzel, S., Lathrop, M., et al. (2009) Control of fetal hemoglobin: new insights emerging from genomics and clinical implications. *Human Molecular Genetics* 18:, 216-223.

[12] Sankaran, V. G., Menne, T. F., Xu, J., et al. (2008) Human fetal hemoglobin expression is regulated by the developmental stage-specific repressor BCL11A. *Science* 322,1839-1842.

[13] Galanello, R., Sanna, S., Perseu, L., et al. (2009) Amelioration of Sardinian $beta^0$ thalassemia by genetic modifiers. *Blood* 114, 3935-3937.

[14] Harteveld, C. L., Refaldi, C., Cassinerio, E., et al. (2008) Segmental duplications involving the alpha-globin gene cluster are causing beta-thalassemia intermedia phenotypes in beta-thalassemia heterozygous patients. *Blood Cells Molecular Diseases* 40, 312-316.

[15] Sollaino, M. C., Paglietti, M. E., Perseu, L., et al. (2009) Association of alpha globin gene quadruplication and heterozygous beta thalassemia in patients with thalassemia intermedia. *Haematologica* 94,1445-1448.

[16] Rivella, S. (2009) Ineffective erythropoiesis and Thalassemias. *Current Opinion in Hematology* 16, 187-194.

[17] Schrier, S. L. (2002) Pathophysiology of thalassemia. *Current Opinion in Hematology* 9,123-126.

[18] Huff, R. L., Hennessy, T. G., Austin, R. E., et al. (1950) Plasma and red cell iron turnover in normal subjects and in patients having various hematopoietic disorders. *Journal of Clinical Investigation* 29, 1041-1052.

[19] Finch, C. A. and Sturgeon, P. (1957) Erythrokinetics in Cooley's anemia. *Blood* 12, 64-73.

[20] Finch, C. A., Deubelbeiss, K., Cook, J. D., et al. (1970) Ferrokinetics in man. *Medicine* 49, 17-53.

[21] Pootrakul, P., Huebers, H. A., Finch, C. A., et al. (1988) Iron metabolism in thalassemia. *Birth Defects Original Articles Service* 23, 3-8.

[22] Cazzola, M. and Finch, C. A. (1989) Iron balance in thalassemia. *Progress in Clinical and Biological Research* 309,93-100.

[23] Centis, F., Tabellini, L., Lucarelli, G., et al. (2000) The importance of erythroid expansion in determining the extent of apoptosis in erythroid precur-sors in patients with beta-thalassemia major. *Blood* 96,3624-3629.

[24] Schrier, S. L. (2002) Pathophysiology of thalassemia. *Current Opinion in Hematology* 9,123-126.

[25] Taher, A., Mehio, G., Ismael, H., et al. (2008) Stroke in thalassemia: a dilemma. *American Journal of Hematology* 83:343.

[26] Pippard, M. J., Callender, S. T., Warner, G. T., et al. (1979) Iron absorption and loading inbeta-thalassaemia intermedia. *Lancet* 2, 819-821.

[27] Pippard, M. J., Callender, S. T., Finch, C. A. (1982) Ferrioxamine excretion in iron-loaded man. *Blood* 60,288-294.

[28] Pootrakul, P., Breuer, W., Sametband, M., et al. (2004) Labile plasma iron (LPI) as an indicator of chelatable plasma redox activity in iron-overloaded beta-thalassemia/HbE patients treated with an oral chelator. *Blood* 104, 1504-1510.

[29] Rachmilewitz, E. A., Weizer-Stern, O., Adamsky, K., et al. (2005) Role of iron in inducing oxidative stress in thalassemia: can it be prevented by inhibition of absorption and by antioxidants? *Annals of the New York Academy of Sciences* 1054,118-123.

[30] Propper, R. D., Cooper, B., Rufo, R. R., et al. (1977) Continuous subcutaenous administration of deferoxamine in patients with iron overload. *New England Journal of Medicine* 297, 418-423.

[31] Olivieri, N. F. and Weatherall, D. J. (2001) Clinical aspects of beta-thalassemia. In: Steinberg, M. H., Forget, B. G., Higgs, D. R., Nagel, R. L., editors. *Disorders of hemoglobin: genetics, pathophysiology and clinical management.* Cambridge University Press; Cambridge, England.

[32] Bannerman, R. M., Keusch, G., Kreimer-Birnbaum, M., et al. (1967) Thalassemia intermedia, with iron overload, cardiac failure, diabetes mellitus, hypopituitarism and porphyrinuria. *American Journal of Medicine* 42, 476-486.

[33] Cossu, P., Toccafondi, C., Vardeu, F., et al. (1981) Iron overload and desferrioxamine chelation therapy in beta-thalassemia intermedia. *European Journal of Pediatrics* 137, 267-271.

[34] Fiorelli, G., Fargion, S., Piperno, A., et al. (1990) Iron metabolism in thalassemia intermedia. *Haematologica* 75, 89-95.

[35] Hershko, C. and Rachmilewitz, E. A. (1979) Mechanism of desferrioxamine-induced iron excretion in thalassaemia. *British Journal of Haematology* 42,125-132.

[36] Hsu, H. C., Lin, C. K., Tsay, S. H., et al. (1990) Iron overload in Chinese patients with hemoglobin H disease. *American Journal of Hematology* 34,287-290.

[37] Erlandson, M. E., Walden, B., Stern, G., et al. (1962) Studies on congenital hemolyticsyndromes. Part IV: gastrointestinal absorption of iron. *Blood* 19, 359-378.

[38] Cazzola, M., Pootrakul, P., Huebers, H. A., et al. (1987) Erythroid marrow function in anemic patients. *Blood* 69, 296-301.

[39] Finch, C. (1994) Regulators of iron balance in humans. *Blood* 84,1697-1702.

[40] Nicolas, G., Bennoun, M., Devaux, I., et al. (2001) Lack of hepcidin gene expression and severe tissue iron overload in upstream stimulatory factor 2 (USF2) knockout mice. *Proceedings of the National Academy of Sciences US* 98,8780-8785.

[41] Nemeth, E., Tuttle, M. S., Powelson, J., et al. (2004) Hepcidin regulates cellular iron efflux by binding to ferroportin and inducing its internalization. *Science* 306, 2090-2093.

[42] Pak, M., Lopez, M. A., Gabayan, V., et al. (2006) Suppression of hepcidin during anemia requires erythropoietic activity. *Blood* 108, 3730-3735.

[43] Peyssonnaux, C., Zinkernagel, A. S., Schuepbach, R. A., et al. (2007) Regulation of iron homeostasis by the hypoxia-inducible transcription factors (HIFs). *Journal of Clinical Investigation* 117, 1926-1932.

[44] Pinto, J. P., Ribeiro, S., Pontes, H., et al. (2008) Erythropoietin mediates hepcidin expression in hepatocytes through EPOR signalling and regulation ofC/EBP{alpha}. *Blood* 111, 5727-5733.

[45] Tanno, T., Bhanu, N. V., Oneal, P. A., et al. (2007) High levels of GDF15 in thalassemiasuppress expression of the iron regulatory protein hepcidin. *Natural Medicine* 13,1096-1101.

[46] Tamary, H., Shalev, H., Perez-Avraham, G., et al. (2008) Elevated growth differentiation factor 15 expression in patients with congenital dyserythropoietic anemia type I. *Blood* 112, 5241-5244.

[47] Kattamis, C. and Kattamis, A. C. (2001) Oxidative stress disturbances in erythrocytes of beta-thalassemia. *Pediatric Hematology and Oncology* 18,85-88.

[48] Celedon, G., Rodriguez, I., España, J., et al. (2001) Contribution of hemoglobin and membrane constituents modification to human erythrocyte damage promoted by peroxyl radicals of different charge and hydrophobicity. *Free Radical Research* 34, 17-31.

[49] Shinar, E., Rachmilewitz, E. A., Lux, S. E. (1989) Differing erythrocyte membrane skeletal protein defects in alpha and beta thalassemia. *Journal of Clinical Investigation* 83, 404-410.

[50] Advani, R., Sorenson, S., Shinar, E., et al. (1992) Characterization and comparison of the RBC membrane damage in severe human alpha and beta thalassemia. *Blood* 79, 1058-1063.

[51] Yuan, J., Kannan, R., Shinar, E., et al. (1992) Isolation, characterization, and immuno-precipitation studies of immune complexes from membranes of beta-thalassemic erythrocytes. *Blood* 79, 3007-3013.

[52] Meral, A., Tuncel, P., Surmen-Gur, E., et al. (2000) Lipid peroxidation and antioxidant status in beta-thalassemia. *Pediatric Hematology and Oncology* 17,687-693.

[53] Tavazzi, D., Duca, L., Grazidei, G., et al. (2001) Membrane-bound iron contributes to oxidative damage of beta-thalassemia intermedia erythrocytes. *British Journal of Haematology* 112,48-50.
[54] Chakraborty, D. and Bhattacharyya, M. (2001) Antioxidant status of red blood cells of patients with beta-thalassemia and E beta-thalassemia. *Clinica Chimica Acta* 305,123-129.
[55] Aessopos, A., Farmakis, D., Karagiorga, M., et al. (2001) Cardiac involvement in thalassemia intermedia: a multicenter study. *Blood* 97,3411-3416.
[56] Telen, M. J. and Kaufman, R. E. (1981) The mature erythrocyte. In: Lee, G. R., Paraskevas, F., Foerster, J., Lukens, J., eds. *Wintrobe's Clinical Hematology*. 10 ed. Baltimore, MD: Lippincott.
[57] Weatherall, D. J. and Clegg, J. B. (2001) Inherited haemoglobin disorders:an increasing global health problem. *Bulletin of the World Health Organization* 79, 704-712.
[58] Modell, B. and Darlison, M. (2008) Global epidemiology of haemoglobin disorders and derived service indicators *Bulletin of the World Health Organization* 86(6), 480-487.
[59] Giordano, P. C., Bouva, M. J., Harteveld, C. L. (2004) A confidential inquiry estimating the number of patients affected with sickle cell disease and thalassemia major confirms the need for a prevention strategy in the Netherlands. *Hemoglobin* 28 (4), 287-296.
[60] Joutovsky, A., Hadzi-Nesic, J., Nardi, M. A. (2004) HPLC Retention time as a diagnostic tool for hemoglobin variants and hemoglobinopathies: a study of 60000 samples in a clinical diagnostic laboratory. *Clinical Chemistry* 50,1736-1747.
[61] Mosca, A., Paleari, R., Ivaldi, G., et al. (2009) The role of haemoglobin A_2 testing in the diagnosis of thalassaemias and related haemoglobinopathies. *Journal of Clinical Pathology* 62(1),13-17.
[62] Bentley, S. A., Ayscue, L. H., Watson, J. M., et al. (1989) The clinical utility of discriminant functions for the differential diagnosis of microcytic anemias. *Blood cells* 15, 575-582.
[63] England, J. M., Bain, B. J., Fraser, P. M. (1973) Differentiation of iron deficiency from thalassaemia trait. *Lancet* 1,1514.
[64] Green, R. and King, R. (1989) A new red cell discriminant incorporating volume dispersion for differentiating iron deficiency anemia from thalassemia minor. *Blood Cells* 5, 481-495.
[65] Mentzer, W. C. Jr. (1973) Differentiation of iron deficiency from thalassaemia trait. *Lancet* 1, 882.
[66] Ricerca, B. M., Storti, S., d 'Onofrio, G., et al. (1987) Differentiation of iron deficiency from thalassaemia trait: a new approach. *Haematologica* 72, 409-413.
[67] Srivastava, P. C. and Bevington, J. M. (1973) Iron deficiency and-or thalassaemia trait. *Lancet* 1, 832.
[68] Sirdah, M., Tarazi, I., Al Najjar, E., et al. (2008) Evaluation of the diagnostic reliability of different RBC indices and formulas in the differentiation of the b-thalassaemia minor from iron deficiency in Palestinian population. *International Journal of Laboratory Hematology* 30(4), 324-330.
[69] Ehsani, M. A., Shahghol, E., Rahiminejad, M. S., et al. (2009) A new index for discrimination between iron deficiency anemia and beta-thalassemia minor: results in 284 patients. *Pakistan Journal of Biological Sciences* 12(5), 473-475.

[70] Junca, J., Flores, A., Roy, C., et al. (1991) Red cell distribution width, free erythrocyte protoporphyrin, and England-Fraser index in the differential diagnosis of microcytosis due to iron deficiency or beta-thalassemia trait. A study of 200 cases of microcytic anemia. *Hematologic Pathology*. 5(1), 33-36.

[71] Jayabose, S., Giamelli, J., Levondoglu-Tugal, O., et al. (1999) Differentiating iron deficiency anemia from thalassemia minor by using an RDW-based index. *Pediatric Hematology and Oncology* 21, 314.

[72] Lafferty, J. D., Crowther, M. A., Ali, M. A., et al. (1996) The evaluation of various mathematical RBC indices and their efficacy in discriminating between thalassemic and nonthalassemic microcytosis. *American Journal of Clinical Pathology* 106, 201-205.

[73] Eldibany, M. M., Totonchi, K. F., Joseph, N. J., et al. (1999) Usefulness of certain red blood cell indices in diagnosing and differentiating thalassemia trait from iron-deficiency anemia. *American Journal of Clinical Pathology* 111,676-682.

[74] Demir, A., Yarali, N., Fisgin, T., et al. (2002) Most reliable indices in differentiation between thalassemia trait and iron deficiency anemia. *Pediatric International* 44,612-616.

[75] Noronha, J. F. A. and Grotto, H. Z. W. (2005) Measurement of reticulocyte and red blood cell indices in patients with iron deficiency anemia and b-thalassemia minor. *Clinical Chemistry and Laboratory Medicine* 43(2), 195-197.

[76] Beyan, C., Kaptan, K., Ifran, A. (2007) Predictive value of discrimination indices in differential diagnosis of iron deficiency anemia and beta-thalassemia trait. *European Journal of Hematology* 78, 524-526.

[77] Ntaios, G., Chatzinikolau, A., Sauli, Z., et al. (2007) Discrimination indices as screening test for b thalassemic trait. *Annals of Hematology* 86,487-491.

[78] Rathod, D. A., Kaur, A., Patel, V., et al. (2007) Usefulness of cell counter-based parameters and formulas in detection of b-thalassemia trait in areas of high prevalence. *American Journal of Clinical Pathology,*128,585-589.

[79] Matos, J. F., Dusse, L. M., Stubbert, R. V., et al. (2013) Comparison of discriminative indices for iron deficiency anemia and β thalassemia trait in a Brazilian population. *Hematology* 18 (3), 169-174.

[80] Chaima, A. S. Red cell indices: differentiation between β -thalassemia trait and iron deficiency anemia and application to sickle-cell disease and sickle-cell thalassemia DOI 10.1515/cclm-2013-0354.

[81] D'Onofrio, G., Zini, G., Ricerca, B. M., et al. (1992) Automated measurement of red blood cell microcytosis and hypochromia in iron deficiency and beta-thalassemia trait. *Archives of Pathology and Laboratory Medicine* 116, 84-89.

[82] Robertson, E. P., Pollock, A., Yau, K. S., et al. (1992) Use of Technicon H*1 technology in routine thalassemia screening. *Medical Laboratory Science* 49, 259-264.

[83] Jiménez, C. V., Minchinela, J., Ros, J. (1995) New indices from the H*2 analyser improve differentiation between heterozygous beta or delta beta thalassaemia and iron deficiency anaemia. *Clinical Laboratory Haematology* 17,151-155.

[84] Brugnara, C. (2003) Iron deficiency and erythropoiesis: new diagnostic approaches. *Clinical Chemistry* 49,1573-1578.

[85] Tassiopoulos, T., Konstantopoulos, K., Tassiopoulos, S., et al. (1997) Erythropoietin levels and microcytosis in heterozygous beta-thalassemia. *Acta Haematologica* 98, 147-149.

[86] Urrechaga, E. (2008) Discriminant value of % Microcytic / % Hypochromic ratio in the differential diagnosis of microcytic anemia *Clinical Chemistry and Laboratory Medicine* 46(12), 1752-1758.

[87] Urrechaga, E. (2009) Red blood cell microcytosis and hypochromia in the differential diagnosis of iron deficiency and β-thalassaemia trait. *International Journal of Laboratory Hematology* 31(5), 528-534.

[88] Ermens, A.A.M., Hoffmann, J.J.M.L., Krockenberger, M., Van Wijk,E.M. (2012) New erythrocyte and reticulocyte parameters on CELL-DYN Sapphire; analytical and preanalytical aspects. *International Journal of Laboratory Hematology* 34, 274-282.

[89] Urrechaga, E., Hoffmann, J. J. M. L., Borque, L., et al. The role of erythrocyte subsets in the differential diagnosis of microcytic anemia. *19th meeting of the Europèan Red Cell Society* (Ijmuiden, October 2013).

[90] Urrechaga, E., Borque, L., Escanero, J. F. (2009) Potential utility of the new Sysmex XE 5000 red blood cell extended parameters in the study of disorders of iron metabolism *Clinical Chemistry and Laboratory Medicine* 47(11), 1411-1416.

[91] Urrechaga, E., Borque, L., Escanero, J. F. (2011) The role of automated measurement of red cell subpopulations on the Sysmex XE 5000 analyzer in the differential diagnosis of microcytic anemia. *International Journal of Laboratory Hematology* 33, 30-36.

[92] Urrechaga, E., Borque, L., Escanero, J. F. (2011) The role of automated measurement of red cell subpopulations in differential diagnosis of microcytic anemia and β thalassemia screening. *American Journal of Clinical Pathology* 135,374-379.

In: Thalassemia
Editor: Makenzie Greene

ISBN: 978-1-63117-954-9

Chapter 3

Computer Aided Diagnosis of Thalassaemias: An Overview

Giovanni Luca Masala*[*] *and Bruno Golosio
POLCOMING Department, Section of Engineering and Information Technologies, University of Sassari, Sassari, Italy

Abstract

The distribution of thalassaemias is global, with particular incidence in areas affected by malaria as the Mediterranean area (Italy, Greece, Turkey, Cyprus) and in southeast Asia (India, Vietnam, Cambodia). Screening of the heterozygous population is fundamental for keeping thalassaemic pathology diffusion under control.

Thalassaemia recognition is based on a first-level analysis performed with haemochromocytometric data and a second-level examination (HbA_2 quantification, globin chain synthesis, and genetic analysis). Many of the latter techniques are finalised to a secure diagnosis of the genetic defect and they are time-consuming and expensive, therefore it would be important to have a Computer Aided Diagnosis (CAD) support based mainly on the haemochromocytometric data and on the simple HbA_2 quantification. Such classification through CAD systems would contribute to the selection of cases that need further examination and could be helpful in laboratory quality control.

Several automated expert systems have been proposed to detect thalassaemias. There are different types of α-thalassaemia resulting from different gene mutations and their distribution is dissimilar in different geographic areas. The CAD systems are often optimized on the α-Thalassaemia and β-Thalassaemia types of the area where the software is built.

In this work an overview of some automated systems used for supporting the diagnosis of different Thalassaemia traits is presented.

[*] Corresponding author: Email: gilmasala@uniss.it.

Introduction

Thalassaemia is an autosomal recessive trait. It occurs therefore in homozygous subjects when both alleles are mutated. The presence of the thalassaemia trait in the heterozygous form does not lead to a pathological condition, so these subjects are commonly considered healthy carriers. Screening of the heterozygous population is fundamental for keeping thalassaemic pathology diffusion under control [1].

In order to make the diagnosis, the blood characteristics must be analysed. A complete blood count is the primary screening test for a laboratory diagnosis of thalassaemia.

A healthy carrier usually has a reduced number of Red Blood Cells (RBCs) in the bloodstream (anaemia), which affects the oxygen transportation to the body tissues. In addition, thalassaemia can cause RBCs to be smaller than the normal or decrease hemoglobin in the RBCs to below-normal levels [2].

However, there is still a limitation in the analysis of data due to a large number of possible candidate characteristics. In addition, there are various types of thalassaemia and thalassaemia traits (persons with the thalassaemia trait do not have the disease but inherit genes that cause the disease).

As a result, a manual diagnostic process can only be carried out by specialists whose decision is based upon an index of mathematically combined values of blood characteristics [3].

Blood Count (CBC) test is the first and the simplest test that can be performed to indicate the thalassaemia's genes existence [3]. The MCV is a highly discriminating feature. In medical practice, a threshold of this parameter is often used to recognise thalassaemia carriers. A threshold value of 77fL was proposed in [4].

Thalassaemia is present in different forms, the best known of which are called α- or β-thalassaemia, depending on whether the mutated genes are for the α- or for the β-chain of haemoglobin respectively. There are different types of α-thalassaemia resulting from different gene mutations. The different types of thalassaemia are not evenly spreads in all the areas of interest of the world affected by malaria.

The α- and β-thalassaemia carrier recognition is based on a first-level analysis performed with haemochromocytometric data and a second-level examination (HbA_2 quantification, globin chain synthesis, and genetic analysis) [5, 6]. As many of the latter techniques, which are finalised to a secure diagnosis of the genetic defect, are time-consuming and expensive, it would be important to have an automated system for diagnostic support doing mainly the haemochromocytometric data and on the simple HbA_2 quantification.

There are no available international reference databases on thalassaemia, where it is possible to find patient with haemochromocytometric data, haemoglobin and diagnoses of thalassaemia genetically verified. In fact the databases used in the literature are characterized by the diffusion of the variants in the area in which they are collected. In this book-chapter the main characteristic of some completed automatic diagnostic systems presented are based on different datasets.

Computer Aided Diagnosis

A simple definition of Computer Assisted Diagnosis (CAD) could be "Application of computer programs designed to assist the physician in solving a diagnostic problem". Such programs are generally based on pattern recognition techniques and classification systems.

The assisted diagnosis makes it easier for the doctor, the analysis of correlations between variables. In addition, as the physician might need to examine routinely a large amount of data (i.e. in screening procedures), he can have moments of distraction or fatigue during diagnosis. Often the lack of consistency of the human observer may be overcome by using CAD schemes as a reminder or “second opinion” or "second look" [7].

Pattern recognition [8] is the research area of Artificial Intelligence that studies the operation and design of systems that recognize patterns in the data. Important application areas are image analysis, biometry classification, speech analysis, DNA sequence identification, man and machine diagnostics, person identification and industrial inspection. The interest in improving the classification systems of data analysis is independent from the context of applications. In fact, in many studies it is often the case to have to recognize and to distinguish groups of various objects, which requires the need for valid instruments capable to perform this task[9]. In Figure 1 a classification system block diagram is shown.

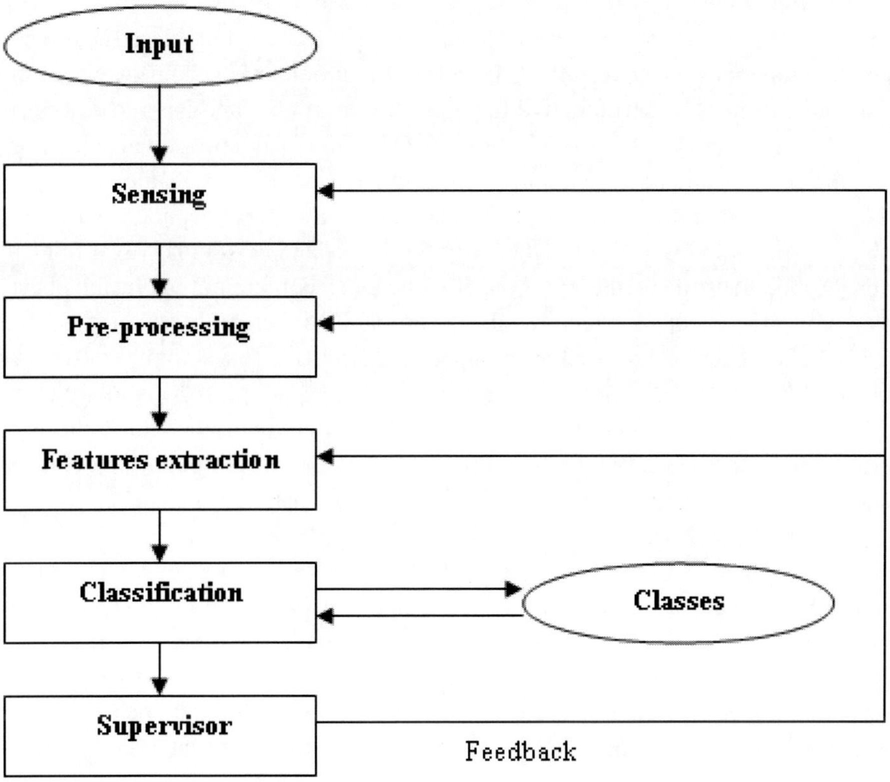

Figure 1. Classification system.

The input to a pattern recognition system is a type of transducer, such as a camera or output of a laboratory instrument. The pre-elaboration module ("pre-processing") has the task to exalt and to adapt the working signal for the purpose of the classification/recognition process.

The module of extraction of the parameters applies a transformation to the signal that reduces the complexity of the information to elaborate and render the system more efficient; an extracted parameter must be obtained in a simple manner and at the same time it must have a high discriminating power. The task of the classifier component of a full system is to use the feature vector provided by the feature extractor and assign the object to a category. The result of the classification process / recognition, during the phase of development and optimization is transmitted to the supervisor.

The function of the supervisor is to evaluate the result in respect to the application, this being the easier way to evaluate the validity of the result. The function of the operator is to measure the error probability.

In literature [8-9] many statistical methods of supervised classification are available. The supervised classification is fundamentally based on the probability theory: it uses the probability density of the values of the feature of the various classes to determine the most probable one. The probability density can be known or estimated on the basis of the training-set whose classes are known. The majority of supervised classifications are implicitly or explicitly based on this concept.

Generally, the approach to linear separable classes, is that classifiers with linear discriminative functions work very well. If instead the problem is not linearly separable then the classifiers with linear discriminative functions are in trouble and have low performances. The method of the Support Vector Machine (SVM) [9, 10] is an optimal evolution of the theory of linear discriminative functions; with the right conditions in the determination of hyperplane separation of the classes, it works also on the non-linear separable cases.

Many classifiers are based on the theory of the Bayesian decision however in many cases the parametric methods of the theory of the Bayesian decision are not applicable, because the available knowledge is not easily expressible in probabilistic terms. In such cases, techniques of simplified classification are used. Such techniques concur, for example, to determine the discriminating functions for various classes beginning from samples. A popular deterministic method is the K-Nearest Neighbours (K-NN) [9]; the input consists of the k closest training examples in the feature space while the output is a class membership. An object is classified by a majority vote of its neighbours, with the object being assigned to the class most common among its k nearest neighbours.

Moreover, there exist other non-algorithmic methods such as artificial neural networks[9, 11]. They were created in order to reproduce typical activities of the human brain such as, perception of images, acknowledgment of shapes, understanding of language, motor coordination, etc. Recent success of artificial neural networks (ANN) are fundamentally used to understand the mechanisms that regulate the nervous system in the hope to realize parallel architectures capable to carry out difficult tasks in respect to sequential architectures. Among the various types of existing neural networks often is used the Multi Layer Perceptron (MLP) adapted for the supervised classification; other ANN with excellent performance in supervised classification are the Radial Basis Function Networks (RBF) and the Probabilistic Neural Network (PNN).

Thalassaemia classification can generally be formulated into a pattern recognition problem. Many of these techniques are used with the aim to analyze haemochromocytometric data to recognize different Thalassaemia traits.

Related Works

Several diagnosis system are proposed in literature; some of them work directly on laboratory facility in semi-automatic mode. The interpretation is made by medical equipments on raw data; in [12] an automatic HPLC analyser for screening haemoglobinopathies is used.

Some proposed system works on image analysis. In [13] a system based on electron microscopy images is presented; in such paper the authors develop a computer vision approach for thalassaemia screening using geometric features characterizing morphology of erythrocytes based on scanning electron microscopy (SEM) images. Erythrocytes were separated from blood samples and chemically processed for SEM imaging at 2000× resolution. Thereafter, marker controlled watershed transform was used to segregate erythrocytes from SEM images. Seventeen geometric features were extracted using various mathematical measures. A neural network MLP was trained for thalassaemia and healthy erythrocytes using these features and tested.

In [14] an Automated image analysis has been used to classify anaemia directly upon the basis of red-blood-cell size. With fast scanning, size-distribution curves were obtained quickly using unstained blood-films. Classification of anaemia and grading of anisocytosis were here all obtained independent of red-blood-cell counting, packed-cell-volume determination, and examination of stained blood-film.

Early works employed statistical methods; in [15] the program HEME using a version of Bayes's theorem compare the probability that the patient has each of 40 diseases currently registered in a table (i.e. iron deficiency, thalassaemia minor, anaemia ...) starting from the findings of a patient.

We found application of clustering techniques in [16] where, on the basis of ferrokinetic parameters, the authors utilized techniques for unsupervised classification (as agglomerative hierarchical cluster analysis and principal coordinate analysis). Two main clusters were found and named anaemia with low potential erythropoiesis and with high potential erythropoiesis, since the most discriminant parameter between them was total erythroid iron turnover, a measure of total erythropoietic activity. A value of total erythropoiesis equal to 4 times the normal was found to discriminate these two types of anaemia in 94% of cases. Within the group with low potential erythropoiesis, three clusters showing different qualitative disturbances of erythropoiesis were singled out. Among patients with high potential erythropoiesis, two clusters were found. A threshold level distinguished between patients having ineffective erythropoiesis or peripheral haemolysis as the major mechanism of anaemia.

In this book chapter we make manly an overview of the automatic systems which perform data analysis on haemochromocytometric parameter.

An implementation of a expert system as a rule-based protocol is presented in [17-19]. In articles an computer base consultation program is developed which is supposed to be able to match the cognitive performance of the expert hematologist. Thalassaemia is not the only target. Findings are used to infer hypothesis by means of the rules, which are in the form of production rules, i.e. *if-then rules*. In [19] the authors provide an important improvement of the system [17-18] through a LISP program based on an epistmological model. The main two features are:

- Diagnosis can be broken down into a network of generic task. A task is a process by which an initial cognitive state (or input information) is transformed into a successive cognitive state.
- The procedure needed to carry out each generic task are epistemolocially classified into three inference types: abduction, deduction, and induction. Inferences represent mental procedures capable of producing new knowledge starting from observed facts and /or previous inferred hypotheses. An epistemological model of diagnostic reasoning is shown in Figure 2.

An hybrid neural-network/rule-based systems [20] have been successfully tested in clinical trials.

The system combining rule-based and artificial neural network(ANN) models was constructed to evaluate microcytic anaemia in a 3-layered program using hematocrit (HCT), mean corpuscular volume (MCV), and coefficient of variation of cell distribution width (RDWcv) as inputs. These measurements are available as standard output on most hematology analyzers. Three categories of microcytic anaemia were considered, iron deficiency (IDA), hemoglobinopathy (HEM), and anaemia of chronic disease (ACD). In the model a single feed forward back propagation network (MLP) is used and provides directly the three possible outputs (IDA,HEM,ACD). In Figure 3 the use-case scheme of the system is shown.

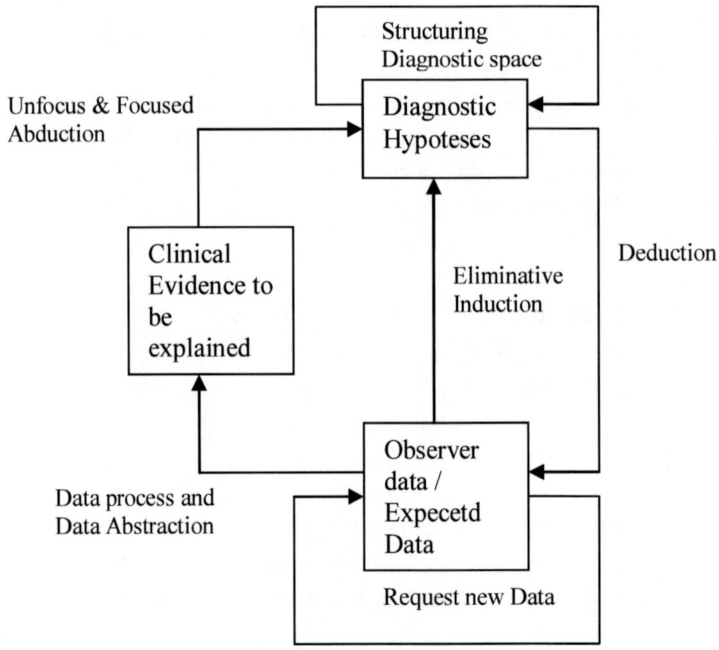

Figure 2. An epistemological model of diagnostic reasoning.

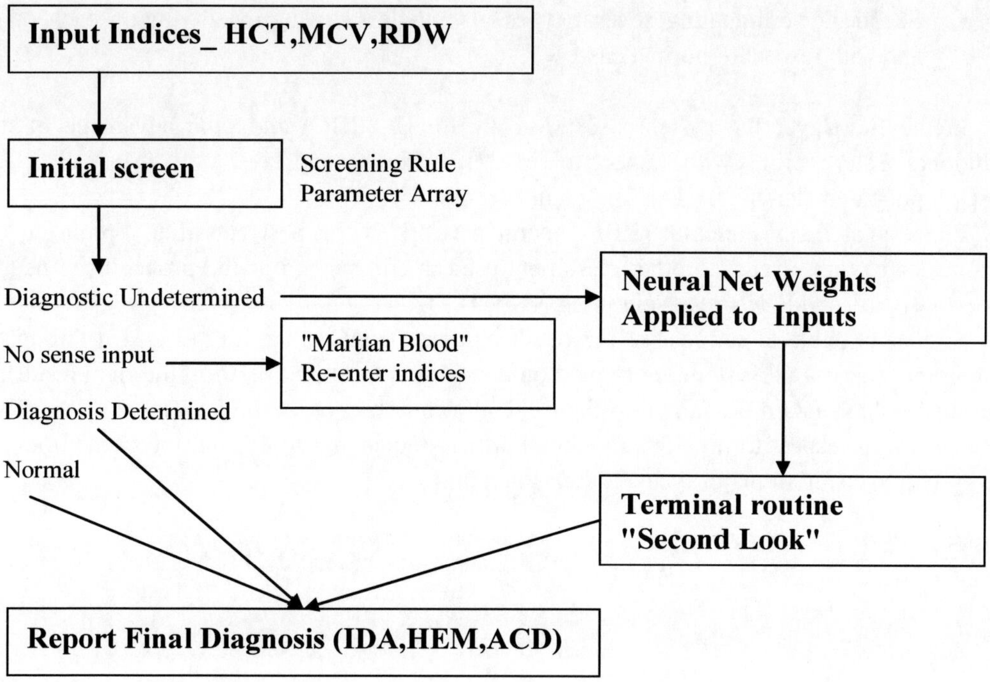

Figure 3. The use-case scheme of the system [20].

In [21] the authors propose as best approach a combination of 3 specialized ANNs, each with 1 output neuron, for the discrimination of the 3 categories, with the following coding of the neurons for the teaching pattern:

- ANN for the discrimination of normals from α carriers: normal = 0, α carrier = 1
- ANN for the discrimination of normals from β carriers: normal = 0, β carrier = 1
- ANN for the discrimination of α carriers from β carriers: α carrier = 0, β carrier = 1

In all cases, a simple feed forward MLP architecture, with 4 input neurons (MCV, Hb, Ht, RBC) and 1 hidden layer, was used. The graphical user interface of the system si very easy and provides the diagnosis and neuron outputs as shown in Figure 4.

In [22] authors propose as model a two-classifiers system based on SVM. On the base of four input (MCV, Hb, Ht, RBC), the first layer is used to differentiate between suspect and normal cases while the second layer, with the same input, is used to discriminate between two different traits (α-thalassaemia carrier against β-thalassaemia carrier). In the ability to recognise type α from type β thalassaemia, the SVM classifier performs similarly to the specialised neural network classifier in terms of specificity and is more accurate in sensivity then MLP in [21]. Figure5 shows the block diagram of the classification steps.

In [1] a novel classification scheme is proposed, which improves the existing systems [21-22], based on two RBF classifiers placed in two cascade layers. This system proposed in the paper [1] divides the recognition problem into two phases:

- First, recognising and separating only β-samples with respect to all others (normals and α-thalassaemia carriers).

- Second, discriminating several types of α-thalassaemia carriers among each other and with respect to normal cases.

In the first layer the system uses (MCV, Hb, Ht, RBC) and take advantage of the additional feature, HbA_2 with respect to [21-22]. In the second layer only (MCV, Hb, Ht, RBC) input parameter are used, as shown in Figure 6.

The Radial Basis Function (RBF) neural network is the best classifier, optimized on training data, with respect to other classifiers used in comparison as the probabilistic neural network (PNN) and K-Nearest Neighbours (KNN).

So it is possible to summarize the result obtained from authors in [1, 21-22] through a histograms because all system are trained on the same dataset and perform the final result on the same gold standard, as shown in Figure 7. We can observe the improvement of the RBF approach with respect to previous models. Further studies aim to expand the capabilities of the system to cover all major types of thalassaemias.

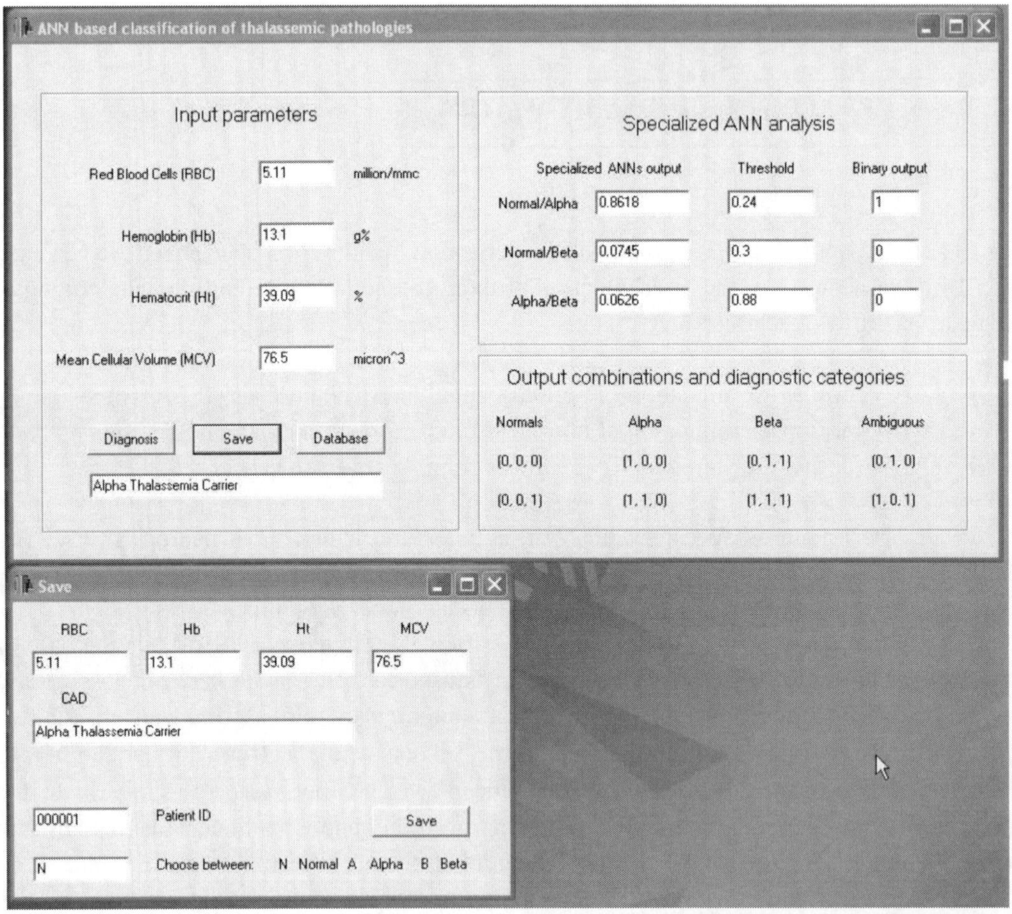

Figure 4. The graphical users interface of the system [21] based on 3 specialized MLP.

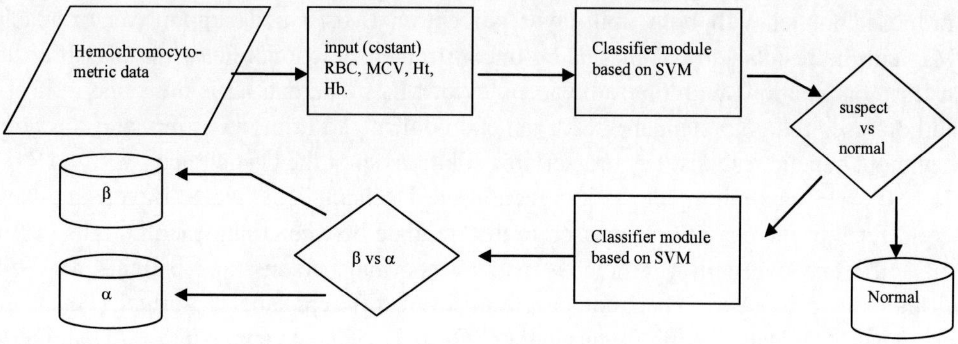

Figure 5. Block Diagram of the system proposed in [22].

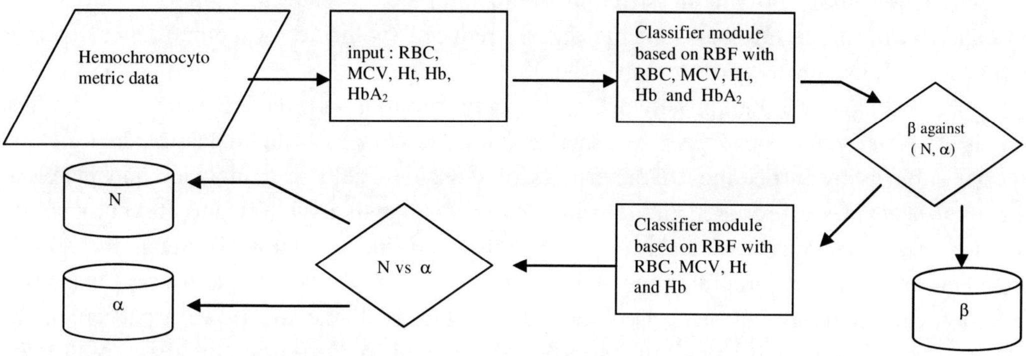

Figure 6. Block Diagram of the system proposed in [1].

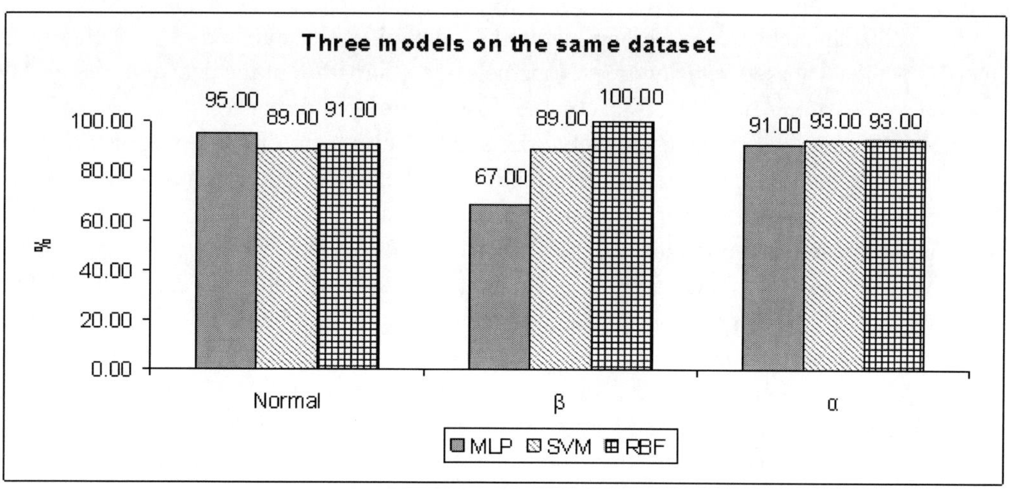

Figure 7. Comparison of the systems [1, 21-22] on the same dataset.

Author of [23] proposed thalassaemia screening using unconstrained functional networks classifier. Functional networks are a generalization of neural networks that combine both knowledge about the structure of the problem, to determine the architecture of the network, and data, to estimate the unknown functional neurons The paper compares the performance of the proposed model with both multilayer perceptron (MLP) and support vector machine (SVM), and the results showed that using unconstrained functional networks classifier takes much less computations with the same accuracy of MLP. The dataset is the same in [21] but the authors uses the gold standard (with genetic confirm) to train classifiers and the normal data (without genetic response) as test set: this solution is not the best choice.

In [24] three data mining classifiers were used: Decision Tree, Naïve Bayes, and Neural Network. Each of the classifiers are used to differentiate between thalassaemia traits patients, with its different levels: iron deficiency patients, normal persons, and patients who suffer from other blood diseases. Their database has seven different labels: Normal, Thalassemia Major (Thal-M), Thalassaemia Intermediate (Thal-I), Thalassaemia Trait (Thal-T), Iron Deficiency (Iron Def), Thalassemia Trait/Iron Deficiency (Thal-T/Iron Def.), and Other which represented any other blood diseases. They use all haemochromocytometric data, age and sex. The Neural Network classifier has more significance result then the other classifiers on dataset with all features and on the dataset reduced (with the most importance features extracted from haemochromocytometric data).

A comparison of a neural network and genetic programming are reported in [25]. The aim is to differentiate between thalassaemic patients, persons with thalassaemia trait and normal subjects by inspecting characteristics of red blood cells, reticulocytes and platelets. But they need in the proposed model more blood testing like Platelet and Reticulocyte. A structured representation on genetic algorithms for non-linear function fitting is the chosen architecture for genetic programming (GP) implementation. The technique uses a binary tree in which each non-terminal node is modelled by a differentiable function. In particular, the use of a second order polynomial in a non-terminal node is made. For comparison, multilayer perceptrons MLP are explored in classification via a neural network. The classification results indicate that the performance of the GP-based decision tree is approximately equal to that of the MLP with one hidden layer. But the MLP with two hidden layers, which is proven to have the most suitable architecture among networks with different number of hidden layers, outperforms the GP-based decision tree. Nonetheless, the structure of the decision tree reveals that some input features have no effects on the classification performance.

Another system based on neural networks and a decision tree is proposed in [26]. The objective of the authors is to identify automatically whether the human subject is a person with abnormal haemoglobin, a person with thalassaemia trait, a thalassaemic patient, or a normal person using haemoglobin typing data from HPLC. The derived data sets contain eight input features or attributes and 14 distinct classes. Each attribute reflects the percentage of haemoglobin at a specific chromatographic retention time. In other words, the attribute set covers multiple types of haemoglobin. Classifiers tested for the task include a neural network MLP, a decision tree and random forests. The study involving stratified 10-fold cross-validation reveals that decision tree is the most suitable classifier for the data that have been preprocessed by attribute discretisation and reduction. Subsequently, decision tree is applied in the clinical trial and further analysis of the classification error indicates that the misclassification among disease classes and the false predictions of severity levels for samples from thalassaemic patients are low. The schematic diagram for the methodology employed in the investigation is shown in Figure 8.

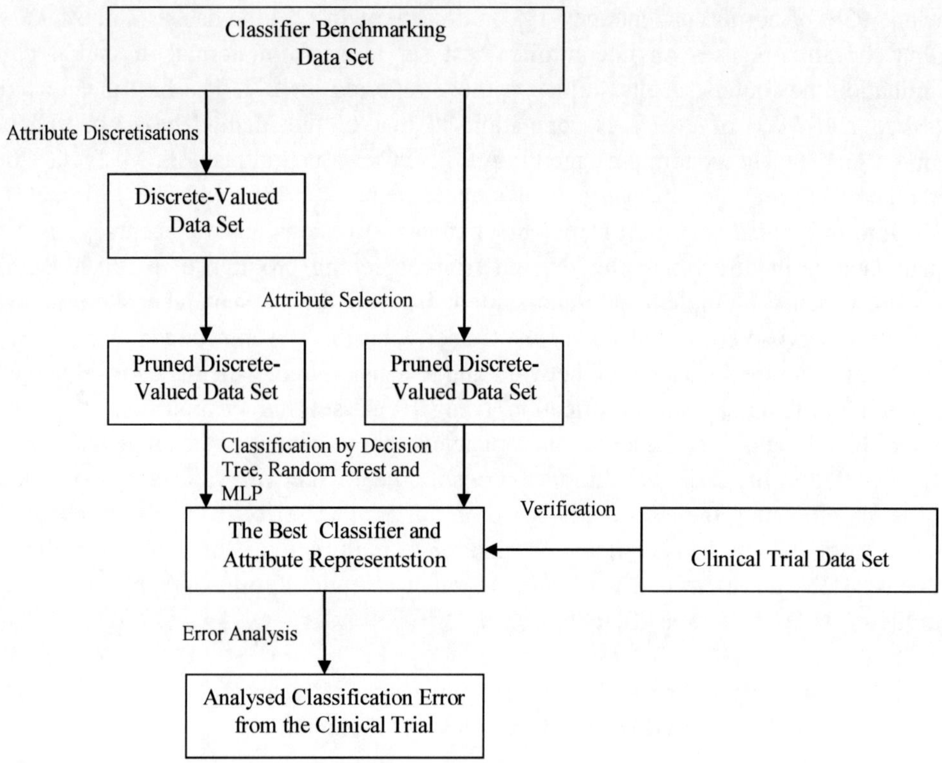

Figure 8. Schematic diagram for the methodology employed in the investigation [26].

Main Results

In this section we report the results of the main systems presented which works in literature on haemochromocytometric data.

The hybrid neural-network/rule-based system described in [20] uses hematocrit (HCT), mean corpuscular volume (MCV), and coefficient of variation of cell distribution width (RDWcv) as inputs. The model's performance was evaluated with actual case data. It was successful in correctly classifying 96.5% of 473 documented cases of microcytic anaemia and anaemia of chronic disease. In [1, 21-22] the dataset consist of 304 clinical records based on a thalassaemia screening carried out by the Ozieri Hospital on Public School's students. Several Public Schools of Northern Sardinia were used in the test. Each 8th grade student (14- to 15-year-old boys and girls) took part in the screening. Although the records can be considered a random sample, subjects with iron deficiency were excluded from the test, as in their case iron levels in the blood must be normalised before thalassaemia diagnosis can be made.

In the system [21], based on three specialised neural MLP, normal individuals are identified with 95% accuracy, while α-carriers with 91% accuracy and β-carriers with 67% accuracy. The system proposed in [22] composed of two SVM cascade classifiers discriminates in the first step normal cases from all carriers, α and β, and in the second step it discriminates α with respect to β carriers. With this system, normal cases are identified with 89% accuracy, α-carriers with 93% accuracy and β-carriers with 89% accuracy. In [1] on the same dataset [21-22] best performances are archived with RBF classifier obtaining 100% of β-carriers, 93% of normal patient and 91% on α-carriers. In [23] the dataset is the same as in [21] but the authors uses an uncontrolled test set to perform normal, α and β carriers discrimination; he founds results similar to those reported in [22]. The best mean accuracy with SVM and MLP of 96.7% is compatible to that of the method based on functional networks (96.4%). The system presented in ref. [24] uses a neural network MLP classifier to differentiate between the normal persons, thalassaemia patients with its different types (Major, Intermediate, Trait), Iron Deficiency patients. It obtains general accuracy of 95.48% on their datasets of 46920 samples derived from screening program of β -thalassaemia in Gaza strip, which was implemented and started since the 9th of September 2000 under full control and supervision of the Thalassaemia Center, Palestine, Avenir foundation.

In [25], the authors use a neural network and a decision tree, which is evolved by genetic programming in thalassaemia classification; using 10 classes and 12 input features extracted from red blood cells, reticulocytes and platelets, they obtain an average classification accuracy of 82%. In [26], the authors propose a neural network and a decision tree in thalassaemia screening; their system is based on thirteen classes of thalassaemia abnormality and one control class by inspecting the distribution of multiple types of haemoglobin in blood specimens, which are identified via high-performance liquid chromatography; they obtain a sensitivity of 93.1% and a specificity of 99.5%.

Table1. Best methods presented in the cited papers on different dataset; * this dataset is used with different test set composition

Best Classifiers	**Input data types**	**Dataset samples**	**Accuracy %**	**Sensitivity % (α, β)**	**Specificity % (Normals)**
Specialized MLP [21]	Hematomocytometric data	304	91.0	86.9	95.0
Two layers SVM[22]	Hematomocytometric data	304	90.6	92.3	89.0
Two layers RBF [1]	Hematomocytometric data	304	92.3	93.0	91.0
MLP and a decision tree, from genetic programming [25]	Hematomocytometric data	300	82.0	-	-
MLP and a decision tree [26]	Liquid chromatography	1000	93.1	93.1	99.5%
Functional neural networks [23]	Hematomocytometric data	304*	96.4%	-	-
MLP[24]	Hematomocytometric data	46920	95.5%	-	-
Hybrid neural-network [20]	Hematomocytometric data	473	96.5%	-	-

In table 1, we summarize the main methods presented in the previous paragraph, highlighting that in this comparison input data available, α and β types and validation methods are different.

Conclusion

This chapter describes Computer Aided Detection Systems for the recognition of thalassaemia carriers distinguishing mainly between α, β and healthy cases. A typical application is on screening programs. The use of Hematomocytometric data, in some of the proposed systems, is suitable because a low-cost approach on data obtained in simple routine analysis is needed for screening programs. Several classification scheme and their performances are also described in different datasets. Complexity of the features of the datasets is low, therefore there is no need for complex feature extraction modules; in general the best results are obtained using classification scheme where artificial neural networks are involved.

References

[1] Masala, GL; Golosio, B; Cutzu, R; Pola, R. A two-layered classifier based on the radial basis function for the screening of thalassaemia (2013) *Computers in Biology and Medicine*, 43 (11), 1724-1731.

[2] Elshami, EH; Alhalees, AM. Automated Diagnosis of Thalassemia Based on DataMining Classifiers. In: The International Conference on Informatics and Applications (ICIA2012). *The Society of Digital Information and Wireless Communication*, 2012, 440-445.

[3] Sun, YJ; Li, HJ; Wang, XY. The diagnostic value about the MCV and red blood cell fragility test in thalassaemia screening (2007). *Chinese Journal of Birth Health & Heredity*, vol. 15, no. 8, 115–116.

[4] Hall, FW; Lundgrin, DB. Screening for alpha-thalassaemia in neonates: routine erythrocyte measurements. *Am J Clin Pathol*, 1987, 87, 389–91.

[5] Thalassaemia Working Party of the British Committee for Standars in Haematology Task Force. Guidelines for investigations of the alpha and beta thalassaemia traits. (1994) *J.Clin Pathol*, 47, 289-95.

[6] British Committee for standards in Haematology. Guideline: the laboratory diagnosis of haemaoglobinopathies (1998) *Br J Haematol*, 101, 783-92.

[7] Masala, GL. Computer aided detection on mammography. World Academy of Science, *Engineering and Technology*, (2006), 15.1, 1-6.

[8] Masala, GL. Pattern recognition techniques applied to biomedical patterns. *Int J Biomed Sci*, (2006), 1.1, 47-55.

[9] Duda, O; Hart, PE; Stark, DG. "*Pattern Classificatio*", second edition, A Wiley-Interscience Publication John Wiley & Sons, 2001.

[10] Vapnik, VN. *Statistical Learning Theory*. Wiley, New York, 1998

[11] Haykin, S. "Neural Networks – A comprehensive foundation", second edition, *Prentice Hall*, 1999.

[12] Galanello, R; et al. Evaluation of an automatic HPLC analyser for thalassemia and haemoglobin variants screening. *Journal of Analytical Methods in Chemistry*, (1995), 17.2, 73-76.

[13] Bhowmick, S; Das, DK; Maiti, AK; Chakraborty, C. Computer-aided diagnosis of thalassemia using scanning electron microscopic images of peripheral blood: A morphological approach (2012) *Journal of Medical Imaging and Health Informatics*, 2 (3), 215-221.

[14] Lund, PR; Barnes, RD. Automated classification of anaemia using image analysis, (1972) *The Lancet*, 300 (7775), 463–464.

[15] Engle, RL; Flehinger, BJ; Allen, S; Friedman, R; Lipkin, M; Davis, BJ; Leveridge, LL. HEME: a computer aid to diagnosis of hematologic disease, (1976), *Bulletin of the New York Academy of Medicine*, 52, 584–600.

[16] Barosi, G; Cazzola, M; Berzuini, C; Quaglini, S; Stefanelli, M. Classification of anemia on the basis of ferrokinetic parameters, (1985), *British Journal of Haematology*, 61, 357–370

[17] Quaglini, S; Stefanelli, M; Barosi, G; Berzuini, A. ANEMIA: an expert consultation system, (1986), *Computers and Biomedical Research*, 19 (1), 13–27.

[18] Quaglini, S; Stefanelli, M; Barosi, G; Berzuini, A. A performance evaluation of the expert system ANEMIA, (1988), *Computers and Biomedical Research*, 21, 307–323,

[19] Lanzola, G; Stefanelli, M; Barosi, G; Magnani, L. NEOANEMIA: a knowledge-based system emulating diagnostic reasoning, (1990), *Computers and Biomedical Research*, 23, 560–582

[20] Birndorf, NI; Pentecost, JO; Coakley, JR; Spackman, KA. An expert system to diagnose anemia and report results directly on hematology forms, (1996), *Computers and Biomedical Research*, 29 (1), 16–26.

[21] Amendolia, SR; Brunetti, A; Carta, P; Cossu, G; Ganadu, ML; Golosio, B; Mura, GM; Pirastru, MG. A real-time classification system of thalassemic pathologies based on artificial neural networks, *Medical Decision Making*, 22 (1), (2002), 18–26.

[22] Amendolia, SR; Cossu, G; Ganadu, ML; Golosio, B; Masala, GL; Mura, GM. A comparative study of k-nearest neighbour, support vector machine and multi-layer perceptron for thalassemia screening, (2003), *Chemometrics and Intelligent Laboratory Systems*, 69 (1), 13–20.

[23] El-sebakhy, EA. Unconstrained Functional Networks Classifier, AIML 05 Conference, 19-21 December 2005, CICC, Cairo, Egyp

[24] Elshami, EH; Alhalees, AM. Automated Diagnosis of Thalassemia Based on DataMining Classifiers. In: The International Conference on Informatics and Applications (ICIA2012). *The Society of Digital Information and Wireless Communication*, 2012, 440-445.

[25] Wongseree, W; Chaiyaratana, N; Vichittumaros, K; Winichagoon, P; Fucharoen, S. Thalassaemia classification by neural networks and genetic programming, (2007), *Information Sciences*, 177 (3), 771-786.

[26] Piroonratana, T; Wongseree, W; Assawamakin, A; Paulkhaolarn, N; Kanjanakorn, C; Sirikong, M; Thongnoppakhun, W; Limwongse, C; Chaiyaratana, N. Classification of haemoglobin typing chromatograms by neural networks and decision trees for thalassaemia screening, (2009), *Chemometrics and Intelligent Laboratory Systems*, 99 (2), 101-110.

In: Thalassemia
Editor: Makenzie Greene
ISBN: 978-1-63117-954-9

Chapter 4

Hematopietic Stem Cell Transplantation for Thalassemia, Price and Prejudice

Lawrence Faulkner*, M.D.
Medical Coordinator Cure2Children Foundation, Florence, Italy

Abstract

Hemoglobinopathies, namely thalassemia and sickle cell disease, are the most frequent life-threatening non-infectious disease of children globally. In many countries, particularly in South Asia, where the majority of the pediatric population of our planet lives, a significant, and increasing, proportion of healthcare-related expenses is employed for the non-curative supportive care of patients with severe thalassemia.

Major advances in effective oral chelators have heralded a new thalassemia era in which patients are expected to have long and productive lives provided access to long-term appropriate care is available. Unfortunately, this is not always the case for most thalassemics, largely due to costs; appropriate life-long supportive therapy is estimated to cost a minimum of 7.000 USD/year, which is higher than the average income in many thalassemia-prone regions. Moreover, drug or transfusion intolerance, blood-borne infections, osteoporosis and pain, pulmonary hypertension and health-related quality of life (HRQoL) remain some open questions.

In parallel with improvements in supportive care also hematopoietic stem cell transplantation (blood and marrow transplantation or BMT) results have substantially improved over the last decade so that a low-risk patients with a compatible sibling is expected to enjoy over 90% cure probability with improved HRQoL. As opposed to supportive care, however, BMT costs have decreased to the point that it is possible to perform a bone marrow transplant for 15.000 USD, i.e. what is needed for 1-2 years of non-curative supportive care, thus making BMT highly cost-effective. Both the transplant community and international accreditation bodies are becoming increasingly aware that expensive and complex hospital infection control standards may not be required and that current reduced-intensity BMT strategies may be offered even on outpatient basis thus

* Email: lawrence.faulkner@cure2children.org.

further cutting costs. The new thalassemia era has also provided the ability to induce negative iron balance, reverse some of the organ damage associated with chronic iron overload, downstage high-risk patients and further decrease transplant-related morbidity and mortality. Finally, it is become increasingly feasible to use partially matched related donors, e.g., mother of father, which are available for the great majority of patients. This latter option might be safer, more accessible, less expensive and as widely applicable as upcoming gene therapy.

Keywords: Thalassemia, Hematopietic stem cell transplantation, Blood and marrow transplantation, Bone marrow transplantation, Cord blood transplantation, Gene therapy, Health-Related Quality of life, Late effects

Introduction

Since the nineties, when effective oral chelation became available, life expectancy as well as health-related quality of life (HRQoL) of individuals with severe thalassemia (ST), defined as inability to keep spontaneous hemoglobin above 7 gm/dL, has improved substantially. At the same time also hematopoietic stem cell transplantation also known as blood and marrow transplantation (BMT) has improved in parallel [1] and its very long term effects. i.e. over 20 years post-BMT, are well know [2]. The bottom line is that nowadays most people with ST are expected to have a long and productive life assuming that optimal supportive care is readily available. So, what is the role of BMT?

Long-term Supportive Care *vs.* Definitive Cure by BMT

Unfortunately it is practically impossible to compare side by side supportive care with BMT because follow up time required for a fair judgment, i.e. probably over 40 years, will make results obsolete and useless. Moreover, this comparison might be very context-dependent, i.e. long-term supportive care (LTSC) implies life-long access to appropriate medical therapy which may not be the case in many low- and middle-income countries (LMICs), where the vast majority of thalassemics live. Last but not least the issue of cost: it is estimated that the minimum yearly cost of adequate LTSC, i.e. the one associated with long-term survival and safe transfusions, is in the range of 7.000 USD/year [3], i.e. well above the average yearly income in most LMICs [4].

Albeit it might be reasonable to assume that most complications related to chronic iron overload should no longer be an issue, the ones related to chronic hemolysis/ineffective erythropiesis such as ospeoporosis, bone pain and pulmonary hypertension [5], might still be significant, not considering drug intolerance and transfusion-associated infections.

In any case BMT-associated risks and long-term results should be "competitive" with best LTSC outcomes. There is increasing evidence that this might be the case, at least in a subset of young people with ST: In a recent report by La Nasa et al. on 109 patients transplanted from a matched related donor with a standard combination of busulfan and cyclophosphamide and followed over 20 years post-BMT, those who were younger than 15 years at transplant, had no comorbidities at BMT and no extensive chronic graft-versus host disease (cGHVD), which occurred in 6% of cases, had HRQoL, employment status and birth rate similar to the general population [2]. The other important issue is whether progress in LTSC will be more rapid than that in BMT; probably not, in fact transplant preparative regimens for hemoglobinopathies are becoming increasing tolerable [6–8] and the BMT paradygm is shifting towards obtaining close to null transplant-related mortality (TRM), very effective cGVHD prevention, and fertility preservation at a potential cost of increased rejection rates. Improvements in supportive care may facilitate obtaining negative iron balance, reverse some of the organ damage [9, 10] and thus downstage high-risk patients and decrease TRM. Hydroxyurea given pre-BMT may also improve outcomes [11]. Second BMT regimens are also becoming increasingly feasible [12], thus decreasing the need for very aggressive first transplant strategies.

Last but not least the issue of financial burden: The total lifetime cost of appropriate supportive care in Taiwan, a high-income country, has been estimated to be in the 360.000 USD range [3] while in LMICs BMT cost as been estimated to be in the 10.000-15.000 USD range [13], thus potentially highly cost-effective.

In spite of increasing evidence of safety and positive impact on long-term HRQoL, at least in children with a compatible donor, BMT remains stigmatized as highly risky by many professionals and institutions taking care of people with ST.

Sources of Transplantable Stem Cells

Bone marrow, mobilized peripheral blood, and cord blood have been used ti cure ST. Most centers currently employ standard bone marrow because it is associated with less cGVHD compared to mobilized peripheral blood collections [14] and with faster engraftment compared to cord blood [15], but there is no strong evidence that marrow is associated with higher cure rates or overall survival. In the "new thalassemia era", however, moderate or severe cGVHD [16], which potentially could affect HRQoL more than ST itself, is not acceptable. The same is true for aggressive preparative regimens required to allow engraftment of cord blood with the associated high likelihood of permanent infertility. Last but not list cost issues: The great majority of appropriate BMT candidates live in LMICs where cost and technical complexities of peripheral blood collection or cord blood banking are often prohibitive. There is no strong indication or rationale to store cord blood from subsequent deliveries of mothers with a thalassemic child, in fact it is better to wait until the healthy compatible newborn is old enough to donate marrow, i.e. 6 to 12 months of age. Standard bone marrow transplant remains the preferred option with cure rates consistently reported to be over 90% in selected young low-risk patients (age < 7 years with no hepatomegaly) with a histocompatible family donor [17, 18]. BMT is also associated with improved quality of life [19] and is increasingly cost-effective [20].

Unrelated marrow donors have been successfully used, but reported incidence of mortality, rejection and chronic GVHD are still significant [18]. Moreover, the extended degree of histocompatibility required makes it very unlikely to find donors for thalassemia patients most of whom belong to ethnic groups under-represented in donor registries [21]. In the European experience, unrelated cord blood has been shown not to be a suitable source of transplantable stem cells for thalassemia major because of high rejection rate and transplant-related morbidity and mortality [22].

Partially matched related donors, e.g., mother or father, have been successfully used for hemoglobinopathies and appear to be safe, high rejection rates, in the 30-40%, however, are still a major problem [8, 23].

The major long-term side effect of BMT is infertility in over 60% of cases while secondary malignancies have not been a major issue as well as growth and development post BMT [2].

BMT Preparative Regimens

No controlled trials have established what is the best BMT strategy for thalassemia. The issue is further complicated by very different outcomes based on risk groups. The "Pesaro" risk stratification based on chelation history, liver size and presence of fibrosis on liver biopsy [24] may have lost significance in the new thalassemia era in which high-risk patients can potentially be downstaged, in fact it might be questionable nowadays to bring a high-risk ST case to BMT before having achieved maximal iron removal, ideally ferritin < 1,000 ng/ml, and organ damage reversal. Moreover, the Pesaro classification was developed largely on patients with regular access to red cell transfusions and may not readily apply to chronically undertransfused children in low-resource settings, in whom hepatomegaly not necessarily reflects severe chronic iron overload and maybe partially corrected with a proper transfusion program or the use of hydroxyurea [25]. Alternative risk group assignment independent of liver biopsy have been proposed in lower-income countries based primarily on age and liver size, so that children younger than 7 years with liver ≤5cm below the costal margin are expected to have over 70% cure rates, irrespective of chelation history or liver fibrosis [26]. Children younger than 7 years with liver ≤2cm below the costal margin may enjoy cure rates greater than 85% [27].

Transplant strategies for ST should provide improved long-term HRQoL and spare fertility as much as possible. Treosulfan-based conditioning regimen has been proposed as ideally suited for patients with thalassemia major [28–30], this drug, however, has largely been used in association with thiotepa, a combination very likely to be associated with permanent sterility in most cases. The gold standard for which there is enough long-term follow up remains the combination of busulfan and cyclophosphamide (BuCy)(2), possibly with the addition of anti-thymocyte globulin (ATG-BuCy) which has been retrospectively shown to substantially reduce rejection rates in large case series [31, 32]. One of the arguments in favor of treosulfan is the lower rate of liver sinusoidal obstructive syndrome (SOS), previously known as veno-occlusive disease of the liver. However, in both the Italian experience (Sodani P., personal communication) and that of the Cure2Children Foundation on over 100 BMTs in Pakistan and India, at least in low- and intermediate-risk patients BuCy has not been associated with high SOS rates [33].

The Issue of Splenectomy Prior to BMT

Enlarged of the spleen is relatively common in ST patients and per se is not associated with higher rejection rates but may increase transfusion requirements and delay engraftment [34]. Retrospective data suggests that splenectomy may be associated with increased transplant-related mortality [34, 35], whether this is an independent risk factor, however, is not clear [26]. Spleen removal may also increase the risk of lymphoproliferative disorders associated with Epstein-Barr virus [36]. At present routine splenectomy prior to BMT for thalassemia should be avoided.

Hepatitis C and BMT

Universal screening for Hepatitis C virus (HCV) was introduced in the early nineties in most affluent countries so that it is unusual to encounter HCV positivity in multiply transfused individuals younger than 20 years. In many developing countries this is not the case and HCV positivity remains a major problem even in children [37, 38] and is associated with both liver fibrosis and hepatocellular carcinoma [39] even though in one third of ST cases HCV can clear spontaneusly [40]. There is no evidence that BMT influences the course of HCV infection and vice versa [41]. Actually, given the additive effect of hepatitis C and iron overload in accelerating liver fibrosis progression [42], HCV positivity might strengthen the indication for BMT. Treatment of active (HCV RNA-positive) infection may be postponed two years post-BMT [41].

Costs and Sustainability

There is general perception that BMT centers need complex engineering standards requiring significant investment, even more so in poor countries where there might be greater risk for opportunistic infections. There is no evidence that the latter is true [43] nor international guidelines call for allogeneic transplant patients, at least those with standard risk features, to be placed in highly protected environments with positive pressure gradients, intensive air exchange and filtration [44]. On the contrary, there is increasing evidence that allogeneic transplant patients may be safely cared for in regular hospital rooms [45] or even as outpatients [46, 47]. Cost-containment is critical in settings where financial constraints directly influence access to cure and thus probability of survival. In the experience of the Cure2Children Foundation (C2C) partner centers in Pakistan and India, where pressure differentials, centralized air filtration, masks, gowns, or shoe covers where not employed, infectious complications observed did not seem to be substantially different from expected [48]. In developing countries BMT may actually improve quality of life for both patients and families by decreasing medical, psychological and financial burdens to a greater extent compared affluent countries and be the best option for many patients with thalassemia due to younger age, increased likelihood to find a related donor because of larger family size and cost-effectiveness. In the C2C-supported BMT network in Pakistan and India hinging on focused training and task-shift strategies within a structured cooperation program, low-risk children younger than 5 years with a matched sibling had a 92% thalassemia-free survival, a result comparable to that obtained in affluent countries [18], with 100% performance score and no extensive chronic GVHD, for an average cost of 10.000 USD per BMT [17, 33]. Within an existing hospital facility, 50,000 USD where sufficient to renovate and fully equip a 2 bedded start up BMT unit. The realistic offer of a definitive cure can also improve compliance with supportive care and engage families in cascade screening and prevention programs: Most mothers of thalassemic children enrolled in C2C-supported BMT network program accepted the offer of free prenatal diagnosis for subsequent pregnancies. Lastly, buccal swab-based HLA-typing technology has greatly facilitated centralized compatibility testing so that patients can be typed locally and referred to BMT centers within South-South cooperation programs offering effective and cost-conscious BMT [49].

BMT and Gene Therapy

The ability to correct the defective globin gene has been the holy grail of the hematologist for decades but unfortunately solid and reproducible results are still pending. However, ST patients are being actively enrolled in gene therapy trials and in another few years a sufficient number for cases may be assessed. Current protocols call for some degree of myelotoxic preparation to facilitate homing and expansion of gene-modified autologous stem cells, generally half maximal dose of busulfan [50], which is actually not substantially different from the one use in reduced intensity BMT strategies. A potential advantage of gene therapy is its universal applicability as compared to BMT which is currently restricted to patients having a matched-related donor, which, depending on family size maybe up to 60% of cases [51]. The increasing safety and feasibility of partially matched related transplantation may extend BMT accessibility to virtually all patients [8, 52], thus narrowing the potential advantages of gene therapy.

Prospects

Most hematologists might currently recommend BMT for a otherwise healthy child younger than 7 years with a HLA-matched sibling while for patients older than 17 most would recommend supportive care, in between lies a gray area still open to debate. A significant proportion of patients with thalassemia on LTSC are married and have children [53]. In terms of fertility preservation transplantation is probably still lagging behind [54] even thought reduced intensity conditioning are increasingly been explored. Use of parental (haploidentical) hematopoietic stem cells is becoming increasingly feasible [8] as well as down staging regimen, thus opening the transplant option to virtually all ST patients. This might the standard that gene therapy will have to confront with.

Emerging therapies such as HbF promoters, antioxidants, arginine, and iron metabolism modifiers, may provide increasingly effective [55] but also potentially underline cost-containment issues. Effective screening and prevention is the ultimate goal but its success depends on government support, awareness and cultural/social acceptance.

Conclusion

Medical progress and knowledge in terms of risks and benefits of LTSC and BMT have improved side by side, nevertheless a substantial body of evidence points to BMT as having a great potential to normalize health-related quality of life and life expectancy in addition to being increasingly cost-effective. Much will depend on the ability to offer tolerable reduced-intensity strategies associated with close to null mortality, no chronic complications and fertility preservation. These goals are increasingly realistic and may decrease prejudice against BMT.

References

[1] Gooley TA, Chien JW, Pergam SA, Hingorani S, Sorror ML, Boeckh M, et al. Reduced mortality after allogeneic hematopoietic-cell transplantation. *N. Engl. J. Med.* 2010 Nov 25;363(22):2091–101.

[2] La Nasa G, Caocci G, Efficace F, Dessì C, Vacca A, Piras E, et al. Long-term health-related quality of life evaluated more than 20 years after hematopoietic stem cell transplantation for thalassemia. *Blood.* 2013 Sep 26;122(13):2262–70.

[3] Ho W-L, Lin K-H, Wang J-D, Hwang J-S, Chung C-W, Lin D-T, et al. Financial burden of national health insurance for treating patients with transfusion-dependent thalassemia in Taiwan. *Bone Marrow Transplant.* 2006 Feb 6;37(6):569–74.

[4] How we Classify Countries | Data [Internet]. [cited 2014 Mar 9]. Available from: http://data.worldbank.org/about/country-classifications

[5] Farmakis D, Aessopos A. Pulmonary hypertension: an emerging risk in hemoglobin disorders. Thalassemia Reports [Internet]. 2012 Jan 13 [cited 2012 Jan 28];1(2s). Available from: http://www.pagepressjournals.org/index.php/thal/article/view/308.

[6] Anurathapan U, Pakakasama S, Rujkijyanont P, Sirachainan N, Songdej D, Chuansumrit A, et al. Pretransplant immunosuppression followed by reduced-toxicity conditioning and stem cell transplantation in high-risk thalassemia: a safe approach to disease control. *Biol. Blood Marrow Transplant.* 2013 Aug;19(8):1259–62.

[7] Hsieh MM, Kang EM, Fitzhugh CD, Link MB, Bolan CD, Kurlander R, et al. Allogeneic hematopoietic stem-cell transplantation for sickle cell disease. *N. Engl. J. Med.* 2009 Dec 10;361(24):2309–17.

[8] Bolaños-Meade J, Fuchs EJ, Luznik L, Lanzkron SM, Gamper CJ, Jones RJ, et al. HLA-haploidentical bone marrow transplantation with post-transplant cyclophosphamide expands the donor pool for patients with sickle cell disease. *Blood.* 2012;120(22):4285–91.

[9] Farmaki K, Tzoumari I, Pappa C, Chouliaras G, Berdoukas V. Normalisation of total body iron load with very intensive combined chelation reverses cardiac and endocrine complications of thalassaemia major. *Br. J. Haematol.* 2010 Feb;148(3):466–75.

[10] Rachmilewitz EA, Giardina PJ. How I treat thalassemia. *Blood.* 2011 Sep 29;118(13):3479–88.

[11] Sodani P, Gaziev D, Polchi P, Erer B, Giardini C, Angelucci E, et al. A new approach for bone marrow transplantation in class 3 thalassemic patients aged less than 17 years. *Blood*. 2004 Mar 23;104(4):1201–3.

[12] Yaqub N, Khalid S, Zahra T, Faulkner L. Second BMT for thalassemia major using post-transplant cyclophosphamide only as GVHD/rejection prophylaxis. 2011.

[13] Hussein MH, El Missiry M, Khalid S, Yaqub N, Gilani SK, Fatima I, et al. Bone marrow transplantation for thalassemia: a global perspective. *Thalassemia Reports*. 2013 Mar 20;3(1s):103–7.

[14] Group SCTC. Allogeneic peripheral blood stem-cell compared with bone marrow transplantation in the management of hematologic malignancies: an individual patient data meta-analysis of nine randomized trials. *J. Clin. Oncol*. 2005;23:5074 – 5087.

[15] Locatelli F, Kabbara N, Ruggeri A, Ghavamzadeh A, Roberts I, Li CK, et al. Outcome of patients with hemoglobinopathies given either cord blood or bone marrow transplantation from an HLA-identical sibling. *Blood*. 2013 Aug 8;122(6):1072–8.

[16] Filipovich AH, Weisdorf D, Pavletic S, Socie G, Wingard JR, Lee SJ, et al. National Institutes of Health consensus development project on criteria for clinical trials in chronic graft-versus-host disease: I. Diagnosis and staging working group report. *Biol. Blood Marrow Transplant*. 2005 Dec;11(12):945–56.

[17] Mehta PA, Faulkner LB. Hematopoietic Cell Transplantation for Thalassemia: A Global Perspective. *Biol. Blood Marrow Transplant*. 2013;19(1 Suppl):S70–3.

[18] Angelucci E. Hematopoietic Stem Cell Transplantation in Thalassemia. *Hematology*. 2010 Dec 1;(1):456–62.

[19] Cheuk DKL, Mok ASP, Lee ACW, Chiang AKS, Ha SY, Lau YL, et al. Quality of life in patients with transfusion-dependent thalassemia after hematopoietic SCT. *Bone Marrow Transplant.* 2008 Sep;42(5):319–27.

[20] Leelahavarong P, Chaikledkaew U, Hongeng S, Kasemsup V, Lubell Y, Teerawattananon Y. A cost-utility and budget impact analysis of allogeneic hematopoietic stem cell transplantation for severe thalassemic patients in Thailand. *BMC Health Serv. Res*. 2010;10:209–21.

[21] Switzer GE, Bruce JG, Myaskovsky L, DiMartini A, Shellmer D, Confer DL, et al. Race and ethnicity in decisions about unrelated hematopoietic stem cell donation. *Blood*. 2013 Feb 21;121(8):1469–76.

[22] Ruggeri A, Eapen M, Scaravadou A, Cairo MS, Bhatia M, Kurtzberg J, et al. Umbilical cord blood transplantation for children with thalassemia and sickle cell disease. *Biol. Blood Marrow Transplant.* 2011 Sep;17(9):1375–82.

[23] Sodani P, Isgro A, Gaziev J, Polchi P, Paciaroni K, Marziali M, et al. Purified T-depleted, CD34+ peripheral blood and bone marrow cell transplantation from haploidentical mother to child with thalassemia. *Blood*. 2010 Feb;115:1296 – 1302.

[24] Lucarelli G, Galimberti M, Polchi P, Angelucci E, Baronciani D, Giardini C, et al. Bone marrow transplantation in patients with thalassemia. *N. Engl. J. Med*. 1990 Feb 15; 322(7):417–21.

[25] Musallam KM, Taher AT, Cappellini MD, Sankaran VG. Clinical experience with fetal hemoglobin induction therapy in patients with β-thalassemia. *Blood*. 2013 Mar 21;121(12):2199–212.

[26] Mathews V, George B, Deotare U, Lakshmi KM, Viswabandya A, Daniel D, et al. A new stratification strategy that identifies a subset of class III patients with an adverse

prognosis among children with beta thalassemia major undergoing a matched related allogeneic stem cell transplantation. *Biol. Blood Marrow Transplant.* 2007;13(8):889–94.

[27] Sabloff M, Chandy M, Wang Z, Logan BR, Ghavamzadeh A, Li C-K, et al. HLA-matched sibling bone marrow transplantation for {beta}-thalassemia major. *Blood.* 2011 Feb 3;117(5):1745–50.

[28] Mathews V, Savani BN. Conditioning regimens in allo-SCT for thalassemia major. *Bone Marrow Transplant.* 2014 Jan 20;

[29] Bernardo ME, Piras E, Vacca A, Giorgiani G, Zecca M, Bertaina A, et al. Allogeneic hematopoietic stem cell transplantation in thalassemia major: results of a reduced-toxicity conditioning regimen based on the use of treosulfan. *Blood.* 2012 Jul 12;120(2):473–6.

[30] Choudhary D, Sharma SK, Gupta N, Kharya G, Pavecha P, Handoo A, et al. Treosulfan-thiotepa-fludarabine-based conditioning regimen for allogeneic transplantation in patients with thalassemia major: a single-center experience from north India. *Biol. Blood Marrow Transplant.* 2013 Mar;19(3):492–5.

[31] Galambrun C, Pondarré C, Bertrand Y, Loundou A, Bordigoni P, Frange P, et al. French multicenter 22-year experience in stem cell transplantation for Beta-thalassemia major: lessons and future directions. *Biol. Blood Marrow Transplant.* 2013 Jan;19(1):62–8.

[32] Goussetis E, Peristeri I, Kitra V, Vessalas G, Paisiou A, Theodosaki M, et al. HLA-matched sibling stem cell transplantation in children with β-thalassemia with anti-thymocyte globulin as part of the preparative regimen: the Greek experience. *Bone Marrow Transplantation.* 2012;47(8):1061–6.

[33] Faulkner L, Yaqub N, Khalid SK, Zhara T, Ansari S, Farzana T, et al. Transplantation in low resource countries. *Thalassemia Reports.* 2011;1(2s):30–3.

[34] Mathews V, George B, Lakshmi KM, Viswabandya A, John JM, Sitaram U, et al. Impact of pretransplant splenectomy on patients with beta-thalassemia major undergoing a matched-related allogeneic stem cell transplantation. *Pediatr. Transplant.* 2009 Mar;13(2):171–6.

[35] Bhatia M, Cairo MS. Splenectomy or no splenectomy prior to allogeneic stem-cell transplantation in patients with severe thalassemia: this is the question. *Pediatr. Transplant.* 2009 Mar;13(2):143–5.

[36] Uhlin M, Norström MM, Mattsson J, Remberger M. Splenectomy prior to allogeneic hematopoietic SCT increases the risk of post-transplant lymphoproliferative disease. *Bone Marrow Transplant.* 2014 Mar;49(3):463–4.

[37] Akhtar S, Moatter T. Hepatitis C virus infection in polytransfused thalassemic children in Pakistan. *Indian Pediatr.* 2004 Oct;41(10):1072–3.

[38] Di Marco V, Capra M, Angelucci E, Borgna-Pignatti C, Telfer P, Harmatz P, et al. Management of chronic viral hepatitis in patients with thalassemia: recommendations from an international panel. *Blood.* 2010 Ottobre;116(16):2875–83.

[39] Borgna-Pignatti C, Vergine G, Lombardo T, Cappellini MD, Cianciulli P, Maggio A, et al. Hepatocellular carcinoma in the thalassaemia syndromes. *Br. J. Haematol.* 2004 Jan;124(1):114–7.

[40] Cunningham MJ, Macklin EA, Neufeld EJ, Cohen AR, The Thalassemia Clinical Research Network. Complications of beta-thalassemia major in North America. *Blood.* 2004 Jul 1;104(1):34–9.

[41] Erer B. Hepatitis C virus infection in thalassemia patients undergoing allogeneic bone marrow transplantation. *Bone Marrow Transplant.* 1994;14(3):369–72.

[42] Angelucci E, Muretto P, Nicolucci A, Baronciani D, Erer B, Gaziev J, et al. Effects of iron overload and hepatitis C virus positivity in determining progression of liver fibrosis in thalassemia following bone marrow transplantation. *Blood.* 2002 Jul 1;100(1):17–21.

[43] George B, Mathews V, Viswabandya A, Srivastava A, Chandy M. Infections in children undergoing allogeneic bone marrow transplantation in India. *Pediatr. Transplant.* 2006 Feb;10(1):48–54.

[44] McGrath E. International Standards for Cellular Therapy Product Collection, Processing and Administration Accreditation Manual, FACT-JACIE 5th edition [Internet]. 2013 [cited 2013 Jun 10]. Available from: http://www.jacie.org/standards/interim-standards

[45] Kumar R, Naithani R, Mishra P, Mahapatra M, Seth T, Dolai TK, et al. Allogeneic hematopoietic SCT performed in non-HEPA filter rooms: initial experience from a single center in India. *Bone Marrow Transplant.* 2009 Jan;43(2):115–9.

[46] Svahn B-M, Remberger M, Myrbäck K-E, Holmberg K, Eriksson B, Hentschke P, et al. Home care during the pancytopenic phase after allogeneic hematopoietic stem cell transplantation is advantageous compared with hospital care. *Blood.* 2002 Dec 15;100(13):4317–24.

[47] Solomon SR, Matthews RH, Barreras AM, Bashey A, Manion KL, McNatt K, et al. Outpatient myeloablative allo-SCT: a comprehensive approach yields decreased hospital utilization and low TRM. *Bone Marrow Transplant.* 2010 Mar;45(3):468–75.

[48] Mohamed El Missiry. Infectious Complications In 96 Matched-Related Bone Marrow Transplants Performed Without Positive Pressure Room Or Centralized Hepa Filtration In Lower Middle Income Countries [Internet]. 2013. Available from: https://ash.confex.com/ash/2013/webprogram/Paper61266.html

[49] El Missiry M, Marwah P, Soni R, Khalid S, Yaqub N, Zara T, et al. HLA-typing by buccal swab to facilitate access to bone marrow transplantation globally: The Cure2Children Foundation preliminary experience. Limassol – Cyprus; 2012.

[50] Payen E, Leboulch P. Advances in stem cell transplantation and gene therapy in the β-hemoglobinopathies. *Hematology.* 2012 Dec 8;2012(1):276–83.

[51] Hajeer AH, Algattan M, Anizi A, Alaskar AS, Jarrar MS. Chances of finding a matched parent-child in hematopoietic stem cell transplantation in Saudi Arabia. *Am. J. Blood Res.* 2012;2(3):201–2.

[52] Bashey A, Zhang X, Sizemore CA, Manion K, Brown S, Holland HK, et al. T-Cell–Replete HLA-Haploidentical Hematopoietic Transplantation for Hematologic Malignancies Using Post-Transplantation Cyclophosphamide Results in Outcomes Equivalent to Those of Contemporaneous HLA-Matched Related and Unrelated Donor Transplantation. *J. Clin. Oncol.* 2013 Apr 1;31(10):1310–6.

[53] Singer ST, Vichinsky EP, Gildengorin G, van Disseldorp J, Rosen M, Cedars MI. Reproductive capacity in iron overloaded women with thalassemia major. *Blood.* 2011 Sep 8;118(10):2878–81.

[54] Rovo A, Tichelli A, Passweg JR, Heim D, Meyer-Monard S, Holzgreve W, et al. Spermatogenesis in long-term survivors after allogeneic hematopoietic stem cells transplantation is associated with age, time interval since transplantation and apparently with absence of chronic GvHD. *Blood*. 2006 Mar 16.

[55] Vichinsky E. Emerging "A" therapies in hemoglobinopathies: agonists, antagonists, antioxidants, and arginine. *Hematology*. 2012 Dec 8;2012(1):271–5.

In: Thalassemia
Editor: Makenzie Greene
ISBN: 978-1-63117-954-9

Chapter 5

Screening and Genotyping of Beta Thalassemia

Sandra Stella Lazarte[1,*], María Eugenia Mónaco[2,†] and Blanca Alicia Issé[1]

[1]Professor Cátedra Bioquímica Clínica I. Facultad de Bioquímica, Química y Farmacia. Universidad Nacional de Tucumán, Argentina
[2]Professor Cátedra Anatomía Humana y Animales de Laboratorio, Facultad de Bioquímica, Química y Farmacia. Universidad Nacional de Tucumán, Argentina

Abstract

Thalassemia comes from a greek word "*thalassa*" meaning the sea and "*amia*" for blood. The term thalassemia was first used in bordering countries of the Mediterranean Sea. Beta thalassemia is characterized by a quantitative deficiency of beta-globin chains and it is caused often for more than 200 punctual mutations than for deletions. The World Health Organization (WHO) has established that the hemoglobinopathies control, particularly the β-thalassemia, as a main priority in health care. In industrialized and in developing countries the strategies use to diagnose the illness are different, but there are three methods which are the most suitable to detect the anomaly: cellulose acetate membrane electrophoresis at alkaline pH, capillary electrophoresis, or high performance liquid chromatography. Screening programs are highly recommended for the identification of thalassemia carriers in countries where thalassemia prevalence is high. The prospective prevention includes identifying β-thalassemia trait carriers and counseling them about mate selection and prenatal diagnosis, to prevent the birth of a child with a major disease. Carrier diagnosis involves the accurate measurement of red blood count (RBC), mean corpuscular hemoglobin (MCH), mean corpuscular volume (MCV), HbA_2 and HbF values.

* Corresponding author: Dr. Sandra Stella Lazarte. Professor Cátedra Bioquímica Clínica I. Facultad de Bioquímica, Química y Farmacia. Universidad Nacional de Tucumán. Argentina. Balcarce 747. San Miguel de Tucumán. Tucumán. Argentina. CP4000. Tel. 54-381-4310994. E. mail: slazarte@fbqf.unt.edu.ar.

† María Eugenia Mónaco: Professor Cátedra Anatomía Humana y Animales de Laboratorio. Facultad de Bioquímica, Química y Farmacia. Universidad Nacional de Tucumán. Argentina. Chacabuco 461. San Miguel de Tucumán. Tucumán. Argentina. CP4000. Tel. 54-381-4247752.

In developing countries a differential diagnosis of iron deficiency anemia is necessary. So, β-thalassemia trait carriers can be detected by screening tests like Naked Eye Single Tube Red Cell Osmotic Fragility Test (NESTROFT), and red cell indices, like Mentzer, Shine and Lal (SLI), Green and King, England and Fraser, RDWI (red blood distribution width index) and others. To increase NESTROFT sensitivity we proposed the spectrophotometer lecture, and for β-thalassemia trait detection, the use of Mentzer (MCV/RBC), SLI (MCV^2 x MCHb x 0.01) and RDWI (MCV x RDW/RBC) indexes. Ultimately, advances in molecular tests have facilitated the prenatal diagnosis of thalassemia and have allowed the genotyping of the β-thalassemia in different geographic areas. The majority of the common mutations tend to cluster within neighboring regions and its distribution depends of the ethnic group. The thalassemia mutations can be identified by PCR-based techniques. In northwestern of Argentina we have recognized the most prevalent mutations by real time PCR. They were a nonsense mutation, Cd39 (C→T), and a RNA processing mutation, IVS-I-1 (G→A).

Definition, Epidemiology and Etiology

Thalassemia is a globin gene disorder that results in a diminished rate of synthesis of one or more of the globin chains and, consequently, a reduced rate of synthesis of the hemoglobin (Hb) or hemoglobins (Hbs) of which that chain constitutes a part. The term thalassemia is derived from the Greek, "*thalassa*" (sea) and "*aima*" (blood). The significantly reduced rate of synthesis of one type of globin chain leads to unbalanced chain synthesis, with an excess of a normal globin chain contributing to the pathological effects, causing either damage to erythroid precursors and ineffective erythropoiesis or damage to mature erythrocytes and hemolytic anemia (Thein, 2002). Normal human adult hemoglobin A (HbA) consists in two pairs of globin chains alpha and beta, $\alpha_2\beta_2$, of which synthesis is normally tightly coordinated to ensure equal production.

In healthy adults, almost 95% of the Hb is HbA with small amounts (<3.5%) of HbA_2 and HbF (<1%) present. The α-globin chain is encoded in duplicate on chromosome 16, and the non-α chains (β, δ, γ) are encoded in a cluster on chromosome 11. β-thalassemia is due to autosomal mutations in the gene encoding β-globin (Weatherall, 2001).

The relative excess of α-chains in β-chain deficiencies will combine with delta (δ) chains to form variable levels of HbA_2 ($\alpha_2\delta_2$) dependent on the severity of the beta chain deficiency. Therefore, β-thalassemia is characterized by increased HbA_2 levels.

The first description of thalassemia was reported by Dr. Thomas Cooley in 1925. There are a multiplicity of genetic mutations in β-thalassemia that give rise to a clinically heterogeneous spectrum ranging from mild anemia with microcytosis (thalassemia minor) and moderate clinical anemia (thalassemia intermedia) to classical, fatal Cooley's anemia (thalassemia major) (Weatherall, 2001).

Currently, about 5% of the world population carries a potentially pathological gene of hemoglobin (ie, healthy people that have inherited a mutant gene from one parent). Each year approximately 300.000 children with thalassemia syndromes (30%) or sickle cell disease (70%) born worldwide. Like healthy carriers (which can reach 25% in some populations) are protected against the deadly effects of malaria, these inherited anemias were initially confined to tropical and subtropical regions. β-thalassemia is more frequent in the Mediterranean Basin, the Middle East and Asia.

The carrier frequency for β-thalassemia in these areas ranges from 1% to 20% (Weatherall, 2001). However, the global increase of migration has introduced hemoglobinopathies in many areas where they were not originally endemic as Northern Europe, North and South America, Caribbean, and Australia (OMS, 2006).

Thalassemia can be classified according to the phenotype or the genotype.

The phenotypes of homozygous or genetic heterozygous compound β-thalassemias include thalassemia major and thalassemia intermedia.

Individuals with thalassemia major usually come to medical attention within the first two years of life and require regular red blood cells transfusions to survive. Thalassemia intermedia includes patients who present later and do not require regular transfusion. Except in the rare dominant forms, heterozygous beta-thalassemia results usually in the clinically silent carrier state and is defined by specific hematological features (Galanello and Origa, 2010). β-thalassemia mutations are divided into two broad categories: β^0 (beta zero) thalassemia and β^+ (beta plus) thalassemia.

Mutations that completely inactivate the β gene resulting in no β globin production cause β^0-thalassemia. Other mutations allow the production of some β globin, and depending on the degree of quantitative reduction in the output of the β chains, are classified as β^+- or β^{++}- ("silent") thalassemia.

The primary determinant of β-thalassemia severity is the type of β allele (β^0, β^+, β^{++}), ameliorated by coinheritance of interacting α-thalassemia (which reduces the pool of free α chains) and coinheritance of an innate ability to increase production of gamma (γ) chains. The additional γ-globin chains will partner the excess α globin to form fetal hemoglobin (HbF, $\alpha_2\gamma_2$) (Thein, 2013).

Subjects with thalassemia major are homozygotes or compound heterozygotes for β^0 or β^+ genes, and subjects with thalassemia intermedia are mostly homozygotes or compound heterozygotes. The heterozygous states for β-thalassemia show a great phenotypic diversity, comparable to that for the inheritance of two β-thalassemia alleles.

In some cases, the β-thalassemia allele is so mild that it is phenotypically "silent", with no anemia or hematological abnormalities (Metaxotou-Mavrommati and Kattami, 1999). In others, the heterozygous state causes a phenotype almost as severe as the major forms, that is, the β-thalassemia allele is dominantly inherited.

Beta Globin Gene Anatomy

β-thalassemias are heterogeneous at the molecular level. Almost 300 disease-causing mutations have been so far identified. The majority of mutations are single nucleotide substitutions or deletions or insertions of oligonucleotides leading to frameshift.

Rarely β-thalassemias result from gross gene deletion (Thein, 2013).

The β globin (*HBB*) gene maps in the short arm of chromosome 11 in a region also containing the δ globin gene, the embryonic epsilon (ε) gene, the fetal $^G\gamma$ and $^A\gamma$ genes, and a pseudogene (ψβ). The five functional globin genes are arranged in the order of their developmental expression (Clark and Thein, 2004) (Figure 1).

The *HBB* gene, which spans 1.6 Kb, contains three exons and both 5' and 3' untranslated regions (UTRs). Globin synthesis is controlled by an adjacent 5' promoter in which a TATA, CAAT, and duplicated CACCC boxes are located.

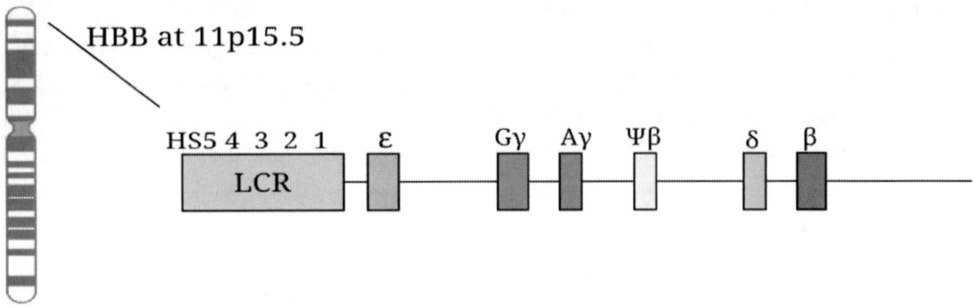

Figure 1. Chromosome localization and structure of β globin gene cluster.

Several transcription factors bind and regulate the function of the *HBB* gene, the most important of which is erythroid Kruppel-like factor 1, which binds the proximal CACCC box, and whose knockout in the mouse leads to a β-thalassemia-like clinical picture (Cao and Galanello, 2010).

In addition deoxyribonuclease (DNase)-hypersensitive sites called Locus Control Region (LCR), 40 kbp (kilobase pairs) 5′ to the embryonic genes, regulate the expression of all β-genes. This region contains four (HS-1 to HS-4) erythroid specific DNAse hypersensitive sites (HSs), which are a hallmark of DNA-protein interaction. Each HS site is constituted by a combination of several DNA motifs interacting with transcription factors, among which the most important are GATA-1. The importance of LCR for the control of the β-like globin gene expression has been discovered by studying a series of naturally occurring deletions that totally or partly remove the HS sites and result in the inactivation of the intact downstream β-globin gene (Thein, 2013)

In this sense it is important to note that point mutations affecting the β-globin expression belong to three different categories: mutations leading to defective β gene transcription (promoter and 5' UTR mutations); mutations affecting messenger RNA (mRNA) processing (splice junction and consensus sequence mutations, polyadenylation, and other 3' UTR mutations); and mutations resulting in abnormal mRNA translation (nonsense, frameshift, and initiation codon mutations) (Cao and Galanello, 2010).

A complete updated list of β-thalassemia mutations is available through the Globin Gene Server Web Site (http://www.globin.cse.psu.edu) (Giardine et al., 2014).

Mutations that completely inactivate the β gene resulting in no β-globin production cause β^0-thalassemia and result from deletion, initiation codon, nonsense, frameshift, and splicing mutations, especially at the splice-site junction.

On the other hand, β^+-thalassemias, are produced by mutations in the promoter area (either the CACCC or TATA box), the polyadenylation signal, and the 5' or 3' UTR or by splicing abnormalities (Cao and Galanello, 2010).

Deletions affecting the β-globin gene are very rare, except for a 619-bp deletion removing the 3' end of the β-globin gene, which is relatively common in Sind and Punjab populations of India and Pakistan. Another group of deletions (complex β-thalassemia), in addition to the β-globin gene, involve also the δ ($\delta\beta^0$-thalassemia), the δ and $^A\gamma$ genes ($^A\gamma\delta\beta^0$-thalassemia), or the whole β-globin gene cluster. Finally, partial or total deletions of the LCR, but leaving the β-globin gene intact, inactivate the β-globin gene (Thein, 2013).

Despite the marked molecular heterogeneity the majority of the common mutations tend to cluster within neighboring regions and its distribution depends of the ethnic group. Thereby, the prevalent molecular defects are limited in each at risk population in which 4–10 mutations usually account for most of the β-globin disease-causing allele (Cao and Galanello, 2010).

Diagnosis of Beta Thalassemia

Today, hemoglobin disorders are generally discovered during a systematic study performed within programs for prevention of thalassemia or sickle cell disease. In several regions (India, Turkey, Iraq, Iran, Gaza Strip, Saudi Arabia, Cyprus, etc.) these are found in premarital screening. In other regions, like west European countries, the research for the main hemoglobin disorders is often limited to populations at risk. It is done either as preconception or neonatal screening programs (Wajcman and Moradkhani, 2011). Thalassemia can also be detected during the study of an unknown origin anemic syndrome.

Opportunistic testing may be initiated by a general practitioner or other medical practitioner, with the informed consent of the patient, or by a hematology laboratory, where an abnormality that requires explanation is detected, e.g., in individuals found to have red cell indices suggestive of thalassemia.

In all cases, a first essential test that needs to be performed is a Complete Blood Count (CBC) looking mostly for anemia, mycrocitosis and hypochromia. If there is microcytosis, appropriate tests for iron deficiency and anemia of chronic disease should be performed and testing for thalassemia considered in patients of appropriate family origin. Depending on agreed local policies, such tests may be initiated by the laboratory. Some laboratories use various published formulae to decide when to initiate such investigations but it should be noted that such formulae are not likely to be reliable in children or pregnant women or in sick patients who may have multiple medical problems influencing the Hb and red cell indices (Ryan et al., 2010). Thalassemia investigations should therefore be considered in any subject that shows unexplained microcytosis and a normal iron profile.

In industrialized and in developing countries the strategies use to diagnose the illness are different, but there are three methods which are the most suitable to detect the anomaly: Cellulose Acetate Membrane Electrophoresis at Alkaline pH (CAE), Capillary Electrophoresis (CE), or High Performance Liquid Chromatography (HPLC).

Diagnostic recommendations regarding the laboratory investigation of thalassemia were first made in 1975 by the International Committee for Standardization in Hematology expert panel on abnormal Hbs and thalassemia. The recommended initial testing included a CBC, electrophoresis of Hb at pH 9.2, and quantification of HbA_2 and HbF. Although CAE has been widely used for many years, the emergence of cation-exchange HPLC, as the method of choice for quantification of HbA_2 and HbF and identification of Hb variants, streamlined the recommended preliminary and follow-up tests for the identification of hemoglobinopathies and thalassemias, and provided rapid and complete diagnostic work-up in a majority of cases. In 2000, Clarke and Higgins (Clarke and Higgins, 2000) suggested that the elements of choice included a CBC, HbH (β_4) test (positive in some α-thalassemias), ferritin, HPLC for HbA_2

and F quantification, and detection of any Hb variants followed by electrophoresis at both alkaline and acid pH.

British Committee for Standards in Haematology recommended in 2010 methods used in screening of thalassemia. They were red cell indices in conjunction with measurement of HbA_2 levels. Routine measuring of blood indices included measurements of Mean Corpuscular Hemoglobin (MCH) and Mean Corpuscular Volume (MCV); it was advised the use of MCH to screen for thalassemia as this parameter is more stable than MCV.

These indices are usually reported for all routine blood counts. It was counselled to quantify HbA_2 by HPLC or microcolumn chromatography (Ryan et al., 2010).

In 2011, Bain suggested to study thalassemia a full blood count and film followed by the application of a primary diagnostic technique like CAE, HPLC or CE with quantification of HbA_2 and HbF.

The choice of methodology and equipment will be based on volume of workload, sample material (liquid blood or dried blood spots), ease of handling, reproducibility, local availability and expertise and cost. Although the consumables for CAE are inexpensive, the labor costs are relatively high and is necessary an expertise evaluation.

When an increase of HbA_2 is observed in CAE, this should be quantified.

Measurement of Cell Blood Count and Hematological Indices

β-thalassemia minor is characterized by reduced MCV and MCH, with increased HbA_2 level. The hematological profile consists of measurements of thered blood cells indices and includes Hb concentration, hematocrit, red blood count (RBC), MCH, MCV, Mean Corpuscular Hemoglobin Concentration (MCHC) and Red Cell Distribution Width (RDW).

Routinely, a blood film accompanies the red cells indices. Thalassemia may have an impact on them, and they are critical to the differential diagnosis of it. The blood count characteristically shows a normal or slightly reduced hemoglobin concentration, elevation of the RBC and reduction of the MCH and MCV (Figure 2).

The MCHC is usually normal when measured by impedance counters (e.g. Coulter or Sysmex instruments), but may be reduced when measured by Bayer light scattering instruments (Bain, 2006). The general classification of thalassemia is hypochromic and microcytic anemia; therefore, the MCV can be considered as a key diagnostic indicator.

The RDW is a measure of the degree of variation in red cell size. In normal subjects, RDW is $< 14.5\%$. Some causes of microcytic anemia, most notably iron deficiency, are characterized by an increase in RDW. The thalassemias, in contrast, tend to produce a uniform microcytic red cell population without a concomitant increase in RDW.

This observation is variable among the thalassemia syndromes, however, with notable increases in RDW in the setting of HbH disease and δβ-thalassemia minor. Therefore, the RDW may provide information useful as an adjunct to diagnosis but is not useful as alone indicator (Clarke and Higgins, 2000). When we use a value of RDW $> 16\%$ to distinguish thalassemia from iron deficiency anemia, the specificity and sensitivity were only 38% and 45%, respectively. Therefore, it is not advisable to use this test to differentiate these anemias (Lazarte et al., 2012 [a]).

The characteristic red cell indices have been used in a number of formulae designed to separate cases of iron deficiency anemia (IDA) from cases of β-thalassemia trait (β-TT)

(Kotwal et al., 1999; Rathod et al., 2007; Ntaios et al., 2008; Okan et al., 2009; Shen et al., 2010; Ferrara et al., 2010; Lazarte et al., 2010-2011). The premise underlying these formulas is that iron deficient erythropoiesis is characterized by red blood cells with decrease hemoglobin concentration and a decreased or normal RBC, whereas individuals who are heterozygous for thalassemia have red cells that are smaller but usually increased in number (Gallivan and Giordano, 2012). Table I shows main indices proposed to discriminate β-TT.

No index has yet been found to offer both sensitivity and specificity of 100%, and it has recommended a different index to each population. In Turkey, Shine and Lal index (SLI) and Green and King index (GKI) offered the best discrimination and RDW Index (RDWI), the worst (Okan et al., 2009). In Greece, GKI shows the highest reliability (Ntaios et al., 2008); while in Palestinian population, GKI and RDWI were the best (Sirdah et al., 2008). Previous work conducted in our laboratory established that the use of the Mentzer Index (MI), SLI and RDWI was more reliable than any other published index (Lazarte et al., 2010-2011; Lazarte et al., 2012[a]) to identify and discriminate β-TT from IDA. But Lafferty et al. (1996) concluded that MCV alone is as effective as the MI and SLI in selecting microcytic patient samples with a high probability of thalassemia minor for thalassemia testing. This cell volume, reported in femtoliters (fL), in most adult populations ranges from 80 to 100 fL. An MCV of 72 fL is maximally sensitive and specific for presumptive diagnosis of thalassemia syndromes (Lafferty et al., 1996). The suspicion of β-TT should be confirmed with specific tests (CAE, HPLC or CE).

RBC $\geq$ 5,0 x 10^{12}/L is also useful as a differential tool because the thalassemias produce a microcytic anemia with an associated increase in the red blood cell number, while the other causes of microcytic anemia, including iron deficiency and anemia of chronic disease, are more typically associated with a decrease in RBC that is proportional to the degree of decrease in Hb concentration.

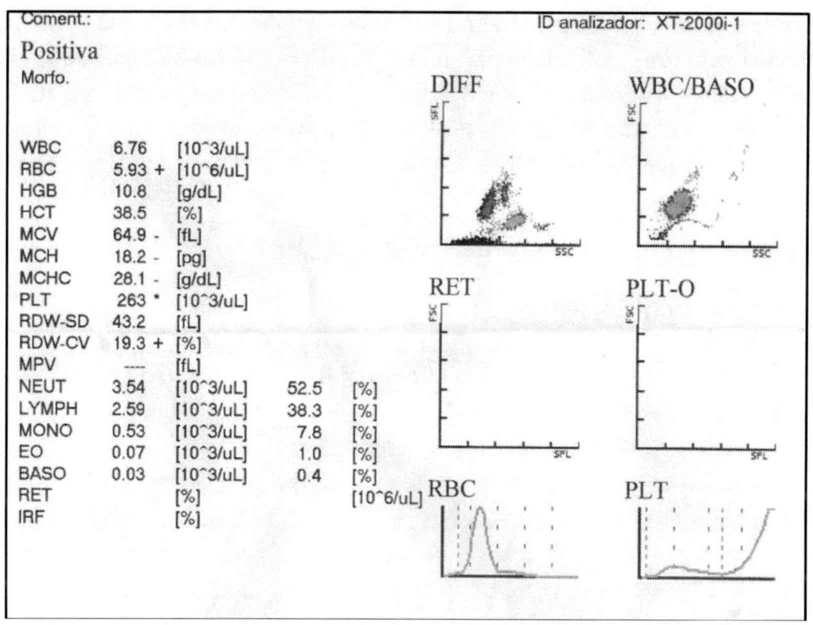

Figure 2. Complete blood count of β-thalassemia carrier obtained in Sysmex XT 2000i Analyzer.

Table 1. Threshold values of the indices used to discriminate between iron deficiency anemia (IDA) and the β-thalassemia trait (β-TT)

INDICES	β-TT	IDA
Red blood count (RBC) ($x10^{12}$/L)	>5,0	<5,0
Mentzer index (MI) = MCV/RBC	<13	>13
Shine and Lal index (SLI) = MCV^2xMCHx0,01	<1530	>1530
England and Fraser index (EFI) = MCV-RBC-5Hb-3,4	Negativo	Positivo
Srivastava index (SI) = MCH/RBC	<3,8	>3,8
RDW [%] (Besman index)	<18	>18
Green and King index (GKI)=MCV^2 x RDW/100 x Hb	<65	>65
Ricerca index (RI)= RDW/RBC	<4,4	>4,4
RDW index (RDWI)= RDW x MCV/RBC	<220	>220

However its sensitivity and specificity was lower than other indices like MI and SLI (Okan et al., 2009; Lazarte et al., 2010-2011).

No significant difference in red blood cells parameters was observed between non-thalassemic fetuses and those with β-TT, HbE trait, homozygous HbE and β-thalassemia/HbE disease (Karnpean et al., 2013). In the neonatal period, babies with β-TT have a normal hemoglobin concentration and normal red cell indices.

Around the age of 3 months, start to appear differences from normal. By 6-12 months of age, the average HbA_2 percentage is higher than in other infants (Wood et al., 1982).

Several authors have reported that mean values for hematological variables (hemoglobin concentration, MCV and MCH) differ significantly between β^+- and β^0-thalassemia trait, but there is considerable overlap (Rosatelli et al., 1992; Rund et al., 1992; López-Escribano, 2009). But other researchers (Stefani et al., 1994; Bragós et al., 2005) did not found significant differences ($p > 0,05$) in red cell indices when compared β^0- and β^+-thalassemia.

The Hb concentration, RBC, hematocrit, MCV, MCH and MCHC are reduced and RDW is increased in β-thalassemia major (β-TM). β-TM is characterized by reduced Hb level (<7 g/ dL), MCV > 50 < 70 fL and MCH > 12< 20 pg. Thalassemia intermedia is characterized by Hb level between 70 and 100 g/L, MCV between 50 and 80 fL and MCH between 16 and 24 pg (Galanello and Origa, 2010).

Blood Smear, Reticulocytes and Bone Marrow Picture

The blood film in β-TT varies from almost normal, with only mild microcytosis, to markedly abnormal (Figure 3). Abnormal features, in addition to microcytosis, include anisocytosis, hypochromia and poikilocytosis. Individuals with a more severe phenotype may have prominent basophilic stippling, target cells and small numbers of irregularly contracted cells.

Elliptocytes are generally more characteristic of iron deficiency than of thalassemia trait, but some thalassemic individuals have prominent elliptocytes. Target cells and basophilic stippling are generally more common in β-thalassemia than in iron deficiency.

Anisochromasia, i.e. variation in the degree of hemoglobinization from one cell to another, is characteristic of iron deficiency and is not usually a feature of uncomplicated β-TT (Bain, 2006). Erythroblasts are normally not seen.

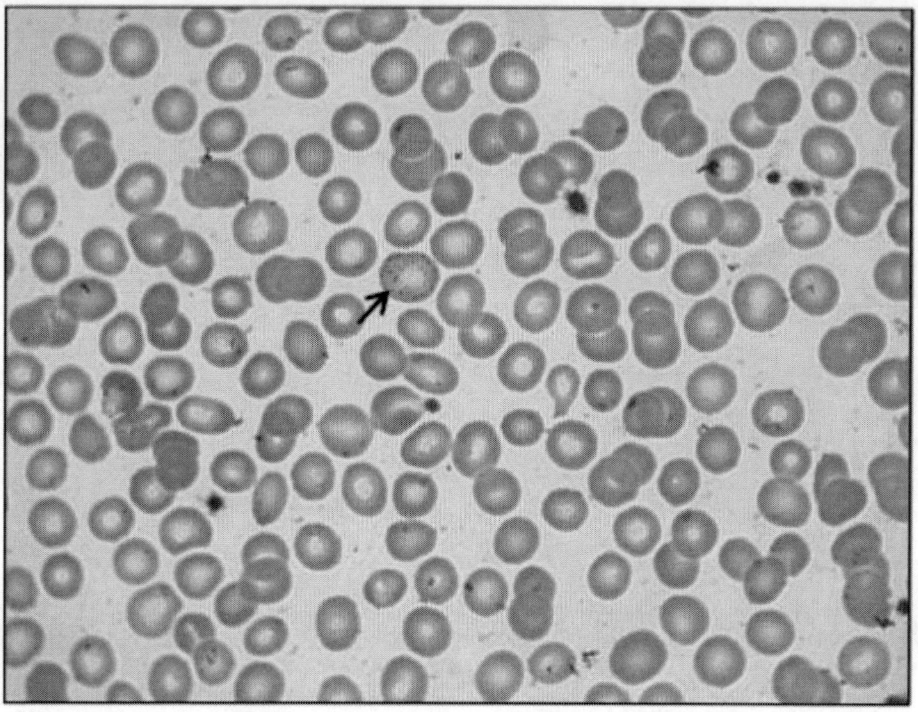

Blood film showing microcytosis, anisochromasia, a teardrop poikilocyte and basophilic stippling (arrow).

Figure 3. Blood film from a patient with β-TT.

In β-TT, the percentage of reticulocytes is normal or may be slightly elevated. The bone marrow aspirate shows increased cellularity as a consequence of erythroid hyperplasia, with a myeloid/erythroid ratio reversed from the normal (3 or 4) to 0.1 or less.

Some erythroblasts show defective hemoglobinization and cytoplasmic vacuolation. An iron stain may show heavy siderotic granulation (Bain, 2006). Bone marrow examination is usually not necessary for diagnosis of affected individuals.

With severe β-thalassemia intermedia (β-TI), the red cell morphology could change dramatically, and anisocytosis and poikilocytosis may be more evident (Gallivan and Giordano, 2012). The blood film of β-TI patients shows features similar to those of typical β-TT, but the abnormalities are more marked. In addition to hypochromia, microcytosis, anisocytosis, poikilocytosis and basophilic stippling, there may be polychromasia and circulating nucleated red blood cells (NRBCs, i.e., erythroblasts). The bone marrow aspirate shows abnormalities of erythropoiesis that are more severe than those of β-TT (Bain, 2006).

Affected individuals with β-TM also show red blood cells morphologic changes, and NRBC (Figure 4). In individuals with β-TM, the hemoglobin level decreases progressively during the first months of life. When the child becomes symptomatic, the hemoglobin level may be as low as 30 to 40 g/L.

Red blood cell morphology is strikingly abnormal, with many microcytes, bizarre poikilocytes, teardrop cells, and target cells. A characteristic finding is the presence of extraordinarily hypochromic, often wrinkled and folded cells (leptocytes) containing irregular inclusion bodies of precipitated α-globin chains (Giardina and Forget, 2009).

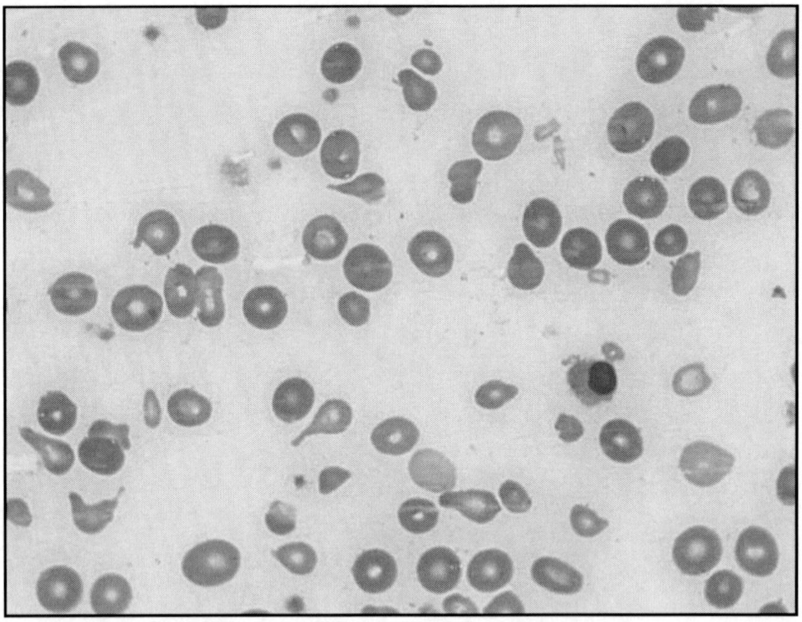

Blood film of a patient with β-TM under maintenance transfusion therapy: many microcytes, bizarre poikilocytes, teardrop cells, and one NRBC.

Figure 4. Blood film from a patient with β-TM.

Nucleated red blood cells are frequently present. The reticulocyte count is 2% to 8% lower than would be expected in view of the extreme erythroid hyperplasia and hemolysis. The low count reflects the severity of intramedullary erythroblast destruction. The white blood cell count is elevated. A moderate polymorphonuclear leukocytosis and normal platelet count are typical unless hypersplenism has developed.

The bone marrow exhibits marked hypercellularity caused by erythroid hyperplasia. The red blood cell precursors show defective hemoglobinization and reduced amounts of cytoplasm (Giardina and Forget, 2009). The number of erythroblasts is related to the degree of anemia and is markedly increased after splenectomy (Galanello and Origa, 2010).

Hemoglobin A_2 and Fetal Hemoglobin Quantification

Diagnosis rests on the detection of an increased HbA_2 percentage. A proportion of cases, around one-third to one-half, also have an increased proportion of HbF.

In most cases of heterozygosis for β^0- or severe β^+-thalassemia, the HbA_2 is between 4% and 5%, whereas when there is heterozygosis for mild β^+-thalassemia there is usually 3.6-4.2% of HbA_2 (Bain, 2006). β-thalassemia carriers are identified by an HbA_2 value $\geq$ 3.5%. However, some carriers have a slight increase in HbA_2. Therefore, a careful determination of the HbA_2 level is necessary to avoid diagnostic pitfalls (Giambona et al., 2009).

HbA_2 is barelly detectable at birth, while the β gene is already active at eigth week of gestation; normal newborns present with 20-30% HbA which gradually increases, while γ gene expression is reduced.

Table 2. Causes of increased and reduced HbA_2 levels

Hb A_2 ↑	Hb A_2 ↓
β-thalassemias	Neonatal period
Sickle cell trait (Hb AS)	"Silent" β-thalassemia alleles
Sickle cell disease (Hb SS)	α-thalassemias
Triplicate α gene	δ-thalassemias
Unstable Hbs	δβ-thalassemia and γδβ-thalassemia
Hereditary Spherocytosis	δ-globin chain variants
Megaloblastic anemias	Lepore Hbs
Hyperthyroidism	Iron deficiency*
Antiretroviral therapy	Lead poisoning
Pseudoxanthoma elasticum	Sideroblastic anemia
Hypertrophic osteoarthropathy	Mieloproliferative disorders

*Recently, Passarello et al. (2012) showed that the presence of iron deficiency did not preclude the detection of classical β carrier in Sicily.

Steinberg and Adams III, 1991; Mosca et al., 2009 [a]; Giambona et al., 2009; Stephens et al., 2012 [a].

HbA_2 levels do not increase synchronously with HbA, but lag behind; the HbA/HbA_2 ratio is about 100 at 32 weeks of gestation and 75 at 45 weeks. The "adult" HbA/HbA_2 ratio of about 40:1 is not reached until at least 6 months of age. This sluggish response of HbA_2 during maturation may reduce its value for the diagnosis of β-thalassemia in young infants (Steinberg and Adams III, 1991). The stable level of HbA_2 is reached after first year of life, and HbF reaches adult levels after the second year.

Therefore it is recommended to perform thalassemia study after the first year of life. But it is important to know that after the third month it would be possible to diagnose a β-thalassemia carrier by the early rise of the HbA_2 fraction, as well as by other variables (MCV and HbF) (Wood et al., 1982; Mosca et al., 2009 [a]).

Table II displays the causes of increased and reduced HbA_2 values. There is many acquired situations where is observed bigger HbA_2 percentage, so that an increased HbA_2 cannot be used as the sole discriminant for β-thalassemia.

All procedures for quantitative determination of HbA_2 are based on the separation of this hemoglobin fraction from HbA, HbF and other hemoglobin variants. The δ chain of HbA_2, contains two additional positive charges compared with the β-chain of HbA. This facilitates its separation by electrophoretic and chromatographic methods that rely on charge differences to resolve proteins from one another (Steinberg and Adams III, 1991).

Several methods have been set up, but only a few are recommended as sufficiently accurate. Traditionally, electrophoresis performed on acetate cellulose strip at alkaline pH has been the method of choice for recognition and quantification of HbA_2 and HbF (Figure 5). Visualization of the Hb bands is made possible by staining with Amido Black or Ponceau Red over a clear background, allowing for quantification of the Hb present by elution of the strip and spectrophotometric estimation.

Quantification of HbA_2 by scanning densitometry is not sufficiently precise to be used in the diagnosis of β-TT and isoelectric focusing (IEF) has not been validated for this purpose (The laboratory diagnosis of haemoglobinopathies, 1998; Bain, 2006).

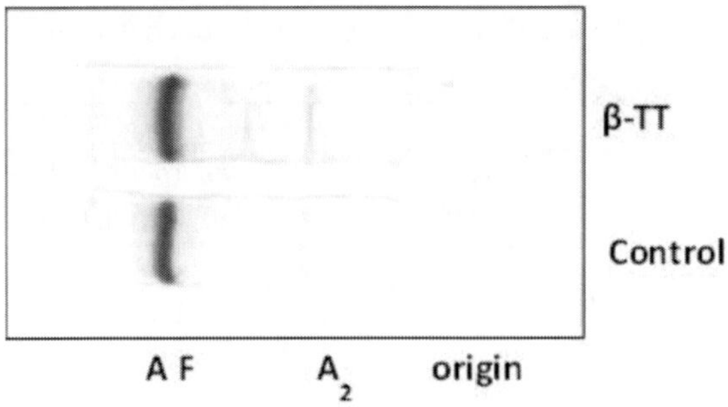

Control sample containing Hbs A and A_2.

Figure 5. Hemoglobin electrophoresis on cellulose acetate at alkaline pH showing increased HbA_2 and HbF.

Another suitable methods for the quantification of HbA_2 include microcolumn cromatography and HPLC. Elution of HbA_2 using macro-column low pressure chromatography with a weak cation-exchange material (such as CM cellulose) or an anion exchange material (such as DEAE cellulose) was a commonly used technique. This procedure, however, is labour intensive and timeconsuming. In 1978, International Committee for Standardization in Haematology (ICSH) recommended ion exchange microcolumn cromatography as a reference method for HbA_2 quantification (ICSH, 1978). Microchromatographic techniques decrease the chromatographic time but sacrifice resolution (Tan et al., 1993).

Moreover, in the presence of HbS, the determination of HbA_2 is not accurate, and it is necessary to use special columns. Finally, in the presence of unstable hemoglobin, HbA_2 may increase only slightly. Therefore, micro-column chromatography should always be combined with hemoglobin electrophoresis to detect hemoglobin variants.

High and low HbA_2 percentages can be distinguished visually on a electrophoretic strip, and this can sometimes be a useful check on microcolumn chromatography results (The laboratory diagnosis of haemoglobinopathies, 1998; Giambona et al., 2009).

Both electrophoretic or conventional chromatographic methods are unable to differentiated HbA_2 from hemoglobin variants such HbE or HbC, that contain similar charge differences (Steinberg and Adams III, 1991).

CAE and HPLC detect other hemoglobinopathies (S, C, E, O_{Arab}, Lepore) that may interact with β-thalassemia. Cation-exchange HPLC was also recommended as the gold standard for population screening of hemoglobinopathies and thalassemias (Clarke and Higgins, 2000). HPLC is a reliable tool that allows accurate determination of HbA_2, HbF and Hb variants such as HbS, HbE, Hb Lepore, HbC, HbD and HbO-Arab. HbA_2 values should always be interpreted together with other findings, such as erythrocyte indices, iron status and familial studies. Some elements may interfere with HbA_2 quantification, including carry-over, column defects, batch-to-batch differences, sample concentration, sample dilution, incorrect calibration, incorrect integration of HbA_2, and sample condition (fresh, old, stored at 4 °C or frozen). Therefore HPLC apparatus must be handled only by well trained personnel, and critical evaluation of the chromatograms, together with calibration and quality control programs run on a regular basis, are essential (Mosca et al., 2009 [b]). Actually, coelution of glycated or modified HbS may slightly increase the observed HbA_2 level (3.8-4.5%), as the presence of Hb Lepore and HbE coeluting with HbA_2 can artificially increase perceived HbA_2 levels (Hb Lepore 10-15%, HbE 22-28%).

But levels of HbA_2 higher than 8% correspond almost always to a mutant Hb such as HbE eluting at the same position (Tan et al., 1993; Giambona et al., 2009).

A technique with excellent separation capacity is capillary electrophoresis (Cotton et al., 1999). The CE is a relatively new system that utilizes the principle of electrokinetic separation of molecules in electrolyte buffer-filled silica capillary. The separation of hemoglobin fractions is achieved in a buffer capillary with a 50 μm inner diameter. The sample is injected in one end, and proteins will migrate to the other end under high-voltage conditions. All the hemoglobin molecules move past a detector that measures the absorbance at 415 nm. An electropherogram (similar to a chromatogram) is thus generated; the percentage of each hemoglobin fraction (HbA, HbF, HbA_2 and any hemoglobin variants) is calculated (Figure 6).

Various types of CE have been developed, but the most common are capillary zone electrophoresis (CZE) and capillary isoelectricfocusing (CIEF) (Giambona et al., 2009; Stephens et al., 2012 [a]). CE patterns were easier to interpret than CAE patterns. While the latter needs technical expertise, the former provides objective results and various settings available for interpretation, recording, and archives. However, the presence of HbA is essential for CE to obtain appropriate zones for verifying the identity of the Hb (Kim et al., 2011).

This method was characterized by a very favorable variance coefficient (CV) for HbA_2 quantification (Cotton et al., 1999) and reliable measurement of HbA_2 values in the presence of HbE and HbD Punjab (Higgins et al., 2009).

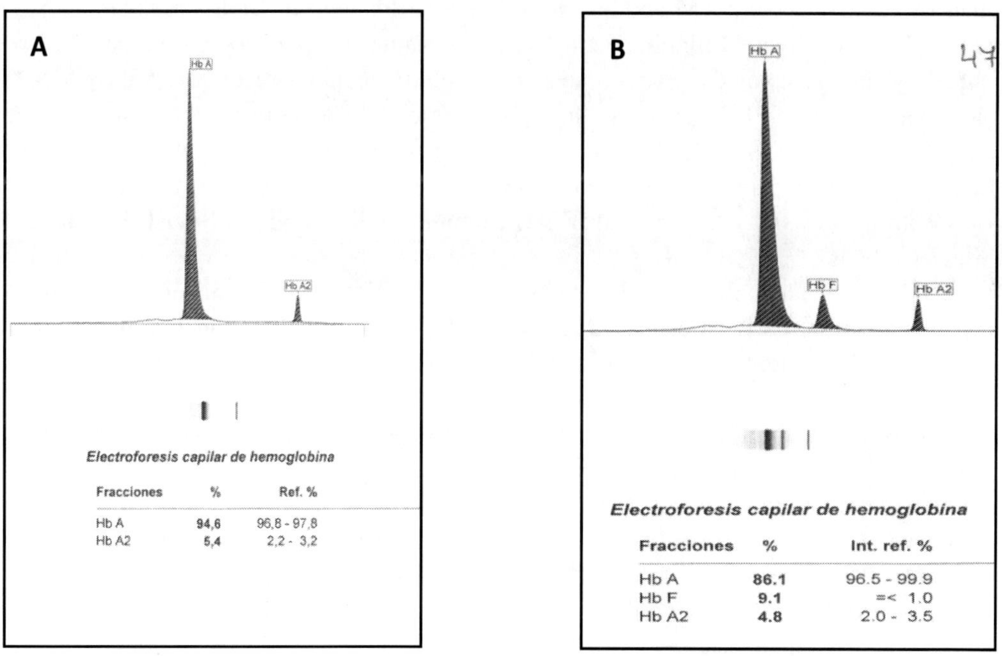

*Cortesy of Dr. Raquel Osatinsky, Consultant Manlab, Diagnóstico Bioquímico y Genómico, Buenos Aires, Argentina.

Figure 6. CE (Sebia Capillarys 2) of β-TT showing: A) increased HbA_2 in adult patient; and B) increased HbA_2 and HbF in a child of 20 months old*.

Hafiza et al. (2012) also observed that the HbE level by CE was much lower than that of HPLC. This finding was anticipated because by HPLC, the HbE and HbA_2 coeluted at the same retention time, while CE measured the actual level of HbE in the sample. CE (Sebia Capillarys 2) offered minimal advantages over the HPLC (Bio-Rad VARIANT II) for the quantification of HbA_2 in the presence of HbS and was not as good for the quantification of HbA_2 in the presence of HbC (Higgins et al., 2009).

Few data are available on the alignment of the different methods used for HbA_2 quantitation and external quality survey results showed a consistent spread of HbA_2 values (Paleari et al., 2007). Paleari et al. (2012) conducted a comparison study among the actual best performing techniques for HbA_2 determination, comprising HPLC (Bio-Rad Variant I, Bio-Rad Variant II, Menarini HA-8160, Tosoh G7, Tosoh G8) and CE (Beckman Coulter MDQ and ProteomeLab PA 800, Sebia Capillarys 2) methods.

The mean within-run imprecision of HbA_2 measurement (expressed as CV, %) was between 0.5% and 4.4% (HPLC) and between 1.2% and 4.4% (CE). Concerning HbF, the mean imprecision at HbF values $\geq$ 1.5% was between 1.2% and 8.2% (as CVs). A poor alignment of routine methods for HbA_2 measurement was found. The need of a better standardization of HbA_2 measurement procedures was underlined (Paleari et al., 2012).

In 1988, the WHO agreed on the value of the 1st International Reference Material for HbA_2 (World Health Organization Expert Committee on Biological Standardization, 1994). This is a stabilized freeze-dried preparation (89/666) prepared from blood obtained from the mother of a patient with β-TM and is held at National Institute of Biological Standards and Controls (NIBSC) South Mimms, Herts, UK. The value assigned to this preparation was obtained by an international collaborative study using the methods recommended by ICSH in 1978 and also by the HPLC equipment that was commercially available at that time.

As it is now 20 years since this international reference material was prepared and validated, another preparation is being developed (Paleari et al., 2010) that will be assayed by mass spectrometry and by the original ICSH recommended methods and by HPLC and CZE as well (Stephens et al., 2012 [a]).

Last recommendations of ICSH for HbA_2 quantification included historical methods of analysis (cellulose acetate electrophoresis with elution or microcolumn chromatography), automated HPLC, automated CE and automated CIEF. CAE and microcolumn chromatography can produce results that are satisfactory for clinical purposes but are time-consuming and need technical expertize. HPLC can give satisfactory results when no hemoglobin variant is present. However, when hemoglobin variants are present, experience is necessary to interpret the chromatograms.

CE and CIEF can also produce satisfactory results if no hemoglobin variant is present, but experience is necessary to interpret the electropherograms (Stephens et al., 2012 [a]).

In the rare "silent" β-TT, both the red cell indices and HbA_2 concentrations may be normal. It is inevitable that most of these cases will be missed in the routine diagnostic laboratory. Only a minority of the point mutations causing β-thalassemia are not associated with a raised HbA_2 level. It appears that β-thalassemia mutations that lead to only mild impairment of β-globin synthesis are accompanied by more modest elevations of HbA_2 than the more severe β-thalassemia-causing mutation (Thein, 2013). For example, in heterozygotes for –101 (C→T), the hematological parameters of 22 subjects investigated were in the normal range, except for rare cases (MCV < 80 fL in two subjects). HbA_2 levels ranged from 3.0 to 4.0%, i.e. slightly or modestly above the norm (Bianco et al., 1997).

Therefore, in population surveys when the HbA_2 is measured only in cases with a MCV below a certain cutoff value (< 80 fL), such individuals may not be detected. Atypical carriers with "very mild" or "silent" β-thalassemia mutations (CBC and HbA_2 levels are borderline/normal) may also include carriers of the triple α-globin gene rearrangement (Giordano et al., 2009).

In "almost silent" β-TT, the red cell indices are abnormal but the HbA_2 percentage is not increased. The hematological phenotype thus resembles that of α-thalassemia trait. A small group of "mild β-thalassemia mutations" results in almost silent β-TT. Such mutations include CAP +1 (A→C) in South Asians (Indians), the African mutation Poly A (T→C) and, occasionally, IVS-I-6 (T→C) in Mediterranean individuals. Both silent and almost silent β-TT can be detected by studies of the rates of globin chain synthesis and by molecular genetic analysis (Old, 2003; Bain, 2006).

Family studies and DNA analysis are strongly recommended to differentiate these atypical β-thalassemia carriers from α-thalassaemia heterozygotes. The measurement of β/α chain synthesis ratio with the assistance of radioactive amino acids needs a more specialized laboratory evaluation. This method is also no longer routinely accessible. Ranjbaran et al. (2013) proposed to determine β/α-globin mRNA ratio by applying relative quantitative real time (qRT)-PCR in such β-thalassemia patients, because no overlapping between minor β-thalassemia and normal group was observed.

Acquired abnormalities can lead to β-TT with a normal HbA_2 concentration. Iron deficiency lowers the HbA_2 percentage both in individuals with no defect of globin genes and in those with thalassaemia trait. The reduced HbA_2 caused by iron deficiency could be due to a reduction in synthesis (transcription and/or translation) of δ-chains or to competition between β and δ-chains for binding the heme group. This is more evident in the presence of a mild β-globin gene mutation. The causes of iron deficiency should always be detected and iron treatment should be implemented. Furthermore, hemoglobin analysis must be repeated for differential diagnosis of β-thalassemia carriers and iron deficiency.

If microcytosis persists after adequate iron supplementation, DNA analysis for β-globin genes should be carried out (Giambona et al., 2009).

The HbA_2 level may be higher in heterozygous β^0-thalassemia than β^+-thalassemia (Rosatelli et al., 1992; Rund et al., 1992; López-Escribano et al., 2013). This is likely to be a result of the greater impairment of β-chain synthesis in β^0-thalassemia. The overlap in values precludes any diagnostic utility of this observation.

HbF is the main hemoglobin component throughout fetal life and at birth, accounting for approximately 80% of total hemoglobin in newborns. HbF is produced from the sixth week of gestation and during the rest of fetal life, replacing the embryonic hemoglobins Gower I, Gower II and Portland. After birth, HbF synthesis rapidly declines and HbF is gradually substituted by HbA in the peripheral blood, so that within the first two years of life, the characteristic hemoglobin phenotype of the adult with very low levels of HbF (less than 1%) is found (Mosca et al., 2009 [b]).

The residual amount of HbF in normal adults is distributed heterogeneously in the red blood cells of which those showing a measurable quantity are dubbed F cells. The level of HbF and the F cell count are strictly correlated and show a similar distribution. The majority of normal adult individuals have usually HbF levels <0.6% of the total Hb (Cao et al., 2011).

The mechanism of persistent γ-chain synthesis in the thalassemias is incompletely understood. Red cell precursors that produce γ-chains are at a selective advantage.

Excess α-chains combine with γ-chains to produce HbF; therefore, the magnitude of α-chain precipitation is less (Divoky et al., 2001).

With good electrophoretic techniques, HbF levels > 2% can be recognizable visually; when an increased level is detected, quantification is required. HPLC, radial immunodiffusion and alkaline denaturation are established methods for the determination of HbF, and capillary electrophoresis is a valid alternative (Cotton et al., 1999). There was good correlation for measurements of HbA, HbF, and HbA_2 between CE and CAE (Kim et al., 2011). Hafiza et al. (2012) showed a significantly lower HbF level by CE than that of HPLC measured from the normal population. This could be due to the presence of HbA_{1c} fractions that could overlap with HbF in HPLC analysis. Although the HbF concentration is not a useful discriminant for β-TT, an increased HbF concentration may be useful for the detection of homozygous β-thalassemia variants, δβ-thalassaemia, hereditary persistence of fetal hemoglobin (HPFH) or β^E/β^{Thal} (Tan et al., 1993). When HPFH are co-inherited with different forms of β-thalassemia, they may lead to greater output of HbF and hence a milder phenotype.

At present, the only internationally recognized standard for HbF is the WHO 1st Reference Material (85/616) that is available from NIBSC, Blanche Lane, South Mimms, Potters Bar, Hertfordshire EN6 3QG, UK (http://www.nibsc.ac.uk), but it was only analysed by the two-minute alkali denaturation technique. The two-minute alkali denaturation technique can produce results that are satisfactory for most clinical purposes but are time consuming and need experience to obtain good results (Stephens et al., 2012 [b]).

Quantification of HbF is not essential for the diagnosis of β-thalassemia, which is dependent on the detection of an increased concentration of HbA_2. Measurement of the HbF in red cell hemolysates is important in the diagnosis of δβ-thalassaemia, HPFH and in the diagnosis of sickle cell disease (SCD), and whilst monitoring the effect of hydroxycarbamide (hydroxyurea) in SCD or β thalassaemia major or intermedia. The distribution of Hb F in red cells is useful in the diagnosis of HPFH and in the assessment of fetomaternal haemorrhage. With the huge increase in throughput of HbA_2 and HbF measurements in hospital laboratories because of both the mandatory and the voluntary screening programmes, automated HPLC or CZE have become the main tool to quantify HbF and HbA_2 in most laboratories in Europe and North America and is being increasingly used in Asia and Africa, and CIEF is also being introduced (Stephens et al., 2012 [b]).

In β-TM, Hb pattern (by CAE or HPLC) varies according to the type of β-thalassemia. In β^0-thalassemia, characterized by the lack of beta globin chain synthesis, HbA is absent, HbF is 95–98%, and HbA_2 is 2-5%. In β^+-thalassemia homozygotes with a residual variable beta globin synthesis or β^0/β^+compound heterozygotes, the Hb pattern shows HbA between 10 and 30%, HbF in the order of 70-90%, and HbA_2 of 2-5% (Cao and Galanello, 2010).

No strict criteria are available for diagnosis of thalassaemia intermedia because this diagnosis is dependent on how a patient develops without transfusion. However, the findings on hemoglobin electrophoresis or HPLC are dependent on the precise underlying genetic defect. The HbA_2 level is likely to be elevated somewhat more than in β-TT and the HbF is elevated (Bain, 2006). Table III sumaries the hematological features of β-thalassemia.

During the last three decades, mass spectrometry (MS), a technique that is widely used in clinical chemistry, laboratory medicine, and research, found its way into the field of Hb analysis. The analysis of HbF has been recently investigated by electrospray-ionization mass spectrometry (ESI-MS), a technique already widely diffused to the analysis of hemoglobin variants also in screening programs.

Table 3. Red blood cells indices and hemoglobin patterns of β-thalassemia

HEMATOLOGICAL PROFILE	β-TT	β-TI	β-TM
Hb [g/L]	Males: 115-153 Females: 91-140	70-100	< 70
MCV [fL]	< 79	50-80	50-70
MCH [pg]	< 27	16-24	12-18
HbA [%]	92-95	*	β^0: 0 β^+: 10-30
HbA_2 [%]	> 3.5	> 4	2-5
HbF [%]	0.5-4	15-45	β^0: 95-98 β^+: 70-90

β-TT: β-thalassemia trait; β-TI: β-thalassemia intermedia; β-TM: β-thalassemia major.

*Depends of type β globin mutation. Not available data.

Cao et al., 2000; Wild and Bain, 2006; Galanello and Origa, 2010; Higgs et al., 2012.

Another methods such as matrix-assisted laser desorption/ionization time-of-flight (MALDI-ToF) or mass-mass spectrometry in which the globin chains are cleaved in small fragments will show a single fragment, or a family of fragments from which the exact substitution could be determined (Wajcman and Moradkhani, 2011).

Controversial reports about HbA_2 quantification by ESI-MS were published. Minor Hb fractions such as HbA_{1C} or HbA_2, which are important for diagnosis of diabetes mellitus or thalassemias, respectively, were unable to be quantified by ESI-MS (Kleinert et al., 2008).

But Daniel et al. (2007) demonstrated the feasibility of electrospray tandem mass spectrometry to measure the δ:β-globin ratio as a surrogate marker of HbA_2.

MS methods (conventional ESI-MS and MALDI-ToF-MS) have two important drawbacks: first, its insufficient resolution that prevents the detection of Hb mutations with small mass differences of the globin chains, and second, MS is only a qualitative technique (Troxler et al., 2012).

Screening of Beta Thalassemia Trait

The thalassemias are found more commonly in certain ethnic groups, lending themselves to effective ethnicity-based population screening. Screening programs include pre-marriage or preconception, antenatal and neonatal programs; they aim to detect both relevant variant hemoglobins, as sickle cell disorders, and relevant thalassemias. Screening programs are introduced when an important health problem is identified and there is a feasible intervention that could prevent a clinical problem or lessen its impact.

In the hemoglobinopathy field, screening programs are aimed either at ameliorating the effects of a condition that has been detected or at lessening the number of births of a baby with a serious disorder (by offering information about carrier status prior to conception or offering termination in the case of an affected pregnancy) (Bain, 2011).

With increasing migration and travel, a genetic disease that was rare in northern Europe, Australia, South and North America is now becoming more common, and systems for genetic counselling, prenatal diagnosis, and life-long medical care are needed.

According to the Thalassemia International Federation, at least 200.000 patients with thalassemia are registered as receiving regular treatment throughout the world. Although the true burden of thalassemia is unknown, the actual number of patients worldwide is probably underestimated and many do not receive any treatment (Higgs et al., 2011).

A policy of detecting carriers and informing them of their risk, and possibilities for reducing it, usually leads to a fall in births and deaths of affected children. Carrier detection can be made retrospectively, following the birth of an affected child, or prospectively. In most countries, the approach develops in three stages. First, retrospectively informing parents with affected children of their 25% recurrence risk allows them to limit family size and, where average family sizes are typically large; this approach can significantly reduce affected birth prevalence. Second, introduction of prenatal diagnosis for couples with affected children enables them to have a family, but has little further effect on affected birth prevalence. Access may also be limited by economic, medical, social or legal factors. Third, information and prospective carrier screening is provided for the whole population. Choice of strategy varies with social attitudes, costs and opportunities within the health system (Modell and Darlison, 2008).

In population screening for β-thalassemia, besides the importance of selecting proper screening tests and techniques, it is also essential to consider the cost of screening. In those programs, is possible to use the red cell indices and test HbA_2 only those with an MCV or MCH below a certain cut-off point. Also, carrier detection is carried out by hematological methods followed by detection mutation by DNA analysis.

A relatively common approach has consisted of a complete blood count to assess the MCV and the MCH. Many recommendations were published about the MCV and HCM cutoffs to consider an individual as potential β-thalassemia carrier. The UK Screening program and British Committee for Standards in Haematology suggested that a diagnosis of β-thalassemia heterozygosity can be made when the MCH is < 27 pg and the HbA_2 is at least 3.5% (Ryan et al., 2010). In Canada, for individuals with MCV < 80 fL or MCH < 27 pg, the next step is hemoglobin electrophoresis or HPLC, quantitation of HbA_2 and HbF, and a blood smear stained for H bodies (Langlois et al., 2008). In India, the cutoff values were MCV (≤ 78.0 fL), MCH (≤ 28 pg) and HbA_2 (>3.8%) for BTT diagnosis (Bhukhanvala et al., 2013).

Generally, an MCH < 27 pg is an indication to quantify HbA_2. Screening by the MCV may be less satisfactory as there is more variation in values between different instruments and, with some instruments, the measured MCV rises with storage of the blood sample (Bain, 2006).

In developing countries, where well-calibrated automated instruments suitable for the measurement of red cell indices may not be available, osmotic fragility can be used for initial screening. The cells of β-TT (and of α-thalassemia trait, iron deficiency and some hemoglobinopathies) are more resistant to lysis when placed in hypotonic solutions than are normal cells. Abnormal osmotic resistance was used in the diagnosis of thalassemia trait in Italy and Greece during the 1930s. Much more recently, the use of a modified naked eye single-tube osmotic fragility test (NESTROFT), as a simple test to screen for thalassemias, has been proposed for use in laboratories in developing countries. Iron deficiency anemia is a recognized cause of false positive tests. Hemoglobin E heterozygosity also leads to a significant proportion of positive tests. The use of a one-tube visual osmotic fragility test reduces the number of samples that have to be referred to a central laboratory for definitive diagnosis (Chow et al., 2005).

In our laboratory the test was performed with a hypotonic saline solution of 4.0 g/L NaCl in phosphate buffer. A tube with 9 g/L NaCl in phosphate buffer corresponding to 0% hemolysis and another tube with distilled water corresponding to 100% hemolysis was also used (Figure 7). The spectrophotometric reading at 540 nm was conducted, and then the percent hemolysis of the sample was calculated. A value < 50% indicated resistance to hemolysis in hypotonic solution. The test proved to be highly sensitive (97%), not very specific (55%), but with a high negative predictive value of 97% (Lazarte et al., 2010-2011). This test was used to detect thalassemia in a group of 91 individuals with hereditary anemias and helped to identify 90% of β-TT (Lazarte et al., 2012 [b]). Recently, Piplani et al. (2013) found a sensitivity of 100%, specificity of 85.47%, a positive predictive value of 66% and a negative predictive value of 100% for NESTROFT. Despite its sensitivity and quickness in around one out of four cases of iron deficiency anemia, this test leads to a false positive result (Singh and Gupta, 2008).

Some silent and "near silent" β-thalassemia alleles will have normal or borderline results for HbA_2, MCH or both. By its nature, silent β-TT will generally only be diagnosed on family studies and subsequent DNA analysis after the birth of a child with β-thalassemia intermedia has already occurred (Bain, 2011).

The techniques to identify specific mutations underlying β-thalassemia in DNA from adults and fetuses are now well established and extensively applied to genetic counselling and prenatal diagnosis (Old, 2003).

Screening Programs

Programs offering screening for *β*-thalassemia heterozygotes have been available for many years around the world.

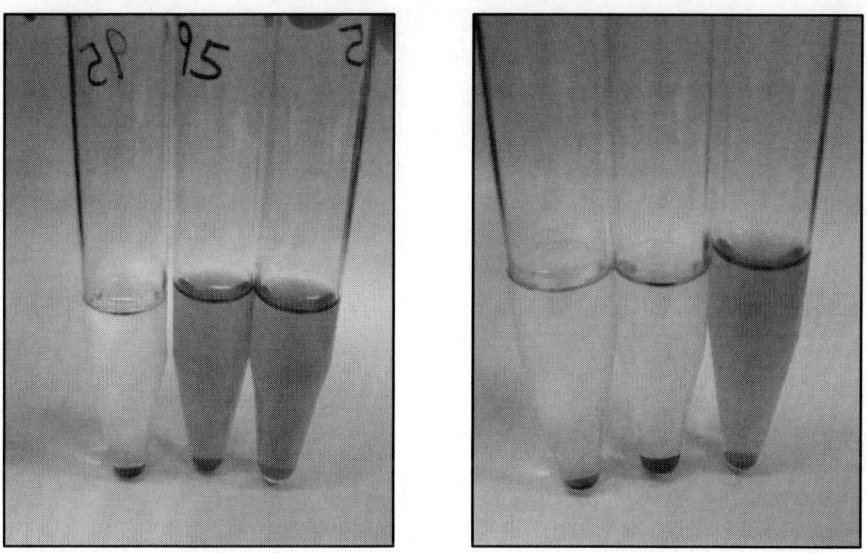

A B

A: Normal; B: β-TT shows resistance at 4,0 g/L NaCl (middle tube). See the text for technical details.

Figure 7. Screening of β-TT by osmotic fragility test modified by Lazarte et al. (2010-2011).

Screening may be a preliminary procedure that identifies persons at elevated risk but does not provide a definitive diagnosis, although sometimes screening results in a definitive identification, as in carrier screening for hemoglobin disorders. Whereas screening applies to populations with unknown risks to individuals, diagnostic testing is offered to individuals and families who are at higher-than-average risk (Wertz et al., 2003).

Interesting guidelines to provide recommendations to physicians, midwives, genetic counsellors, and clinical laboratory scientists involved in pre-conception or prenatal care regarding carrier screening for thalassemia and hemoglobinopathies, was developed by the Prenatal Diagnosis Committee of the Canadian College of Medical Geneticists and the Genetics Committee of the Society of Obstetricians and Gynecologists of Canada.

Their recommendations include carrier screening of women if she and/or her partner are identified as belonging to an ethnic population whose members are at higher risk of being carriers. If both partners are found to be carriers of thalassemia or an Hb variant, or of a combination of thalassemia and hemoglobin variant, they should be referred for genetic counselling, and prenatal diagnosis through DNA analysis, using cells obtained by chorionic villus sampling or amniocentesis, should be offered (Langlois et al., 2008).

Premarital screening for carrier status for common disorders in a community allows couples a fuller range of options than post-marital screening. All such screening, however, should be voluntary, with the cooperation of the community, and preceded by full education. Premarital screening should not be required by law, as this violates personal autonomy (Wertz et al., 2003). But in Iran, after a 5-year pilot screening, the Iranian Ministry of Health approved in 1996 a mandatory national screening protocol (screening and genetic counseling) for premarital testing (Zeinalian et al., 2013).

Table IV displays the results of pre-marriage programs developed in Iraq, Iran, United Arab Emirates, Turkey, Saudi Arabia and Gaza Strip.

Around 1.1% of couples worldwide are at risk for having children with a hemoglobin disorder, i.e. sickle cell disease or thalassemia, and 2.7 per 1000 conceptions are affected.

Prevention is making only a small impression: affected birth prevalence is estimated at 2.55 per 1000. Most affected children born in high-income countries survive with a chronic disorder, while most born in low-income countries die before the age of 5 years: hemoglobin disorders contribute the equivalent of 3.4% of mortality in children aged less than 5 years worldwide or 6.4% in Africa (Modell and Darlison, 2008).

Prenatal diagnosis for pregnancies at increased risk is possible by analysis of DNA extracted from fetal cells obtained by amniocentesis or chorionic villus sampling. Analysis of fetal cells in maternal blood and analysis of fetal DNA in maternal plasma for the presence of the father's mutation are currently under investigation (Harteveld et al., 2009).

When both parents are carriers there is a 25% risk at each pregnancy of having children with homozygous thalassemia.

However, because pregnancy termination is unacceptable to some persons (even when the fetus is affected), methods were developed, beginning in the early 1990s, to perform diagnostic testing before implantation (Rund and Rachmilowitz, 2005).

During last three decades there has been much progress in the methods for fetal sampling, and most notably in the molecular technologies for analyzing parental and fetal DNA samples. New approaches focus on new sources of fetal genetic material for analysis, in combination with the application of new technologies.

Table 4. Prevalence of β-TT and SCD in couples screened in premarital programs

COUNTRY	β-TT [%]	SCD [%] (trait or cases)	Number of couples
Iraq (Al Allawi et al., 2013)	3.98	0.07	54132
Iran (Zeinalian et al., 2013)	0.31	ND	703082
United Arab Emirates (Belhoul et al., 2013)	4.56	2.9	3210
Turkey (Uysal et al., 2013)	4.96	0.33	19277
Saudi Arabia (Memish and Saeedi, 2011)	1.8	4.5	786070
Gaza Strip (Tarazi et al., 2007)	2.9	ND	19712

ND: not determined.

Table 5. Diagnosis of β-thalassemia by DNA analysis in prenatal programs

COUNTRY	Number of samples	β-TM [%]	β-TT [%]	Normal
China (He et al., 2014)	1058	23.7	46.8	29.5
Taiwan (Peng et al., 2013)	1240	21.5*	50.2†	28.3
Turkey (Mendilcioglu et al., 2011)	407	25.8	49.4	24.8
Iran (Nikuei et al., 2008)	106	17.0	60.4	22.6

*Also includes α-thalassemia hydrops and HbE/β-thalassemia.
†Also includes α-thalassemia trait and αβ-thalassemia trait.

New sources of fetal (embryonic) genetic material includes embryo-biopsy samples within the context of preimplantation genetic diagnosis (PGD) and free fetal DNA in the circulation of the pregnant mother, as an approach for non-invasive prenatal diagnosis (NIPD). Both PGD and NIPD are limited by the minimal quantity of fetal (embryonic) sample available for analysis and thus require the application of new technologies with extremely high sensitivity, combined with stringent sample preparation and handling, to optimize accuracy and minimize contamination (Harteveld et al., 2009). However, techniques using DNA in maternal plasma to exclude thalassemia in the fetus are applicable only to couples for whom the paternal and maternal mutations are different (Rund and Rachmilowitz, 2005).

Without doubt the scientific community will continue to strive towards new means of achieving an accurate, rapid result as early in pregnancy as possible, in order to maximize the reproductive choices of prospective parents (Harteveld et al., 2009).

Systematic carrier screening with the option of prenatal diagnosis is established in parts of Asia (in parts of China, including Hong Kong Special Administrative Region [SAR], Macao SAR, some southern regions and the province of Taiwan, parts of India, the Islamic Republic of Iran, the Maldives and Singapore), parts of the Caribbean and most of southern Europe (except Albania). In Australia, much of northwest Europe, New Zealand and North America, prenatal diagnosis is available and antenatal carrier screening is standard practice (Modell and Darlison, 2008).

Table V shows the results of antenatal programs of China, Taiwan, Turkey and Iran.

These programs have been very effective, as indicating by increasing knowledge on thalassemia and its prevention by the target population and by the marked decline of the incidence of thalassemia major (Cao, 2002).

The aggregated global data suggest a 16% reduction in births of children with thalassemia and a 4% reduction in births of children with sickle-cell disorders. The greater part of the estimated reduction is attributed to reduced reproduction by informed at-risk couples, rather than prenatal diagnosis (Modell and Darlison, 2008).

Genetic Diagnosis - DNA Analysis

It is significant to emphasize that in some cases the identification of asymptomatic carriers for the β-TT can present particular interpretative difficulties looking at the biological and hematological situation only. Also, the typical phenotype of the β-TT, essentially characterized by reduced MCV, MCH, and increased HbA_2, may be modified by several coinherited genetic factor such as simultaneous inheritance of heterozygous β-thalassemia and α-thalassemia or heterozygous β-thalassemia and δ-thalassemia, which may cause problems in carrier identification (Bain, 2006). That reasons justify the molecular analysis of the globin genes. These allow to make a definitive diagnosis of the causative mutations and thus to inform to the clinician and patients for management and counselling. Moreover, couples at risk of having an affected child can be offered genetic counselling and reproductive options including prenatal diagnosis which involves fetal sampling to determine the fetal genotype (Harteveld et al., 2009). The key to identifying the globin gene mutations in carriers and affected patients is an understanding of the genotype/ phenotype relationships of the various globin gene mutations and the effects of interaction when several mutations are coinherited. Often the quickest way to identify the mutations in an affected patient is to study the hematology of the patient's parents and other family members, and to screen them for single mutations. Carrier screening and mutation identification also forms one of the cornerstones of any prevention program for the hemoglobin disorders. The strategy for carrier screening and mutation analysis is based on that fact that although heterozygotes are symptom free, they present specific hematologic characteristics that are useful for their identification (Old, 2003; Clark and Thein, 2004; Patrinos et al., 2005). The majority of known thalassemia mutations and abnormal hemoglobin variants can be identified by PCR-based techniques, which are appropriate for genotyping carriers and, in most cases, fetal DNA for classical prenatal diagnosis. The sensitivity and specificity of PCR has revolutionized the molecular diagnostic field. It has almost eliminated the use of radioactive isotopes for detecting sequences and has enabled diagnosis to be made on much smaller quantities of DNA. The main source of DNA is peripheral leucocytes obtained from anticoagulated peripheral blood, preferably with ethylene-diamine-tetraacetic acid (EDTA). Fetal DNA is mainly isolated from chorionic villi obtained through ultrasound-guided transcervical aspiration or ultrasound-guided transabdominal aspiration (Patrinos et al., 2005). Fetal DNA can also be prepared from amniotic fluid cells directly or after culture. Noninvasive methods of prenatal diagnosis utilize DNA from fetal cells in maternal circulation (Cheung et al., 1996) or free circulating fetal DNA in maternal blood (Chiu et al., 2002).

The noninvasive methods, however, are still under development and are not offered routinely for the hemoglobinopathies.

Molecular methods aimed at characterizing the mutations in hemoglobinopathies are traditionally separated into two categories: "direct" mutation detection methods, and "indirect" methods (Harteveld et al., 2009).

"Direct" mutation methods are PCR-based techniques which have been designed for identifying a known mutation. They include methods such as Allele Specific Oligonucleotide probes (ASO) and Amplification Refractory Mutation System (ARMS) for point mutations and gap-PCR for specific deletions. PCR-based approaches for scanning or screening for unknown mutations ("indirect" methods) take advantage of altered conformation of single-stranded DNA and include Denaturing Gradient Gel Electrophoresis (DGGE) and Denaturing High Pressure Liquid Chromatography (DHPLC). These indirect methods require the use of a subsequent method to specifically characterize any nucleotide variation found. Direct sequencing is capable of detecting any point mutation within a gene region.

Other methods like Multiplex Ligation-dependent Probe Amplification (MLPA) for the detection of deletions, real-time PCR and high resolution Melting Curve Analysis (HRMA) for the detection of point mutation, whose use is becoming more widespread in recent years, are discussed below. Finally, evolving technologies including DNA microarray techniques and pyrosequencing ("next-generation sequencing") are briefly described.

Allele-Specific Oligonucleotide (ASO) Hybridization and Reverse Dot-Blot

The method is based on the principle of specific hybridization of two oligonucleotide probes, one complementary to the mutant sequence and the other to the normal sequence (Ristaldi et al., 1989). The ASO's differ from each other by a single base change designed to be in the center of the ASO to maximize instability of any mismatch.

Genomic DNA is specifically amplified using specific primers encompassing the mutation and the PCR product bound to a nylon membrane in the form of dots (Saiki et al., 1989). The ASO's are 5'-endlabelled with 32P-dATP, biotin or horseradish peroxide and the PCR dot sequentially hybridized with the mutant and wild type ASO's. The genotype of the DNA sample is read by the presence or absence of hybridization signal from the mutant and wild type probes. The technique is reliable and has been used with great success specifically in populations where there are one or two predominant mutations (Ristaldi et al., 1989).

However, traditional protocols are laborious and can only screen one mutation at a time. To overcome this, a method of reverse dot-blotting has been developed in which pairs of cold mutant and wild type ASO's are fixed as dots or slots to nylon membrane strips (Saiki et al., 1989). Amplified genomic DNA, encompassing the region containing the putative mutations, is labelled by use of end-label primers or the internal incorporation of biotinylated dUTP and then hybridized to the strips. The reverse dot-blot allows the simultaneous detection of multiple β-thalassemia mutations and has been successfully applied for prenatal diagnosis, especially for populations with a limited number of common mutations (Winichagoon et al., 1999).

Besides in-house protocols, several commercial kits are available (Viennalab Strip Assay™ for 21 α- and 47 β-globin gene deletions and point mutations; www.Viennalab.com and BioRad mDx® BeTha Gene 1 and 2 kits; www.bio-rad.com).

Both have limited applications as the panel detects a limited number of mutations and the kits are expensive and demonstrate batch-to-batch variation.

Allele-Specific Priming – Amplification Refractory Mutation System (ARMS-PCR)

Primer-specific amplification is based on the principle that a perfectly matched primer is much more efficient at annealing and directing primer extension than a mismatched primer.

The most widely used method is the ARMS in which allele-specific amplification relies on the specificity of the 3' terminal nucleotide. A common PCR primer is used with either a primer complementary to the target mutation or, in a separate reaction, with a primer complementary to the wild-type sequence, allowing the differentiation of normal wild-type, versus heterozygote, versus homozygous mutant (Murugesan et al., 2012). To monitor false-negative results because of failure of the amplification reaction itself, an internal PCR control which amplifies another region of the genome should be included in the reaction.

ARMS is extremely fast (Old et al., 1990; Tan et al., 1994), requiring only a single PCR step, followed by agarose gel electrophoresis. A disadvantage is that the ARMS reaction requires stringent standardization and optimization of reaction conditions for each primer set, and if the assays are not well optimized there is a risk of false positive or negative results.

ARMS has been improved by development of a single tube assay (Ye et al., 2001), where both the mutant and the wild type alleles are detected simultaneously in the same reaction. More than one mutation can also be screened for at the same time in a single reaction by multiplexing the ARMS primers coupled with a common primer (Mirasena et al., 2008; Mahadik, 2012). Multiplex ARMS requires stringent optimization of primer annealing conditions and primer concentrations.

In the context of prenatal diagnosis, a simple and rapid ARMS assay is appropriate when the mutations in both parents are previously identified (Ahmed, 2007).

However, in populations with a wide mutation spectrum or for multi-ethnic populations, when couples present during pregnancy with previously undetermined genotypes, ARMS is not an ideal first-line method for characterizing the parental mutations.

Gap-PCR

Gap-PCR is used to detect deletions for which the location of the breakpoints is known. Primers complementary to the 5′and 3′ breakpoint regions amplify a deletion-specific fragment that spans the deletion breakpoint when it is present. For small deletions such as the 619 bp deletion, a common cause of β-thalassemia in Asian Indians, differential amplification products are generated in the mutant and wild type. When the deletion is vast (> 2 kb) it is technically difficult to generate a product in the wild type. As a control, a primer can be included that anneals within the deleted sequence to generate an additional product with one of the other primers flanking the deletion. In this way, false negatives are monitored in the wild type and indicate if an individual is heterozygous for the deletion (Clark and Thein, 2004).

Tritipsombut et al. (2012) reported an improvement of this technique; they detected eight common β-globin cluster deletions in Southeast Asian countries by a simple molecular technique based on a single-tube multiplex Gap-PCR. Unlike the β-thalassemia, deletions and rearrangements are a common cause of α-thalassemia, for this reason Gap-PCR and multiplex Gap-PCR are routinely used to analyze them (Chong et al., 2000; Tan et al., 2001). With respect to prenatal diagnosis, Gap-PCR is useful to detect the more common deletions in both the α and β-gene clusters, and has been especially applied for prenatal diagnosis to detect the deletions causing α^0-thalassemia to prevent Hb Bart's Hydrops Fetalis Syndrome (Yap et al., 2009). However, results with Gap-PCR should be verified by an alternative method, like MLPA, since the method is vulnerable to allele drop-out due to sporadic nucleotide changes that may occur within the primer regions.

Denaturing Gradient Gel Electrophoresis (DGGE)

Denaturing Gradient Gel Electrophoresis or DGGE, as originally described by Myers et al. (1987), allows the separation, and thus detection, of DNA molecules of up to a few hundred base-pairs that differ by as little as a single nucleotide. This method relies on the mutant sequence altering the mobility of the PCR product on a gel compared with the wild type, and require further analysis to resolve the causative mutation, direct sequencing. The electrophoretic separation is based upon the melting properties of the double-stranded DNA molecule, which separate (melt-out) under conditions of increased temperature or under the influence of an increasing gradient of denaturant in a polyacrylamide gel. The use of a "GC-tail" on the 5′ end of one of the PCR primers creates a region of very high melting temperature at one end of the amplicon, facilitating the potential detection of mutations across the entire region of interest. In heterozygote samples, denaturation and reannealing of single stranded molecules during PCR lead to the formation of homo and heteroduplexes, giving up to 4 bands visible per heterozygous sample.

DGGE has been useful in some laboratories for screening of β-thalassemia mutations, for carrier detection and prenatal diagnosis (Losekoot et al., 1990; Fodde and Losekoot, 1994).

This screening technique simply shows the presence of a mutation which has to be definitively identified by another method such as direct sequencing to confirm the identity of the nucleotide variations.

Denaturing High-Performance Liquid Chromatography (DHPLC)

DHPLC is based on the detection of heteroduplex molecules by ion-pair reverse-phase liquid chromatography under partially denaturing conditions. This method allows for the automated detection of single base DNA substitutions as well as small insertions and deletions (O'Donovan et al., 1998). When using heteroduplex analysis by DHPLC under partially-denaturing conditions, heteroduplexes are retained less than their corresponding homoduplexes on a unique DNA separation matrix. DHPLC uses unpurified PCR products that are subjected to a final denaturing/reannealing step to ensure adequate formation of the heteroduplex.

Analysis time for such a procedure is, typically, within 10 min per sample, depending upon the configuration of the instrument, with heteroduplex profiles being easily distinguished from homoduplex analogues.

DHPLC has been extensively used for mutation screening of the β-globin genes, not only for its high sensitivity and efficiency, but also because of its cost effectiveness (Li et al., 2008). The technique is capable of distinguishing between the heteroduplex elution profile of common β-thalassemia mutations showing 100% sensitivity and specificity, although, as for DGGE, mutation confirmation by a second method is warranted, especially since the elution patterns may be complicated by polymorphisms. Once the parental chromatographs have been determined, the protocol can be reliably applied to prenatal diagnosis (Colosimo et al., 2003).

Multiplex Ligation-Dependent Probe Amplification (MLPA)

Multiplex ligation-dependent probe amplification is a recently described method that can detect mid-size deletions down to a few hundred bases or single exon level. Each probe consists of two oligonucleotides that bind adjacent to each other at the target sequence. A ligation reaction takes place and all intact probes are amplified in a PCR using one single set of labelled primers as all probes have the same primer recognition ends.

Thus, through the use of universal PCR primers the efficiency of the similarly sized ligated probe-pairs the PCR step is semi-quantitative, and in this way MLPA can detect deletions or duplications across the locus. Amplification products differ in size, which can be separated by electrophoresis using a standard sequencer. The peak height/area of a probe represents the amount of amplification product, which is in turn proportional to the copy number of target sequence recognized by the probe in the sample.

This technique is fast and easy to perform, requiring only standard instruments in a routine molecular diagnostic laboratory (Schouten et al., 2002).

Supported by the recent availability of commercial kits for detecting copy number variations across the α- and β-globin gene clusters (MRC-Holland and ServiceXS), MLPA is being applied in an increasing number of diagnostic laboratories. For example, So et al. (2009) using a commercial MLPA kit to screen a 106 Chinese patients founded 17 deletions in the β-globin cluster in 17 patients: 8 of Chinese $(^{A}\gamma\delta\beta)^{0}$ thalassemia (deletion 100 kb), 7 of Southeast Asian (Vietnamese) deletion (27 kb) and 2 of Thai $(^{A}\gamma\delta\beta)^{0}$ thalassemia (deletion 79 kb). MLPA allowed to study and elucidate these complex genotypes and correlated them with phenotypic data.

As a new technology it has not yet been widely applied for prenatal diagnosis, although, since it is a robust method, this is likely to change. In this way, Miri-Moghaddam et al. (2013) and Chen et al. (2013) have reported the use of this method in prenatal diagnosis of β- and α-thalassemia, respectively.

Real-Time PCR - Hybridization Probes

Real-time PCR (RT-PCR) is a variation of regular PCR in which amplification and detection are coupled in a single step, which facilitates the detection of amplicons as they are produced.

RT-PCR integrates microvolume rapid-cycle PCR with fluorometry, allowing a real-time fluorescent monitoring of the amplification reaction for quantitative PCR and/or characterization of PCR products for rapid genotyping, precluding any post-PCR sample manipulation (Figure 8). The method is based on the use of fluorescently labeled hybridization probes which hybridize to adjacent internal sequences within target amplified DNA, one of which covers the region expected to contain the mutation(s) (Tubbs, 2012).

Once approximated, the donor fluorescent dye emits light at a wavelength in the absorption spectra of the second fluorescent dye and reports successful hybridization by the emission of fluorescent light specific to the reporter fluorophore (reaction known as FRET: fluorescence resonance energy transfer) (Harteveld et al., 2009).

Hybridization probes have perhaps their greatest utility in detection of single point mutations through the use of melting curve analysis as a post-PCR step. During the process of melting curve analysis, the products are melted and quickly cooled, and then the reaction mixture is slowly reheated with simultaneous detection of fluorescence that reflects the temperature at which the DNA target/probe duplex is disassociated. The midpoint of the melt curve is equivalent to the melting temperature (Tm), which will of course be at a lower temperature for an amplicon that contains a mismatch between the specific probe and the target (Tubbs, 2012). Thus, if a mutation is present, the melting point will occur at a lower temperature than for the duplexes that are exactly complementary to the sequence of the probe. A single base mismatch under the "mutation probe" results in a Tm shift of 5-10°C, it allowing easy distinction between wild type and mutant alleles.

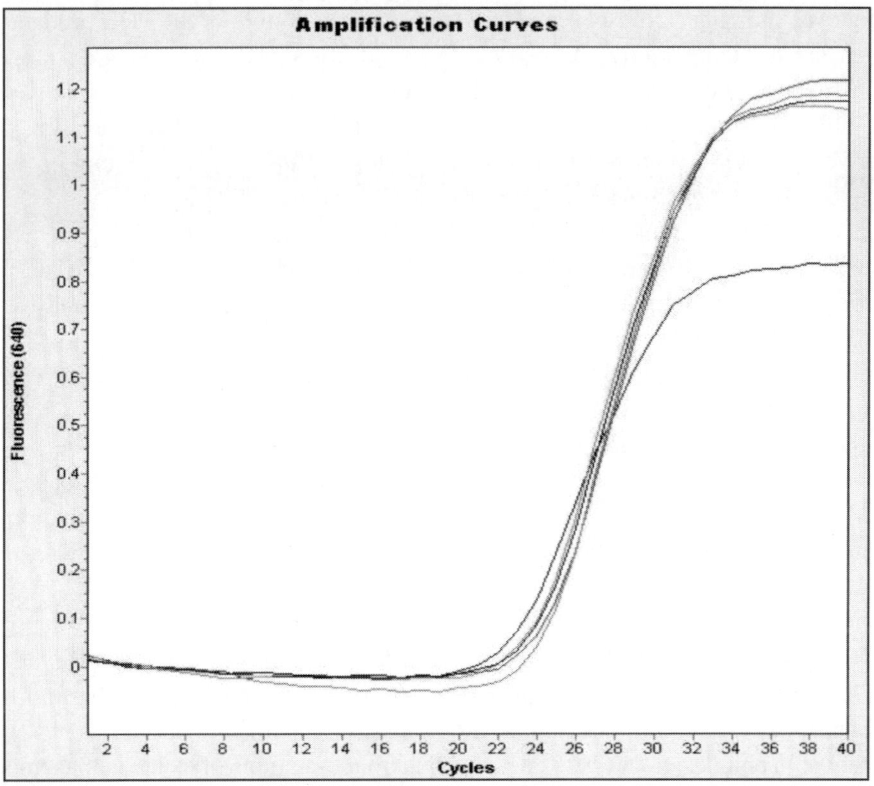

Figure 8. Amplification curves obtained in LightCycler™ system - Roche Molecular Biochemicals.

The ability to detect base mismatches under the low Tm probe and the use of two different colored probes (LightCycler™ system - Roche Molecular Biochemicals) allows more than one mutation to be screened in a single PCR reaction (Harteveld et al., 2009).

This technology, although it is expensive and difficult to standardize, is very fast, simple, and high throughput, and allows the reliable detection of several mutations simultaneously both carrier screening and prenatal diagnosis (Vrettou et al., 2003; Hung et al., 2010). Concerning with FRET approach, in our laboratory we have successfully used an analogous LightCycler method to define the profile of β-thalassemic mutations in the province of Tucumán (Argentina northwestern). The most frequent mutations were Cd39 (C→T), IVS-I-1 (G→A) and IVS-I-110 (G→A). The data showed that the main source of β-thalassemia alleles in Tucumán is the Mediterranean region as the most frequent mutations in this region are at codon 39 of the second exon and at positions 1, 6 and 110 of the first intron (Figure 9) (Burgos and Mónaco, 2012).

High Resolution Melting Analysis (HRM)

High-resolution melting is a new gene scan tool that quickly performs the Polymerase Chain Reaction (PCR) and identifies sequence alterations without requiring post-PCR treatment. Analogous to the principle of DGGE, the melting profile of a PCR product depends on its GC-content, the length and the sequence composition; changes in melting profile will occur when mutations are present and heteroduplexes are formed. This is monitored by saturating dyes showing fluorescence when intercalated in double strand PCR products.

Increasing the temperature causes double strand DNA to become single-stranded. The transition from double to a single strand in the presence of fluorescent dyes actively intercalating double-stranded DNA leads to signal modification. The HRM analysis melting profile gives a specific sequence-related pattern allowing discrimination between wild-type sequences and homozygote–heterozygote variants (Reed et al., 2007).

It is a closed-tube scanning method, which does not require any processing after PCR, but it does require the use of specialized equipment like the LightScanner® (Idaho Technology), or modified real-time thermal cyclers, such as the LightCycler 480 (Roche) and the Rotor-Gene 6000 (Corbett) (Herrmann et al., 2007).

Unlike other scanning methods, HRM analysis offers a faster and more convenient closed-tube method of assessing the presence of mutations and gives a result that can be further investigated if it is of interest.

Besides, the closed-tube system reduces the risk of contamination (Er and Chang, 2012).

HRM analysis was used by Shih et al. (2009) and He et al. (2010) for mutations in the HBB gene, and the results of the HRM analysis were completely consistent with those by direct DNA sequencing.

In the context of prenatal diagnosis, Pornprasert and Sukunthamala (2010) reported use the SYTO9 and SYBR GREEN1 high-resolution melting analysis for diagnosis of β-thalassemia/HbE, from DNA samples which were extracted from amniotic fluid or cord blood of 11 pregnancies whose fetuses were at risk for β-thalassemia/HbE.

Moreover, Yenilmez et al. (2013) detected paternal mutations of sickle cell anemia and β-thalassemia in cell-free fetal DNA using HRM analysis.

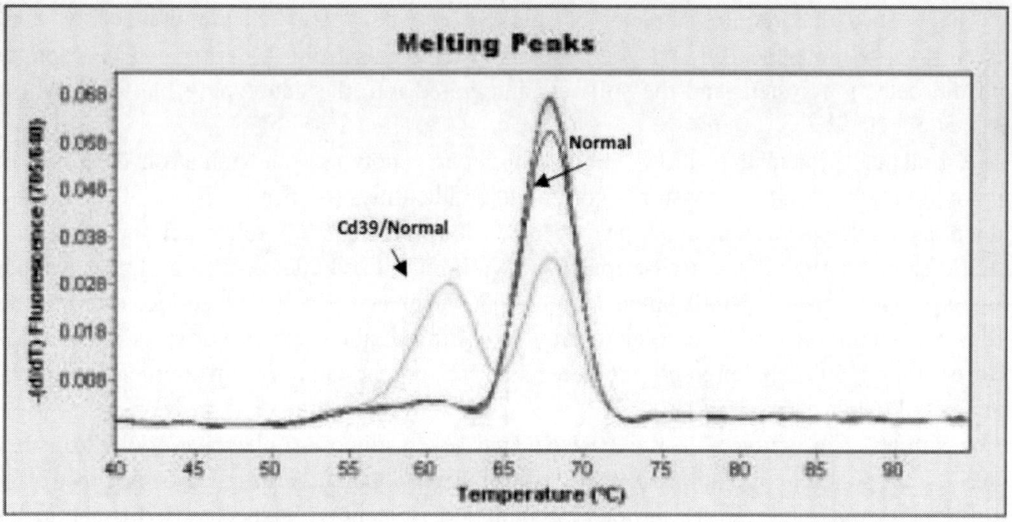

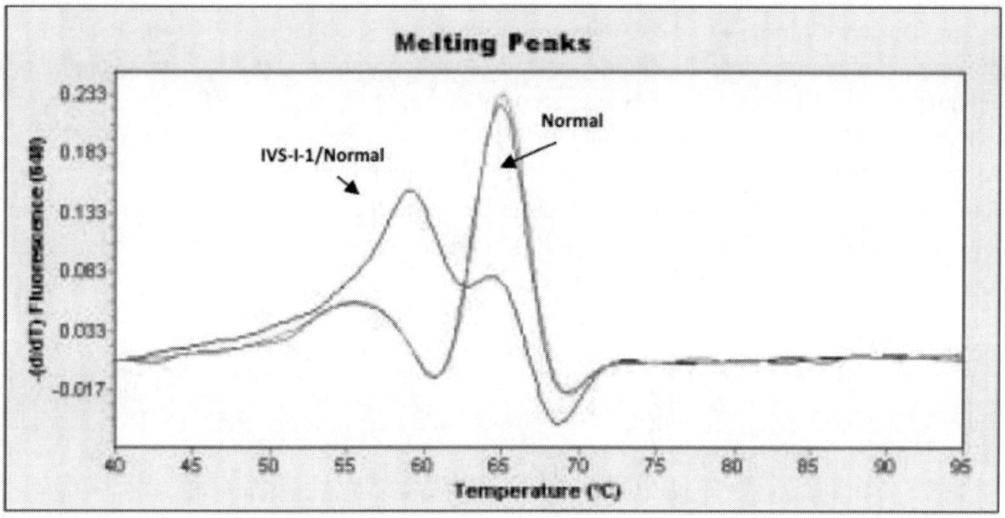

Figure 9. Melting curves for the two most frequent mutations, i.e. Cd39 and IVS-I-1, observed in Tucumán, Argentina.

High-Throughput Globin Gene Mutation Screening ("Evolving Technologies")

Recent developments in automation and miniaturization technologies have created new standards and changed the philosophy of molecular diagnostics in the post-genomic era. DNA microarrays (DNA chips) have become synonymous with high-throughput mutation detection and large-scale DNA sequencing. DNA microarrays as a means of resequencing genes, for which a reference sequence is known, to scan for all possible sequence variation or mutation is another possible development (Clark and Thein, 2004; Patrinos et al., 2005). Microarray-based diagnostics are evolving technologies that have the potential for optimal and cost-effective genotyping.

Diagnostics that require a panel of markers can be genotyped simultaneously using microarrays. Sample-specific and genotype-specific signals from the array can be captured with the detection system and the software integrated into the genotyping platform (Murugesan et al., 2012).

A practical system that allows high-throughput genotyping and mutation detection by employing allele-specific extension on oligonucleotide arrays has been reported. This method, known as allele-specific arrayed primer extension (AS-APEX); relies on the sequence-specific extension by reverse transcriptase of two immobilized allele-specific oligonucleotide primers (approximately 30-40 bp in length) that differ at their 30-nucleotide, defining the alleles. Based on this principle, a microarray consisting of allele specific primers to detect the most common 15 non deletion α gene defects and 23 β gene mutations in southeast Asia was constructed (Chan et al., 2004).

A similar microarray, with the 10 *HBB* and seven glucose-6-phosphate dehydrogenase (G6PD) common gene mutations in the Mediterranean population, has also been constructed for β-thalassemia and G6PD deficiency mutation screening, respectively (Thalassochip microarray) (Gemignani et al., 2002).

The ThalassoChip was updated with new probes and now has the ability to detect 57 β-globin gene mutations and 3 single nucleotide polymorphisms (SNPs) in a single test. (Shammas et al., 2010).

Pyrosequencing is rapidly gaining popularity as a resequencing methodology for detecting known mutations and polymorphisms in small well defined regions (Clark and Thein, 2004). It is a real -time assay, which is based on the detection of released pyrophosphate (PPi) during DNA synthesis. It relies on individual nucleotides being sequentially added to an extended primer that releases pyrophosphate during nucleotide incorporation. This pyrophosphate is converted to a light signal using ATP sulphurylase and luciferase, and is proportional to the quantity of nucleotides incorporated (Ronaghi, 2001).

A cascade of enzymatic reactions follow, which generate visible light in proportion to the number of nucleotides incorporated. As the system adds the four deoxyribonucleotide triphosphates one at a time and measures the light signals as each is incorporated, it ensures the identification of the added nucleotide and thus the sequence of the template. The sequence is read in real time and is semi-quantitative making it quick and highly suitable for heterozygote identification.

Pyrosequencing technology is relatively new, and has only recently been implemented, thus a single-nucleotide polymorphism genotyping (including an integrated single-cell-through-sequencing assay) to detect a mutation at the globin IVS-I-110 was development by Salk et al. (2006). With respect to prenatal diagnosis, Timbs et al. (2012) reported the genotyping of 148 chorionic villi and 29 uncultured amniotic fluid DNA samples by pyrosequencing. They founded 100% concordance with the fetal diagnosis result obtained by ARMS-PCR or DNA sequencing. Pyrosequencing revealed an 83% decrease in diagnostic failures using uncultured amniocyte DNA samples. Overall, they founded pyrosequencing to be simpler, more robust, quicker, and less expensive than conventional sequencing and ARMS making it a good choice for rapid prenatal diagnosis of thalassemia and sickle cell disease.

The pyrosequencing technology is already time and cost-competitive, compared to existing sequencing methods, and given the potential for further developments and improvements in chemistry, instrumentation, and integration with sample preparation, it could be a promising alternative for resequencing of the compact human globin gene loci.

Conclusion

The choice of molecular techniques to perform diagnostics for hemoglobinopathies largely depends on the prevalence and mutation spectrum in the population to be examined. In general, the knowledge of the population-specific mutation spectrum supports the selection of the most appropriate methods for molecular analysis. Regarding these data, relevant information is recorded in the HbVar database (http://www.globin.cse.psu.edu/hbvar).

However, with the advent of global migration, multiethnic societies present with a larger variety of mutations and complex combinations of different mutations. Then, population-specific diagnostic approaches are becoming less reliable, and other diagnostic strategies are required than those applied in geographically isolated areas where only a limited number of mutations are causing thalassemia (Harteveld, 2013).

Before one selects a method to detect globin gene mutations in a diagnostic laboratory, scientific, financial-economical, legal and ethical issues must be considered. Although not every methodological platform is applicable in every laboratory involved in molecular testing for thalassemias, the golden rule is to use at least two different methods that are technically sound and yield unambiguous results, so that consistency and accuracy are ensured.

Also, each laboratory should be quality accredited by international or local recognized organizations e.g., to comply with competent genetic testing procedures and personnel qualifications. With respect to ethical issues each thalassemia patient needs to understand why the test is being offered, as well as its implications for disease prevention and management, and the patient's psychosocial well-being. Written informed consent should be obtained from the patient, parent, or guardian prior to the test, and strict confidentiality regarding the patient's genetic and/or medical records and test results must always be ensured (Patrinos et al., 2005)

Finally, it seems important to emphasize that, in all cases, it is essential to evaluate the hematological parameters in relation to the biochemical and molecular results to exclude the presence of more complex genotypes than the one found in the first place.

If these three elements do not perfectly match, other traits can be present making risk assessment more complex (Harteveld, 2013). Thus, any clinician confronted with findings suggestive of a hemoglobinopathy should consult with their clinical laboratory about analysis of the hematological profile and/or globin gene profile that might aid thalassemia diagnosis for better-quality disease management.

References

Ahmed, S. Prenatal diagnosis of beta-thalassemia: 12 years' experience at a single laboratory in Pakistan. *Prenat. Diagn.* 2007;27(13):1224-7.

Al-Allawi, N. A., Jalal, S. D., Ahmed, N. H., Faraj, A. H., Shalli, A., Hamamy, H. The first five years of a preventive programme for haemoglobinopathies in Northeastern Iraq. *J. Med. Screen.* 2013;20(4):171-6.

Bain, B. Haemoglobinopathy diagnosis: Algorithms, lessons and pitfalls. *Blood Rev.* 2011; 25:205-13.

Bain, B. The α, β, δ and γ thalassaemias and related conditions. In: *Haemoglobinopathy Diagnosis*, Second Edition. Blackwell Publishing Ltd. Malden, Massachussetts, US. 2006; pp. 63-138.

Belhoul, K. M., Abdulrahman, M., Alraei, R. F. Hemoglobinopathy carrier prevalence in the United Arab Emirates: first analysis of the Dubai Health Authority premarital screening program results. *Hemoglobin*. 2013;37(4):359-68.

Bhukhanvala, D., Seliya, V., Shah, A., Gupte, S. Study of parents of β-thalassemia major children to determine cutoff values of hematological parameters for diagnosis of β-thalassemia trait and assessment of anemia in them. *Indian J. Med. Sci*. 2013;67(5-6): 117-22.

Bianco, I., Cappabianca, M. P., Foglietta, E., Lerone, M., Deidda, G., Morlupi, L., et al. Silent thalassemias: genotypes and phenotypes. *Haematologica*. 1997;82(3):269-80.

Bragós, I. M., Noguera, N. I., Raviola, M. P., Milani, A. C. Genética molecular de beta talasémicos heterocigotas. Interrelación con parámetros hematológicos. *Rev. Cubana Hematol. Inmunol. Hemoter*. 2005;21(1).

Burgos, M., Mónaco, M. E. Bases moleculares de la β-talasemia en la provincia de Tucumán. *Revista da XX Jornadas de Jovens Pesquisadores da AUGM*, Universidad Federal de Paraná (BRASIL). 2012:263-9.

Cao, A., Galanello, R., Origa, R. *Beta-Thalassemia*. 2000 Sep. 28 [updated 2013 Jan. 24]. In: Pagon, R. A., Adam, M. P., Bird, T. D., Dolan, C. R., Fong, C. T., Smith, R. J. H., Stephens, K., editors. GeneReviews™ [Internet]. Seattle (WA): University of Washington, Seattle; 1993-2013. Available from http://www.ncbi.nlm.nih.gov/books/NBK1426/

Cao, A., Galanello, R. Beta-thalassemia. *Genet. Med*. 2010;12(2):61-76.

Cao, A., Moi, P., Galanello, R. Recent advances in β-thalassemias. *Pediatr. Rep*. 2011;3(2):e 17.

Cao, A. Carrier screening and genetic counselling in beta-thalassemia. *Int. J. Hematol*. 2002; 76 Suppl. 2:105-13.

Chan, K., Wong, M. S., Chan, T. K., Chan, V. A thalassaemia array for Southeast Asia. *Br. J. Haematol*. 2004;124(2):232-9.

Chen, Y. J., Yang, X. H., Zeng, X. Q., Qiao, L. L. The application of multiplex ligation-dependent probe amplification technology in diagnosis and prenatal diagnosis of α-thalassemia. *Zhonghua Xue Ye Xue Za Zhi*. 2013;34(7):591-4.

Cheung, M. C., Goldberg, J. D., Kan, Y. W. Prenatal diagnosis of sickle cell anaemia and thalassaemia by analysis of fetal cells in maternal blood. *Nat. Genet*. 1996;14(3):264-8.

Chiu, R. W., Lau, T. K., Leung, T. N., Chow, K. C., Chui, D. H., Lo, Y. M. Prenatal exclusion of beta thalassaemia major by examination of maternal plasma. *Lancet*. 2002; 360 (9338):998-1000.

Chong, S. S., Boehm, C. D., Higgs, D. R., Cutting, G. R. Single-tube multiplex-PCR screen for common deletional determinants of alpha-thalassemia. *Blood*. 2000;95(1):360-2.

Chow, J., Phelan, L., Bain, B. J. Evaluation of single-tube osmotic fragility as a screening test for thalassemia. *Am. J. Hematol*. 2005;79(3):198-201.

Clark, B. E., Thein, S. L. Molecular diagnosis of haemoglobin disorders. *Clin. Lab. Haematol*. 2004;26(3):159-76.

Clarke, G. M., Higgins, T. N. Laboratory Investigation of Hemoglobinopathies and Thalassemias: Review and Update. *Clin. Chem*. 2000;46(8):1284-90.

Colosimo, A., Guida, V., Scolari, A., De Luca, A., Palka, G., Rigoli, L., et al. Validation of dHPLC for molecular diagnosis of beta-thalassemia in Southern Italy. *Genet. Test*. 2003, 7(3):269-75.

Cotton, F., Lin, C., Fontaine, B., Gulbis, B., Janssens, J., Vertongen, F. Evaluation of a capillary electrophoresis method for routine determination of hemoglobins A_2 and F. *Clin. Chem*. 1999;45(2):237-43.

Daniel, Y. A., Turner, C., Haynes, R. M., Hunt, B. J., Dalton, R. N. Quantification of hemoglobin A_2 by tandem mass spectrometry. *Clin. Chem*. 2007;53(8):1448-54.

Divoky, V., Mrug, M., Thornley-Brown, D., Divoka, M., Prchal, J. T. Non-anemic homozygous beta(0) thalassemia in an African-American family: association of high fetal hemoglobin levels with beta thalassemia alleles. *Am. J. Hematol*. 2001;68(1):43-50.

Er, T. K., Chang, J. G. High-resolution melting: applications in genetic disorders. *Clin. Chim. Acta*. 2012;414:197-201.

Ferrara, M., Capozzi, L., Russo, R., Bertocco, F., Ferrara, D. Reliability of red blood cells indices and formulas to discriminate between beta thalassemia trait and iron deficiency in children. *Hematol*. 2010;15(2):112-5.

Fodde, R., Losekoot, M. Mutation detection by denaturing gradient gel electrophoresis (DGGE). *Hum. Mutat*. 1994;3(2):83-94.

Galanello, R., Origa, R. Beta-thalassemia. *Orphanet. J. Rare Dis*. 2010;5:11.

Gallivan, M., Giordano, P. Analysis of hemoglobinopathies, hemoglobin variants and thalassemias. In: Kottke-Marchand, K. and Davis, B. H. eds. *Laboratory Hematology Practice*. Wiley Blackwell Publishing Ltd. Chichester, UK. 2012; pp: 562-85.

Gemignani, F., Perra, C., Landi, S., Canzian, F., Kurg, A., Tõnisson, N., et al. Reliable detection of beta-thalassemia and G6PD mutations by a DNA microarray. *Clin. Chem*. 2002;48(11):2051-4.

Giambona, A., Passarello, C., Renda, D., Maggio, A. The significance of the hemoglobin A_2 value in screening for hemoglobinopathies. *Clin. Biochem*. 2009;42(18):1786-96.

Giardina, P. J., Forget, B. G. Chapter 41: Thalassemia syndromes. In: Hoffman, R., Benz, E. J., Shattil, S., Furie, B., Silberstein, L. B., McGlave, P., et al. *Hoffman: Hematology: Basic Principles and Practice*, 5th ed. Churchill Livingstone Elsevier. Philadelphia, US. 2009.

Giardine, B., Borg, J., Viennas, E., Pavlidis, C., Moradkhani, K., Joly, P., et al. Updates of the HbVar database of human hemoglobin variants and thalassemia mutations. *Nucleic Acids Res*. 2014;42 (Database issue).

Giordano, P. C., Bakker-Verwij, M., Harteveld, C. L. Frequency of alpha-globin gene triplications and their interaction with beta thalassemia mutations. *Hemoglobin*. 2009;33:124-131.

Hafiza, A., Malisa, M. Y., Khirotdin, R. D., Azlin, I., Azma, Z., Thong, M. C., et al. HbA_2 levels in normal, beta-thalassaemia and haemoglobin E carriers by capillary electrophoresis. *Malays. J. Pathol*. 2012;34(2):161-4.

Harteveld, C. L., Kleanthous, M., Traeger-Synodinos, J. Prenatal diagnosis of hemoglobin disorders: present and future strategies. *Clin. Biochem*. 2009;42(18):1767-79.

Harteveld, C. L. State of the art and new developments in molecular diagnostics for hemoglobinopathies in multiethnic societies. *Int. J. Lab. Hematol*. 2013. [Epub. ahead of print].

He, S., Li, D., Lai, Y., Zhang, Q., Que, T., Tang, Y., et al. Prenatal diagnosis of β-thalassemia in Guangxi Zhuang Autonomous Region, China. *Arch. Gynecol. Obstet.* 2014;289(1):61-5.

He, X., Sheng, M., Xu, M., Xiong, C., Ren, Z. Rapid identification of common β-thalassemia mutations in the Chinese population using duplex or triplex amplicon genotyping by high-resolution melting analysis. *Genet. Test Mol. Biomarkers.* 2010;14(6):851-6.

Herrmann, M. G., Durtschi, J. D., Wittwer, C. T., Voelkerding, K. V. Expanded instrument comparison of amplicon DNA melting analysis for mutation scanning and genotyping. *Clin. Chem.* 2007;53(8):1544-8.

Higgins, T. N., Khajuria, A., Mack, M. Quantification of HbA_2 in patients with and without beta-thalassemia and in the presence of HbS, HbC, HbE, and HbD Punjab hemoglobin variants: comparison of two systems. *Am. J. Clin. Pathol.* 2009;131(3):357-62.

Higgs, D. R., Engel, J. D., Stamatoyannopoulos, G. Thalassaemia. *Lancet.* 2012;379(9813): 373-83.

Hung, C. C., Chen, S. U., Lin, S. Y., Fang, M. Y., Chang, L. J., Tsai, Y. Y., et al. Preimplantation genetic diagnosis of beta-thalassemia using real-time polymerase chain reaction with fluorescence resonance energy transfer hybridization probes. *Anal. Biochem.* 2010; 400(1):69-77.

International Committee for Standardization in Haematology. Recommendations for selected methods for quantitative estimation of Hb A_2 and for Hb A_2 reference preparation. *Br. J. Haematol.* 1978;38(4):573-8.

Karnpean, R., Fucharoen, G., Fucharoen, S., Ratanasiri, T. Fetal red blood cell parameters in thalassemia and hemoglobinopathies. *Fetal Diagn. Ther.* 2013;34(3):166-71.

Kim, J. E., Kim, B. R., Woo, K. S., Kim, J. M., Park, J. I., Han, J. Y. Comparison of capillary electrophoresis with cellulose acetate electrophoresis for the screening of hemoglobinopathies. *Korean J. Lab. Med.* 2011;31(4):238-43.

Kleinert, P., Schmid, M., Zurbriggen, K., Speer, O., Schmugge, M., Roschitzki, B., et al. Mass spectrometry: a tool for enhanced detection of hemoglobin variants. *Clin. Chem.* 2008;54(1):69-76.

Kotwal, J., Saxena, R., Choudhry, V. P., Dwivedi, S. N., Barghava, M. Erythrocyte indices for discriminating thalassaemic and non-thalassaemic microcytosis in Indians. *Nat. Med. J. India.* 1999;12(6):266-7.

Lafferty, J. D., Crowther, M. A., Ali, M. A., Levine, M. The evaluation of various mathematical RBC indices and their efficacy in discriminating between thalassemic and non-thalassemicmicrocytosis. *Am. J. Clin. Pathol.* 1996;106(2):201-5.

Langlois, S., Ford, J. C., Chitayat, D., Désilets, V. A., Farrell, S. A., Geraghty, M., et al.; CCMG Prenatal Diagnosis Committee; SOGC Genetic Committee. Carrier screening for thalassemia and hemoglobinopathies in Canada. *J. Obstet. Gynaecol. Can.* 2008;30(10): 950-71.

Lazarte, S., Haro, C., Jimenez, C., Ledesma Achem, E., Burgos, M., Mónaco, M. E., Issé, B. Es útil el índice hematimétrico ADE en el diagnóstico diferencial de anemia ferropénica y talasemia?" In: *Libro XXIX Jornadas Científicas*. Asociación de Biología de Tucumán. Horco Molle (Tucumán), Argentina. 2012[a]; pp. 105.

Lazarte, S., Leri de Nofal, M., Jimenez, C., Haro, C., Burgos, M., Issé, B. Red cell osmotic resistance in the hereditary anemias diagnosis in Tucumán, Argentina. *Acta Bioquím. Clín. Latinoam.* 2012[b];46(4):645-53.

Lazarte, S., Leri de Nofal, M., Rossi, E., Jiménez, C., Ledesma Achem, E., Issé, B. Diagnóstico diferencial de anemia ferropénica y rasgo beta talasémico: Valor predictivo de las pruebas de cribado. *Arch. Bioq., Quím. y Farm.-Tucumán*. 2010-2011;XXI(1):8-17.

Li, Q., Li, L. Y., Huang, S. W., Li, L., Chen, X. W., Zhou, W. J., et al. Rapid genotyping of known mutations and polymorphisms in beta-globin gene based on the DHPLC profile patterns of homoduplexes and heteroduplexes. *Clin. Biochem*. 2008;41(9):681-7.

López-Escribano, H., Parera, M. M., Guix, P., Castro, J. A., Ramon, M., Picornell, A. Utility and importance of accurate Hb A_2 measurements for defining a strategy for β-thalassemia screening: experience in the Balearic Islands, Spain. *Hemoglobin*. 2013;37(6):593-8.

López-Escribano, H. Estudio genético de portadores de beta talasemia mediante la técnica de PCR a tiempo real en la Isla de Mallorca. Roche Diagnostics Informa. Especial 4as *Jornadas de Residentes*. Ed Roche Diagnostics S.L. 2009; pp. 4-19.

Losekoot, M., Fodde, R., Harteveld, C. L., van Heeren, H., Giordano, P. C., Bernini, L. F. Denaturing gradient gel electrophoresis and direct sequencing of PCR amplified genomic DNA: a rapid and reliable diagnostic approach to beta thalassaemia. *Br. J. Haematol.* 1990;76(2):269-74.

Mahadik. C. T. Experience with multiplex ARMS (MARMS)-PCR for the detection of common β-thalassemia mutations in India. *Cardiovasc. Hematol. Agents Med. Chem.* 2012;10(1):14-24.

Memish, Z. A., Saeedi, M. Y. Six-year outcome of the national premarital screening and genetic counseling program for sickle cell disease and β-thalassemia in Saudi Arabia. *Ann. Saudi Med.* 2011;31(3):229-35.

Mendilcioglu, I., Yakut, S., Keser, I., Simsek, M., Yesilipek, A., Bagci, G., Luleci, G. Prenatal diagnosis of β-thalassemia and other hemoglobinopathies in southwestern Turkey. *Hemoglobin*. 2011;35(1):47-55.

Metaxotou-Mavrommati, A., Kattamis, C. Molecular, haematological and clinical studies of the -101 C --> T substitution of the beta-globin gene promoter in 25 beta-thalassaemia intermedia patients and 45 heterozygotes. *Br. J. Haematol.* 1999;107(4):699-706.

Mirasena, S., Shimbhu, D., Sanguansermsri, M., Sanguansermsri, T. Detection of beta-thalassemia mutations using a multiplex amplification refractory mutation system assay. *Hemoglobin*. 2008;32(4):403-9.

Miri-Moghaddam, E., Zadeh-Vakili, A., Nikravesh, A., Sistani, S. S., Naroie-Nejad, M. Sistani population: a different spectrum of β-thalassemia mutations from other ethnic groups of Iran. *Hemoglobin*. 2013;37(2):138-47.

Modell, B., Darlison, M. Global epidemiology of haemoglobin disorders and derived service indicators. *Bull. World Health Organ*. 2008;86(6):480-7.

Mosca, A., Paleari, R., Ivaldi, G., Galanello, R., Giordano, P. C. The role of haemoglobin A_2 testing in the diagnosis of thalassaemias and related haemoglobinopathies. *J. Clin. Pathol*. 2009[a];62(1):13-7.

Mosca, A., Paleari, R., Leone, D., Ivaldi, G. The relevance of hemoglobin F measurement in the diagnosis of thalassemias and related hemoglobinopathies. *Clin. Biochem*. 2009[b]; 42(18):1797-801.

Murugesan, G., Jan, S., Han, J.-Y. Single nucleotide polymorphisms in molecular diagnostics. In: Kottke-Marchand, K. and Davis, B. H. eds. *Laboratory Hematology Practice*. Wiley Blackwell Publishing Ltd. Chichester, UK. 2012; pp: 168-80.

Myers, R. M., Maniatis, T., Lerman, L. S. Detection and localization of single base changes by denaturing gradient gel electrophoresis. *Methods Enzymol*. 1987;155:501-27.

Nikuei, P., Hadavi, V., Rajaei, M., Saberi, M., Hajizade, F., Najmabadi, H. Prenatal diagnosis for beta-thalassemia major in the Iranian Province of Hormozgan. *Hemoglobin*. 2008; 32 (6):539-45.

Ntaios, G., Chatzinikolaou, A., Saouli, Z., Girtovitis, F., Tsapanidou, M., Kaiafa, G., et al. Discrimination indices as screening test for beta-thalassemic trait. *Ann. Hematol*. 2008;87 (1):61-2.

O'Donovan, M. C., Oefner, P. J., Roberts, S. C., Austin, J., Hoogendoorn, B., Guy, C., et al. Blind analysis of denaturing high-performance liquid chromatography as a tool for mutation detection. *Genomics*. 1998;52(1):44-9.

Okan, B., Cigiloglu, A., Cifci, S., Yilmaz, M., Pehlivan, M. Red cell indices and functions differentiating with the β-thalassaemia trait from those with iron deficiency anaemia. *J. Int. Med. Res*. 2009;37:25-30.

Old, J. M., Varawalla, N. Y., Weatherall, D. J. Rapid detection and prenatal diagnosis of beta-thalassaemia: studies in Indian and Cypriot populations in the UK. *Lancet*. 1990;336 (8719):834-7.

Old, J. M. Screening and genetic diagnosis of haemoglobin disorders. *Blood Rev*. 2003; 17 (1):43-53.

Organización Mundial de la Salud (OMS). *Talasemias y otras hemoglobinopatías*. EB 118/5. Ginebra, 2006. Available from http://apps.who.int/gb/archive/pdf_files/EB118/B118_5-sp.pdf.

Paleari, R., Giambona, A., Cannata, M., Leto, F., Maggio, A., Mosca, A. IFCC Working Group Standardization of HbA_2. External quality assessment of hemoglobin A_2 measurement: data from an Italian pilot study with fresh whole blood samples and commercial HPLC systems. *Clin. Chem. Lab. Med*. 2007;45:88-92.

Paleari, R., Gulbis, B., Cotton, F., Mosca, A. Interlaboratory comparison of current high-performance methods for HbA_2. *Int. J. Lab. Hematol*. 2012;34(4):362-8.

Passarello, C., Giambona, A., Cannata, M., Vinciguerra, M., Renda, D., Maggio, A. Iron deficiency does not compromise the diagnosis of high HbA_2 β thalassemia trait. *Haematologica*. 2012;97(3):472-3.

Patrinos, G. P., Kollia, P., Papadakis, M. N. Molecular diagnosis of inherited disorders: lessons from hemoglobinopathies. *Hum. Mutat*. 2005;26(5):399-412.

Peng, C. T., Liu, S. C., Peng, Y. C., Lin, T. H., Wang, S. J., Le, C. Y., et al. Distribution of thalassemias and associated hemoglobinopathies identified by prenatal diagnosis in Taiwan. *Blood Cells Mol. Dis*. 2013;51(3):138-41.

Piplani, S., Manan, R., Lalit, M., Manjari, M., Bhasin, T., Bawa, J. NESTROFT - A Valuable, Cost Effective Screening Test for Beta Thalassemia Trait in North Indian Punjabi Population. *J. Clin. Diagn. Res*. 2013;7(12):2784-7.

Pornprasert, S., Sukunthamala, K. SYTO9 and SYBR GREEN1 with a high-resolution melting analysis for prenatal diagnosis of β^0-thalassemia/hemoglobin-E. *Eur. J. Haematol*. 2010;85(5):424-9.

Ranjbaran, R., Okhovat, M. A., Mobarhanfard, A., Aboualizadeh, F., Abbasi, M., Moezzi, L., et al. Analysis of β/α globin ratio by using relative qRT-PCR for diagnosis of beta-thalassemia carriers. *J. Clin. Lab. Anal*. 2013;27(4):267-71.

Rathod, D. A., Kaur, A., Patel, V., Patel, K., Kabrawala, R., Patel, V., et al. Usefulness of cell counter-based parameters and formulas in detection of β-thalassemia trait in areas of high prevalence. *Am. J. Clin. Pathol.* 2007; 128:585-89.

Reed, G. H., Kent, J. O., Wittwer, C. T. High-resolution DNA melting analysis for simple and efficient molecular diagnostics. *Pharmacogenomics*. 2007;8(6):597-608.

Ristaldi, M. S., Pirastu, M., Rosatelli, C., Monni, G., Erlich, H., Saiki, R., et al. Prenatal diagnosis of beta-thalassaemia in Mediterranean populations by dot blot analysis with DNA amplification and allele specific oligonucleotide probes. *Prenat. Diagn.* 1989;9 (9): 629-38.

Ronaghi, M. Pyrosequencing sheds light on DNA sequencing. *Genome Res.* 2001;11(1):3-11.

Rosatelli, C., Leoni, G. B., Tuveri, T., Scalas, M. T., Mosca, A., Galanello, R., et al. Heterozygous beta-thalassemia: relationship between the hematological phenotype and the type of beta-thalassemia mutation. *Am. J. Hematol.* 1992;39(1):1-4.

Rund, D., Filon, D., Strauss, N., Rachmilewitz, E. A., Oppenheim, A. Mean corpuscular volume of heterozygotes for beta-thalassemia correlates with the severity of mutations. *Blood.* 1992;79(1):238-43.

Rund, D., Rachmilewitz, E. Beta-thalassemia. *N. Engl. J. Med.* 2005;353(11):1135-46.

Ryan, K., Bain, B. J., Worthington, D., James, J., Plews, D., Mason, A., et al. British Committee for Standards in Haematology, Significant haemoglobinopathies: guidelines for screening and diagnosis. *British J. Haematol.* 2010;149:35-49.

Saiki, R. K., Walsh, P. S., Levenson, C. H., Erlich, H. A. Genetic analysis of amplified DNA with immobilized sequence-specific oligonucleotide probes. *Proc. Natl. Acad. Sci. US.* 1989;86(16):6230-4.

Salk, J. J., Sanchez, J. A., Pierce, K. E., Rice, J. E., Soares, K. C., Wangh, L. J. Direct amplification of single-stranded DNA for pyrosequencing using linear-after-the-exponential (LATE)-PCR. *Anal. Biochem.* 2006;353(1):124-32.

Schouten, J. P., McElgunn, C. J., Waaijer, R., Zwijnenburg, D., Diepvens, F., Pals, G. Relative quantification of 40 nucleic acid sequences by multiplex ligation-dependent probe amplification. *Nucleic Acids Res.* 2002;30(12):e57.

Shammas, C., Papasavva, T., Felekis, X., Christophorou, C., Roomere, H., Synodinos, J. T., et al. ThalassoChip, an array mutation and single nucleotide polymorphism detection tool for the diagnosis of β-thalassaemia. *Clin. Chem. Lab. Med.* 2010;48(12):1713-8.

Shen, C., Jiang, Y. M., Shi, H., Liu, J. H., Zhou, W. J., Dai, Q. K., et al. Evaluation of indices in differentiation between iron deficiency anemia and beta-thalassemia trait for Chinese children. *J. Pediatr. Hematol. Oncol.* 2010;32(6):218-22.

Shih, H. C., Er, T. K., Chang, T. J., Chang, Y. S., Liu, T. C., Chang, J. G. Rapid identification of HBB gene mutations by high-resolution melting analysis. *Clin. Biochem.* 2009;42(16-17):1667-76.

Singh, S. P., Gupta, S. C. Effectiveness of red cell osmotic fragility test with varying degrees of saline concentration in detecting beta thalassaemia trait. *Singapore Med. J.* 2008;49 (10):823-6.

Sirdah, M., Tarazi, I., Al Najjar, E., Al Haddad, R. Evaluation of the diagnostic reliability of different RBC indices and formulas in the differentiation of the beta-thalassaemia minor from iron deficiency in Palestinian population. *Int. J. Lab. Hematol.* 2008;30 (4): 324-30.

So, C. C., So, A. C., Chan, A. Y., Tsang, S. T., Ma, E. S., Chan, L. C. Detection and characterization of beta-globin gene cluster deletions in Chinese using multiplex ligation-dependent probe amplification. *J. Clin. Pathol.* 2009;62(12):1107-11.

Stefanis, L., Kanavakis, E., Traeger-Synodinos, J., Tzetis, M., Metaxotou-Mavromati, A., Kattamis, C. Hematologic phenotype of the mutations IVS1-n6 (T→C), IVS1-n110 (G→A), and CD39 (C→T) in carriers of beta-thalassemia in Greece. *Pediatr. Hematol. Oncol.* 1994;11(5):509-17.

Steinberg, M. H., Adams, III J. G. Hemoglobin A_2: Origin, Evolution, and Aftermath. *Blood.* 1991;78(9):1265-77.

Stephens, A. D., Angastiniotis, M., Baysal, E., Chan, V., Davis, B., Fucharoen, S., et al. International Council for the Standardisation of Haematology (ICSH). ICSH recommendations for the measurement of haemoglobin F. *Int. J. Lab. Hematol.* 2012[b];34(1):14-20.

Stephens, A. D., Angastiniotis, M., Baysal, E., Chan, V., Fucharoen, S., Giordano, P. C., et al.; International Council for the Standardisation of Haematology (ICSH). ICSH recommendations for the measurement of haemoglobin A_2. *Int. J. Lab. Hematol.* 2012[a]; 34(1):1-13.

Tan, A. S., Quah, T. C., Low, P. S., Chong, S. S. A rapid and reliable 7-deletion multiplex polymerase chain reaction assay for alpha-thalassemia. *Blood.* 2001;98(1):250-1.

Tan, G. B., Aw, T. C., Dunstan, R. A., Lee, S. H. Evaluation of high performance liquid chromatography for routine estimation of haemoglobins A_2 and F. *J. Clin. Pathol.* 1993; 46(9):852-6.

Tan, J. A., Tay, J. S., Lin, L. I., Kham, S. K., Chia, J. N., Chin, T. M., et al. The amplification refractory mutation system (ARMS): a rapid and direct prenatal diagnostic technique for beta-thalassaemia in Singapore. *Prenat. Diagn.* 1994;14(11):1077-82.

Tarazi, I., Al Najjar, E., Lulu, N., Sirdah, M. Obligatory premarital tests for beta-thalassaemia in the Gaza Strip: evaluation and recommendations. *Int. J. Lab. Hematol.* 2007;29(2): 111-8.

The laboratory diagnosis of haemoglobinopathies. *Br. J. Haematol.* 1998;101(4):783-92.

Thein, S. L. The Molecular Basis of β-Thalassemia. *Cold Spring Harb. Perspect. Med.* 2013; 3:a011700.

Thein, S. L. β-thalassaemia prototype of a single gene disorder with multiple phenotypes. *Int. J. Hematol.* 2002;76(Suppl. 2):96-104.

Timbs, A. T., Rugless, M. J., Gallienne, A. E., Haywood, A. M., Henderson, S. J., Old, J. M. Prenatal diagnosis of hemoglobinopathies by pyrosequencing: a more sensitive and rapid approach to fetal genotyping. *Hemoglobin.* 2012;36(2):144-50.

Tritipsombut, J., Phylipsen, M., Viprakasit, V., Chalaow, N., Sanchaisuriya, K., Giordano, P. C., et al. A single-tube multiplex gap-polymerase chain reaction for the detection of eight β-globin gene cluster deletions common in Southeast Asia. *Hemoglobin.* 2012;36(6):571-80.

Troxler, H., Kleinert, P., Schmugge, M., Speer, O. Advances in hemoglobinopathy detection and identification. *Adv. Clin. Chem.* 2012;57:1-28.

Tubbs, R. R. Development of amplification-based molecular genetic testing in hematology. In: Kottke-Marchand, K. and Davis, B. H. eds. *Laboratory Hematology Practice.* Wiley Blackwell Publishing Ltd. Chichester, UK. 2012; pp: 155-167.

Uysal, A., Genc, A., Taşyürek, N., Türkyilmaz, B. Prevalence of β-thalassemia trait and abnormal hemoglobin in premarital screening in the province of Izmir, Turkey. *Pediatr. Hematol. Oncol.* 2013;30(1):46-50.

Vrettou, C., Traeger-Synodinos, J., Tzetis, M., Malamis, G., Kanavakis, E. Rapid screening of multiple beta-globin gene mutations by real-time PCR on the LightCycler: application to carrier screening and prenatal diagnosis of thalassemia syndromes. *Clin. Chem.* 2003; 49(5):769-76.

Wajcman, H., Moradkhani, K. Abnormal haemoglobins: detection and characterization. *Indian J. Med. Res.* 2011;134:538-46.

Weatherall, D. J. Phenotype-genotype relationships in monogenic disease: lessons from the thalassemias. *Nature Rev. Gen.* 2001;2(4):245-55.

Wertz, D. C., Fletcher, J. C., Berg, K. Review of Ethical Issues in Medical Genetics. Report of Consultants to WHO. Human Genetics Programme. Management of Non communicable Diseases. WHO. 2003. Available from http://www.who.int/genomics/publications/ en /ethical_issuesin_medgenetics%20report.pdf.

Wild, B., Bain, B. Investigation of abnormal haemoglobins and thalassaemia. In: Lewis, S. M., Bain, B. J., Bates, I. *Dacie and Lewis Practical Haematology*. Tenth Ed. Churchill Livingstone Elsevier. Philadelphia, US. 2006; pp. 271-310.

Winichagoon, P., Saechan, V., Sripanich, R., Nopparatana, C., Kanokpongsakdi, S., Maggio, A., et al. Prenatal diagnosis of beta-thalassaemia by reverse dot-blot hybridization. *Prenat. Diagn.* 1999;19(5):428-35.

Wood, W. G., Weatherall, D. J., Hart, G. H., Bennett, M., Marsh, G. W. Hematologic changes and hemoglobin analysis beta thalassemia heterozygotes during the first year of life. *Pediatr. Res.* 1982;16(4 Pt 1):286-9.

Yap, C., Wang, W., Tan, A. S., Tan, W. C., Lim, M. N., Chong, S. S. Successful preimplantation genetic diagnosis of Hb Bart's hydrops fetalis in Singapore after fresh and frozen embryo replacement cycles. *Ann. Acad. Med. Singapore*. 2009;38(10):910-3.

Ye, S., Dhillon, S., Ke, X., Collins, A. R., Day, I. N. An efficient procedure for genotyping single nucleotide polymorphisms. *Nucleic Acids Res*. 2001;29(17):E88-8.

Yenilmez, E. D., Tuli, A., Evrüke, I. C. Noninvasive prenatal diagnosis experience in the Çukurova Region of Southern Turkey: detecting paternal mutations of sickle cell anemia and β-thalassemia in cell-free fetal DNA using high-resolution melting analysis. *Prenat. Diagn.* 2013:1-9.

Zeinalian, M., Nobari, R. F., Moafi, A., Salehi, M., Hashemzadeh-Chaleshtori, M. Two decades of pre-marital screening for beta-thalassemia in central Iran. *J. Community Genet.* 2013;4(4):517-22.

In: Thalassemia
Editor: Makenzie Greene

ISBN: 978-1-63117-954-9

Chapter 6

Molecular Therapies for Treatment of Thalassemia

Eleni Papanikolaou*
Laboratory of Biology, University of Athens School of Medicine,
Athens, Greece

Abstract

Although in the original design for developing molecular therapies for monogenic diseases thalassemia was presented as the main candidate, yet genetic treatments were only available through two clinical trials only a few years ago with very few patients being enrolled in these studies. The reason for this inconsistency is mainly because molecular/genetic treatments must prove themselves to be safer than the current symptomatic therapies than include transfusion and iron chelation.

This review presents the current status of gene therapy for hemoglobin disorders, reviews the recent results and discusses how the knowledge gained from these trials can be used to develop a safe and effective gene therapy approach for the treatment of β-thalassemia. It also elaborates the next trend in molecular therapies for thalassemia that include manipulation of induced plupipotent stem cells (iPSCs) and gene editing.

Keywords: Gene therapy, insertional mutagenesis, retroviral integration, nucleases, Hematopoietic Stem Cells (hHSCs); lentiviral vector; bone marrow, thalassemia, sickle cell disease

* Correspondence should be addressed to: Papanikolaou Eleni, Lecturer of Gene Therapy, Laboratory of Biology, School of Medicine, University of Athens, 176 Michalakopoulou St., 11527, Athens, Greece. Email: elpapanik@med.uoa.gr, epapanik@bioacademy.gr.

Introduction

The β-thalassemias are inherited anemias caused by mutations that reduce or suppress production of the β-globin chain of hemoglobin being most prevalent in the Mediterranean region, the Middle East, the Indian subcontinent and South East Asia, representing a serious health problem. Current therapies include chronic transfusions in combination with life-long iron chelation, hydroxyurea for the induction of fetal hemoglobin (HbF) and supportive care. However, the complications of iron overload, together with the sequelae of the anemia and ineffective erythropoiesis, are major causes of morbidity and mortality in these patients [1]. Finally, although regular blood transfusions in combination with aggressive iron chelation have remarkably delayed the onset of iron-related organ failure and improved mortality, many patients continue to be affected by cardiac disease, delayed pubertal maturation and eventually develop endocrine failure. A matched allogeneic hematopoietic stem cell (HSC) transplant is curative, but restricted by the availability of matched related donors and has potential serious complications [1].

Gene therapy is essentially autologous bone marrow transplantation (BMT) of genetically modified, i.e. corrected cells. Specifically, hematopoietic stem cells ($CD34^+$) are removed from the patient, transduced *in vitro* with the therapeutic globin lentiviral vector (*ex vivo* gene therapy), and returned to the patient intravenously [1]. Autologous transplantation of gene corrected cells is to date, the only radical treatment outperforming allogeneic bone marrow transplantation in terms of response, morbidity, and mortality. Therefore, the safe genetic engineering and engraftment of hematopoietic stem cells is the key to effectively treat thalassemia.

Gene Therapy by Addition of Globin Genes via Retroviral Vectors

A critical step in the development of gene therapy for blood disorders was the research that focused on identifying the most effective vector system for gene transfer. In the early 1980s, investigators successfully demonstrated the stable γ-retroviral vector transfer of a marker gene into the chromosomal DNA genome of hemopoietic stem cells in murine models [2]. Retroviral vectors are especially utilized in blood disorder gene therapy because of their ability to integrate their genome into the host's genome and can therefore stably deliver the therapeutic gene which in turn, is theoritically expressed throughout life. Later, several attempts were made to utilize this vector type to transfer globin genes, driven by the endogenous β-globin promoter, into the HSCs of mice but resulted in poor gene-transfer efficiency and low expression of the globin transgene [3]. During this same period, powerful DNA-enhancer elements from the β-globin locus control region (LCR) located on human chromosome 11 were identified as necessary for the nearby globin genes to be expressed at very high levels [4], but when these elements or portions thereof were placed into the oncoretroviral globin vector design, poor vector production and genetic instability of the viral vector genome were observed [5].

A significant breakthrough in the field of globin gene therapy occurred in 2000 when Sadelain and colleagues developed and utilized a globin lentiviral vector based on HIV [6]. This vector type was able to transmit a much larger LCR configuration along with the β-globin gene without rearrangement and could be produced in sufficient titer to allow gene transfer at a high level in β-thalassemic mice. This resulted in significant disease amelioration of the mouse thalassemic model. Thus, the lentiviral vector configuration that confered greater stability and higher titers combined with the lentiviral innate superior transduction efficiency of HSCs advanced the utilization of lentiviral vectors in the globin gene therapy field. Moreover, the vector used in the specified study laid the basis for the final vector configuration that is currently employed in the first US clinical trial for gene therapy of thalassemia conducted by the Sadelain group [7]. By utilizing lentiviral vectors, several other research groups have also achieved phenotypic correction of thalassemia either in murine or in *in vitro* human models [8-11].

Most of the researchers in the globin gene therapy field have constructed viral vectors bearing β-globin as the therapeutic transgene, since it is the genetic defect in this gene which lies at the root of decreased β-globin expression. Experiments have been conducted in murine thalassemia models and in thalassemic $CD34^+$ hematopoietic stem cells. In the thalassemic mouse model, as previously mentioned, Sadelain and colleagues using vector TNS9 have shown that chimeric hemoglobin molecules incorporating human β-globin comprised about 21% of the total hemoglobin [6]. Imren et al. [12] showed that the lentiviral driven β-globin expression reached approximately 32% of the total hemoglobin while the respective amount from the GLOBE vector ranged from 14-37% as evidenced by the group of Ferrari [13]. Leboulch and colleagues subsequently demonstrated that lentiviral-mediated stem cell transfer of an anti-sickling variant of the human β-globin chain resulted in hematologic correction and diminished end-organ damage in murine SCD [9]. Globin lentiviral vectors have also been used to transfer a β-globin gene into primitive human hematopoietic cells that are capable of establishing hematopoiesis in immunodeficient mice [10, 15]. Correction of the β-thalassemia phenotype in human cells was also demonstrated by the establishment of effective erythropoiesis in erythroid cultures *in vitro* [8, 10, 11], either by the use of a γ-globin lentiviral vector by [8, 11] or by the use of a β-globin lentiviral vectors [10, 15].

β-thalassemia is characterized by reduced levels of β-globin chain production. However, the synthesis of α-globin continues to be normal in β-thalassemia, resulting in the accumulation of excess unmatched α-globin chains in the erythroid precursors that precipitate forming inclusion bodies, causing damage to the red blood cell (RBC) membrane, destruction and finally apoptosis [16]. Thus, factors that reduce the degree of chain imbalance such as an innate ability to increase fetal hemoglobin (HbF, $\alpha_2\gamma_2$), as in the HPFH phenotype, have an ameliorating effect on the disease. Hence, gene therapy of β-thalassemia based on γ-globin addition via viral vectors or γ-globin gene reactivation displays a considerable advantage. For the aforementioned reasons the groups of D. Persons [11] and N.P. Anagnou [8] are using γ-globin lentiviral vectors to treat thalassemia in a gene therapy context. Most commonly, persistent γ-globin expression is caused by a number of naturally occurring deletions at the 3' end of the β-globin locus. One of the hypotheses that have been proposed for the persistent γ-globin expression resulting from these deletions predicts that the deletions juxtapose distal enhancer elements in proximity to the γ-genes leading to their activation. Examples include the HPFH-1, HPFH-2, HPFH-3, and HPFH-6 deletions. Sequences located immediately downstream to their 3' breakpoints have been shown to act as enhancers in transient transfection assays and in transgenic mice [1]. Also, the addition of the HPFH-2 breakpoints to γ-globin transgenes extended gene expression beyond the early fetal liver stage, suggesting that HPFH breakpoints have the capacity to alter the developmental regulation of γ–globin [8]. The HPFH phenotype can also be caused by point mutations in the promoters of fetal Aγ and Gγ genes such as the -117 single point mutation in the Aγ-gene promoter (-117 HPFH) [8].

Gene Editing for Treatment of Thalassemia

The latest trend in thalassemia gene therapy involves the notion of genome editing: Just as editing text involves adding, removing, or replacing words, genome editing is an approach in which the genome sequence is directly changed by adding, replacing, or removing DNA bases in targeted and specific genome areas (http://www.stanford.edu/group/hopes/cgi-bin/wordpress/2013/10/genome-editing/). This is feasible due to sequence-specific nucleases which introduce double-strand breaks that lead to small chromosomal deletions via nonhomologous end joining (NHEJ)–mediated repair [17]. Such nucleases are transcription activator-like effector nucleases (TALENs), zinc-finger nucleases (ZFNs) and nucleases of the CRISPR/Cas9 system.

In the recent study by Bauer et al. [18] a novel powerful tissue- and developmental stage–specific enhancer located within the second intron of BCL11A was identified. The enhancer promotes expression of BCL11A gene, which encodes a repressor that silences γ-globin genes in adult human erythroid cells (only during the course of erythropoiesis and not hemopoiesis). Consequently, removal of this erythroid-specific enhancer reduced the amount of BCL11A, thereby allowing expression of γ-globin genes. This exquisite specificity inevitably points to genome editing as a plausible approach to lasting corrective cell-specific therapy for certain hemoglobinopathies such as thalassemia. It is only because of the nature of the physiology of globin switching that it is possible to make such a correction since it involves specifically γ-globin expression via endogenous reactivation.

Genome editing approaches have been so far tested in the β-thalassemia and α-thalassemia context through TALENs [19] and zinc finger nucleases [20] respectively, but were based on the generation of iPSCs followed by correction through homologous recombination. The main issue here is the relatively low frequency of homologous recombination. Therefore, the evolution of genetic approaches for treatment of thalassemia includes isolation of $CD34^+$ hematopoietic stem cells from thalassemic patients, gene-editing for targeted deletion of the BCL11A erythroid enhancer and re-infusion to the patient. The only study so far, describing the effects of genome editing as well as the therapeutic outcome upon targeted deletion of specific erythroid regulatory elements has been presented in the latest ASH meeting, held in New Orleans last December. This highly promising and at the very least, impressive study was the fruitful collaboration of George Stamatoyannopoulos' group in UW and Sangamo Biosciences and employed genome editing through zinc finger nucleases [21]. This study involved the targeted deletion of the wider genomic region of BCL11A and not only the erythroid-specific repressor. Although approximately 75% of alleles were modified and it appeared to confer a normalization of the β-like to α-globin ratio to ~1.0 in RBCs obtained from genome-edited $CD34^+$ cells from two individuals with β-thalassemia major, still there are several parameters that need to be taken into account before this approach reaches the clinic.

- First, gene transfer of ZFNs occurred through mRNA introduction in $CD34^+$ cells through electroporation. Electroporation (or electropermeabilization) is a process that can induce transient openings in cell plasma membrane by executing external electric field on cells, increasing thus the permeability of cell membrane. Although the transfection efficiency is depedent on the cell line and the buffer used, the kinetics of pore resealing after electroporation indicate that it is a random process and it is generally agreed that the resealing of the membrane requires seconds to minutes [22]. Generally, cell survival is not a concern when working with bacterial cells, but can be a major issue with mammalian cells. The viability of mammalian cells depends on the resealing of electric-field-induced pores in cell membrane after electroporation and the extent of excess leakage of intracellular molecules during electroporation [22]. These were the main reasons that initial studies with electroporation led to very low transfection efficiencies and cell viability, severely limiting the development of this technology. Although the emergence of nucleofection provided an efficient means for transfecting cells *in vitro*, it still presents serious disadvantages, such as the very high cost involved and last, but not least, the unknown strength of the electrical field used and the unknown electroporation buffer composition. This technique has been widely used to transfect large number of cells and is an especially attractive method in DNA vaccine technology for cancer and in the ongoing Phase 2 and Phase1/2 clinical trials to evaluate the safety and efficacy of a novel ZFP Therapeutic® for the treatment of HIV/AIDS by employing gene editing technology to knock out the CCR5 co-receptor of HIV in T-cells of HIV-infected individuals [23] by Sangamo.
- Second, it is unclear how exactly are off-target effects detected after gene editing with the specific ZFNs in the context of thalassemia and whether they are only detected by the surveyor assay or additional methods. This is a major issue for thalassemia since off-target effects have been previously observed during the CCR5 knock out strategy. Specifically, these ZFNs showed a tenfold lower preference for the CCR2 gene (the closest paralogue to the CCR5 target in the genome) and revealed an off-target event that occurs once in every 20.000 events, located in the intron of the ABLIM2 gene (actin binding lIm protein family, member 2) involved in central nervous system development and maintenance [24]. The tenfold lower preference for the CCR2 gene can be a major issue for thalassemia due to the homology of all hemoglobin related genes.

Therefore, although it might be both ethical and almost mandatory to utilize such methods in HIV-infected individuals or patients suffering from cancer, it is an entirely different issue to apply this technique to thalassemic patients for the following reasons: a) Thalassemia per se in a non-malignant situation that does not result in hematologic cancer of any type (unlike other anemias), b) the current symptomatic treatments that include transfusion and iron chelation are very well tolerated and standardized among thalassemic patients and c) any new molecular/genetic strategy must prove to be safer than the current symptomatic therapies. After all, these are the main reasons that, although in the original design for developing molecular therapies for monogenic diseases thalassemia was presented as the main candidate, yet, genetic treatments were available through only two clinical trials with very few patients being enrolled.

On the other hand, other more versatile methods with better predictability of off-target effects could be utilized in the future for the succesful gene editing approach for thalassemia such as the Crispr/Cas system [25].

Induced Pluripotent Stem Cells

The generation of induced pluripotent stem (iPS) cells enables for the first time the derivation of unlimited numbers of patient-specific stem cells [26] and holds great promise for regenerative medicine. Recent studies have explored the potential of iPS cell generation combined with gene and cell therapy for disease treatment in mice and humans. Ye and colleagues have previously shown that iPS cells can be generated from cells derived from skin fibroblasts, amniotic fluid or chorionic villus sampling of patients with ß-thalassemia [27]. In other words, it is now possible to reprogram the patient's own somatic cells into stem cells and correct their ß-globin gene. Furthermore, homologous recombination experiments demonstrated that it is possible to correct the mutated ß-globin gene in iPSCs derived from thalassemic patients [28]. The ultimate goal would be to engraft patients with these corrected iPSCs and generate healthy red cells. However, for the promise of iPS cell technology in therapeutic applications to be fully realized, clinically translatable methodologies for the introduction of therapeutic genes into human iPS cells will be needed. Moreover, major issues need to be addressed such as: a) what is the best way to generate iPS cells efficiently with minimal genotoxicity due to the reprogramming process and/or without genotoxic alteration that might occur through the repair process. b) Which are the best iPS clones suitable for clinical investigation i.e. how one can address the genetic, epigenetic, tumorigenic, and differentiation potential of individual iPS clones? c) To what extend is it possible to generate engraftable HSCs from IPs cells capable of conferring sustained hematopoietic reconstitution in transplanted recipients? d) Is it possible to scale up the differentiation culture processes and absolutely ensure the depletion of cells with the potential of teratoma formation? Last, but not least, as very well stated by Ettinger and Flotte "the emergence of all the potential promise of these innovative molecular therapies is coinciding with a future in which the costs of new therapies may be the major determinate of whether they will be available to patients" [29].

Somatic cell reprogramming opens the door to many genetic engineering approaches, including screening for retroviral integrations in potential genomic safe harbors [30] and targeted gene delivery, including nuclease-based approaches [19]. However, although the advent of iPS cells is far from clinically relevant and simultaneously poses a number of fascinating biologic questions and generates issues that concern their differentiation potential and propensity to transform as very well stated by Riviere et al. [31], yet the recent publications by Obokata and colleagues manifests a very versatile and easy way to generate iPS cells [32] with increased differentiation capacity [33]. It is therefore anticipated that generation of iPS cells will be further advanced from a plethora of tissues and cells, thus making their eventual use in the clinic more feasible and relevant mainly because of the novel technique that does not include any kind of genetic manipulation.

The Current Gene Therapy Clinical Trials for Thalassemia

A phase I/II clinical trial of β-globin gene therapy for β-thalassemia is currently being conducted by the group of Leboulch and his colleagues in France in collaboration with bluebird bio [34]. The primary objective of this trial is to determine the toxicity and the safety of the approach. The secondary objectives are to evaluate the proportion of genetically modified nucleated blood cells, the expression of the therapeutic hemoglobin in blood, and the potential hematological and clinical benefits. The study initially utilized vector the *insulated* LentiGlobin HPV569 which was based on founding work conducted by Prof. P. Leboulch [9, 12]. Three patients have been treated so far in this study: Subject 1002 and 1003 were treated in 2006 and 2007 while Subject 1004 was treated in November 2011. The first thalassemia patient treated, at 28 years of age, experienced a period of aplasia that lasted longer than expected. Although no adverse events occurred, untransduced cells kept as a back-up were required to be administered to avoid infectious and hemorrhagic complications during this prolonged high-risk period. The second patient in the study with severe thalassemia, who underwent a complete procedure without the necessity of injection of back-up cells, was an 18-years old male suffering from severe anemia due to the combined HbE/βo thalassemia genotype requiring regular transfusions (about 160 mL of packed erythrocytes/kg/year) since the age of 3. He received $4x10^6$ $CD34^+$ cells/kg [35]. Twenty months after gene therapy, the patient did not suffer any side effects associated with the procedure as a whole. The proportion of lentiviral-modified blood nucleated cells rose progressively to 6% after 12 months, while the requirement for transfusion declined progressively and transfusions were no longer necessary after 12 months. The concentration of therapeutic hemoglobin in blood reached 2.8 g/dL equivalent to 1⁄3 of total hemoglobin 7 months after the last transfusion or 19 months after gene therapy. At twenty-eight months post-therapy, hemoglobin levels have been stabilised at 9.5 g/dL [1] with high reticulocyte counts, suggesting that the genetically modified erythroid cells compensated only partially for the deficits of red cells and hemoglobin [1]. Importantly, the patient reported good wellbeing, free of transfusions and frequent blood tests. He is able to perform his full-time job without any signs of fatigue. However, despite the clinical improvement of this patient, it was reported that the patient was found to have a relative clonal dominance [35]. Of the 10% of lentiviral-modified cells, one clone, identified as having an integration site in the third intron of the HMGA2 gene, was present in excessive proportion relative to the contributions of other clones, as identified by their genomic vector integration sites. Expression of HMGA2 is largely restricted to embryonic and stem cells while the RNA is normally degraded by Let-7 miRNAs binding to multiple targets in Exon 5. In this case, there has been an occasional over-expression of a truncated HMGA2 mRNA (E1 – E3) upon rearrangement within the long Intron 3 due to loss of target sites for Let-7 miRNA [34]. Also, one of two insulators was deleted in the HMGA2 insertion. However, the patient has been stable for approximately 7 years, free of transfusions and is doing well. In summary, this historical patient, who underwent *ex vivo* globin gene transfer for a severe genetic disease, provided the proof of principle of this therapeutic approach. This case also validates somatic gene transfer using a lentiviral SIN vector with chromatin insulators for transducing long-term repopulating hematopoietic stem cells.

The third patient to undergo complete transfusion of genetically corrected $CD34^+$ cells was a 23-year old woman, suffering from HbE/βo-thalassemia major who has been transfusion dependent since her second month of life. Transplantation was performed in November of 2011 and was uneventful. Engrafted neutrophils were detected by day 22 post transplantation and the patient was presented with delayed platelet reconstitution but without related complications. She is clinically stable with improving hematologic parameters, has returned to full time work and the early gene marking is similar to the previously treated patient.

However, both of these two patients showed very low vector copy number per cell, starting from 0.02 VCN/cell in neutrophils. This fact, combined with the gradual decrease in the vector-producing hemoglobin and the loss of the insulator element in several sites of integration prompted bluebird bio to re-design the vector format. The novel vector, termed LentiGlobin BB305, preserves the internal vector sequences and globin gene and regulatory sequences identical but also presents the following differences compared to the parental LentiGlobin HPV569:

- insulators were removed
- 5' HIV U3 promoter/enhancer replaced with a 5' CMV promoter/enhancer and therefore, that is no longer necessary in lentiviral vector manufacturing.

Based on the above information bluebird bio is not planning to treat any additional patient with LentiGlobin HPV569. The LentiGlobin BB305 is being currently assessed in terms of hemoglobin expression and transduction efficiency in $CD34^+$ Sickle Cell Anemia cells, in *in vitro* immortalization (IVIM) assays for genotoxicity, and in β-thalassemic ($Hbb^{th1/th1}$) mice [34]. Preliminary results showed that the new Lentiglobin vector exhibited improved titer, significantly higher transduction efficiency in $CD34^+$ cells, produces equivalent globin expression per vector copy, and is generally safe as demonstrated by the IVIM assays and by the study in the thalassemic mice.

Last, but not least, the group of Michel Sadelain in New York, obtained in 2012 the first US Food and Drug Administration (FDA) approval to proceed to a clinical study in adult subjects with β-thalassemia major [7]. To date, 5 patients have been enrolled and the first three have been treated, i.e. have been transplanted with the transduced HSCs after non-myeloablative conditioning. Engraftment data are available for the first two patients. Patient 1 is a 23 year old female with a ß039 – IVS1,110 mutation and patient 2 is an 18 year old female with a ß039 –IVS1,6 mutation. Both patients underwent mobilization of peripheral blood stem cells (PBSCs) with filgrastim and mobilized 25 x 10^6 and 9.9 x 10^6 CD34 cells/Kg, respectively. $CD34^+$ PBSCs were transduced with the lentiviral vector TNS9.3.55 encoding the normal human beta-globin gene (Thalagen™). The average vector copy number (VCN) in bulk $CD34^+$ cells for these two patients was respectively 0.39 and 0.21 copies per cell. Both patients underwent non-myeloablative cytoreduction with busulfan administered at 2 mg/Kg/dose x 4 doses (total 8 mg/Kg), followed by reinfusion of 11.8 x 10^6 and 8.4 x 10^6 $CD34^+$ cells/Kg, respectively. Both patients tolerated cytoreduction well and recovered their blood counts. While they continue to be transfusion dependent, both patients show a gradual rise in vector copy number in peripheral blood white blood cells and neutrophils, steadily increasing by 1-2% every month, reaching an average VCN of 5-7% 3-6 months after transplantation.

Conclusion

Gene therapy with autologous transplantation of transduced human HSCs is an exciting approach for potential cure of hemopoietic disorders that requires further laboratory and clinical evaluation to determine its safety and efficacy. Despite the drawbacks and uncertainties, researchers in the field remain optimistic that, with continued concerted efforts, HSC gene transfer to treat β-thalassemia will become a useful therapeutic option, while the recent advances hold promise for the outcome of curative stem cell-based therapies.

References

[1] Papanikolaou E, Anagnou NP (2010). Major challenges for gene therapy of thalassemia and sickle cell disease. *Curr. Gene. Ther.* (5): 404-412.

[2] Williams DA, Lemischka IR, Nathan DG, Mulligan RC: Introduction of new genetic material into pluripotent haematopoietic stem cells of the mouse. *Nature* (1984) 310:476-480.

[3] Bender MA, Gelinas RE, Miller AD: A majority of mice show long term expression of a human β-globin gene after retrovirus transfer into hematopoietic stem cells. *Mol. Cell Biol.* 1989; 9: 1426-34.

[4] Grosveld F, van Assendelft GB, Greaves DR, Kollias G: Position independent, high-level expression of the human β-globin gene in transgenic mice. *Cell* (1987) 51:975-985.

[5] Forrester WC, Novak U, Gelinas R, Groudine M: Molecular analysis of the human β-globin locus activation region. *Proc. Natl. Acad. Sci. USA* (1989) 86: 5439-5443.

[6] May C, Rivella S, Callegari J, Heller G, Gaensler KM, Luzzatto L, Sadelain M: Therapeutic haemoglobin synthesis in β-thalassaemic mice expressing lentivirus-encoded human β-globin. *Nature* (2000) 406:82-86.

[7] Boulad F, Riviere I, Wang X, Bartido S, Prockop SE, Barone R, Moi P, Maggio A, and Sadelain M. First US Phase I Clinical Trial Of Globin Gene Transfer For The Treatment Of Beta-Thalassemia Major. Paper No 716, 55th Annual ASH Meeting, December 2013.

[8] Papanikolaou E, Georgomanoli M, Stamateris E, Panetsos F, Karagiorga M, Tsaftaridis P, Graphakos S, Anagnou NP. The new self-inactivating lentiviral vector for thalassemia gene therapy combining two HPFH activating elements corrects human thalassemic hematopoietic stem cells. *Hum. Gene. Ther.* (2012) 23: 15-31.

[9] Pawliuk R, Westerman KA, Fabry ME, Payen E, Tighe R, Bouhassira EE, et al: Correction of sickle cell disease in transgenic mouse models by gene therapy. *Science* (2001) 294:2368-2371.

[10] Puthenveetil G, Scholes J, Carbonell D, Qureshi N, Xia P, Zeng L, et al. Successful correction of the human β-thalassemia major phenotype using a lentiviral vector. *Blood* (2004) 104:3445-3453.

[11] Wilber A, Hargrove PW, Kim YS, Riberdy JM, Sankaran VG, Papanikolaou E, et al. Therapeutic levels of fetal hemoglobin in erythroid progeny of β-thalassemic CD34+ cells after lentiviral vector-mediated gene transfer. *Blood* (2011) 117: 2817-2826.

[12] Imren S, Payen E, Westerman KA, Pawliuk R, Fabry ME, Eaves CJ, et al. Permanent and panerythroid correction of murine β-thalassemia by multiple lentiviral integration in hematopoietic stem cells. *Proc. Natl. Acad. Sci. USA* 2002; 99: 14380-85.

[13] Miccio A, Cesari R, Lotti F, Rossi C, Sanvito F, Ponzoni M, et al. In vivo selection of genetically modified erythroblastic progenitors leads to long-term correction of β-thalassemia. *Proc. Natl. Acad. Sci. U. S. A.* 2008; 105: 10547-52.

[14] Imren S, Fabry ME, Westerman KA, Pawliuk R, Tang P, Rosten PM. High-level β-globin expression and preferred intragenic integration after lentiviral transduction of human cord blood stem cells. *J. Clin. Invest*. 2004; 114: 953-62.

[15] Roselli EA, Mezzadra R, Frittoli MC, et al. Correction of β-thalassemia major by gene transfer in haematopoietic progenitors of pediatric patients. *EMBO Mol. Med.* 2010; 2(8):315-28.

[16] Mathias LA, Fisher TC, Zeng L, Meiselman HJ, Weinberg KI, Hiti AL et al. (2000). Ineffective erythropoiesis in β-thalassemia major is due to apoptosis at the polychromatophilic normoblast stage. *Exp. Hem*. (28): 1343-1353.

[17] Lee HJ, Kim e, and Kim JS (2010). Targeted chromosomal deletions in human cells using zinc finger nucleases. *Genome Res*. (20): 81–89.

[18] Bauer DE, Kamran SC, Lessard S, Xu J, Fujiwara Y, Lin C, Shao Z, Canver MC, Smith EC, Pinello L, Sabo PJ, Vierstra J, Voit RA, Yuan GC, Porteus MH, Stamatoyannopoulos JA, Lettre G, Orkin SH (2013). An erythroid enhancer of BCL11A subject to genetic variation determines fetal hemoglobin level. *Science* (342): 253-257.

[19] Ma N, Liao B, Zhang H, Wang L, Shan Y, Xue Y, Huang K, Chen S, Zhou X, Chen Y, Pei D, Pan G. Transcription activator-like effector nuclease (TALEN)-mediated gene correction in integration-free β-thalassemia induced pluripotent stem cells. *J. Biol. Chem.* (2013) 288: 34671-34679.

[20] Chang CJ, Bouhassira EE. Zinc-finger nuclease-mediated correction of α-thalassemia in iPS cells. *Blood* (2012) 120: 3906-3914.

[21] Reik A, Chang KH, Stehling-Sun S, Zhou Y, Lee GK, Truong L, Wood T, Zhang Z, Luong A, Chan A, Liu PQ, Miller JC, Paschon DE, Guschin DY, Zhang L, Yannaki E, Giedlin MA, Rebar EJ, Gregory PD, Urnov FD, Papayannopoulou T, and Stamatoyannopoulos G. Targeted Gene Modification In Hematopoietic Stem Cells: A Potential Treatment For Thalassemia and Sickle Cell Anemia. Paper No 434, 55th Annual ASH Meeting, December 2013.

[22] Rols MP, Teissié J. Electropermeabilization of mammalian cells. Quantitative analysis of the phenomenon. *Biophys J.* (1990) 58: 1089-1098.

[23] http://www.clinicaltrials.gov/ct2/show/NCT01044654?term=hiv+and+sangamo&rank=1.

[24] Urnov FD, Rebar EJ, Holmes MC, Zhang HS, Gregory PD. Genome editing with engineered zinc finger nucleases. *Nat. Rev. Genet*. (2010) 11: 636-646.

[25] Hsu PD, Scott DA, Weinstein JA, Ran FA, Konermann S, Agarwala V, et al. DNA targeting specificity of RNA-guided Cas9 nucleases. *Nat. Biotechnol*. (2013) 9: 827-832.

[26] Yu J, et al. Induced pluripotent stem cell lines derived from human somatic cells. *Science* (2007) 318:1917–1920.

[27] Ye L, Chang JC, Lin C, Sun X, Yu J, Kan YW. Induced pluripotent stem cells offer new approach to therapy in thalassemia and sickle cell anemia and option in prenatal diagnosis in genetic diseases. *PNAS* (2009) 106: 9826-9830.

[28] Wang Y, Zheng CG, Jiang Y, Zhang J, Chen J, Yao C, Zhao Q, Liu S, Chen K, Du J, Yang Z, Gao S. Genetic correction of β-thalassemia patient-specific iPS cells and its use in improving hemoglobin production in irradiated SCID mice. *Cell Res.* (2012) 22: 637-648.

[29] Ettinger, W.H., Flotte, T.R., 2011. The role of gene and cell therapy in the era of health care reform. Hum. *Gene Ther.*, 22: 1307-1309.

[30] Papapetrou EP, Lee G, Malani N, Setty M, Riviere I, Tirunagari LM, Kadota K, Roth SL, Giardina P, Viale A, Leslie C, Bushman FD, Studer L, Sadelain M. Genomic safe harbors permit high β-globin transgene expression in thalassemia induced pluripotent stem cells. *Nat. Biotechnol.* (2011) 29: 73-78.

[31] Rivière I, Dunbar CE, Sadelain M. Hematopoietic stem cell engineering at a crossroads. *Blood.* (2012) 119: 1107-1116.

[32] Obokata H, Wakayama T, Sasai Y, Kojima K, Vacanti MP, Niwa H, Yamato M, Vacanti CA. Stimulus-triggered fate conversion of somatic cells into pluripotency. *Nature* (2014) 505: 641-647.

[33] Obokata H, Sasai Y, Niwa H, Kadota M, Andrabi M, Takata N, Tokoro M, Terashita Y, Yonemura S, Vacanti CA, Wakayama T. Bidirectional developmental potential in reprogrammed cells with acquired pluripotency. *Nature* (2014) 505: 676-680.

[34] http://osp.od.nih.gov/sites/default/files/1164_bluebirdbio.pdf.

[35] Cavazzana-Calvo M, Payen E, Negre O, Wang G, Hehir K, Fusil F, Down J, Denaro M, Brady T et al. Transfusion independence and HMGA2 activation after gene therapy of human β-thalassaemia. *Nature.* (2010) 467: 318-322.

In: Thalassemia
Editor: Makenzie Greene
ISBN: 978-1-63117-954-9

Chapter 7

Developments in the Molecular Diagnosis of Beta-Thalassaemia

***Sherry S. Y. Ho*[1*], *Angela N. Barrett*[2], *Mahesh Choolani*[2] and *Evelyn S. C. Koay*[1,3]**

[1]Departments of Laboratory Medicine, Molecular Diagnosis Centre, National University Hospital, Singapore

[2]Departments of Obstetrics & Gynaecology, Yong Loo Lin School of Medicine, National University of Singapore, Singapore

[3]Departments of Pathology, Yong Loo Lin School of Medicine, National University of Singapore, Singapore

Abstract

Beta-thalassaemia (OMIM #613985) is the most common autosomal recessive disorder worldwide. In 2007, 42,409 global conceptions are affected by beta-thalassaemia and half of these occurred in Southeast Asia. To date, there are more than 800 variants in the beta-globin gene out of which more than 280 cause beta-thalassaemia with varying phenotypes (http://globin.bx.psu.edu/hbvar). Molecular diagnosis of these mutations are necessary for establishing proper treatment, disease prognosis and family planning. The development of molecular diagnostic methods to detect beta-thalassaemia is largely dependent on the prevalence and spectrum of mutations in the population. Direct sequencing is the gold standard to detect point mutations in or near the beta-globin gene which cause >90% of beta-thalassaemia defects. Multiplex ligation-dependent probe amplification (MLPA) detects deletions or duplications by quantitative amplification of multiple probe pairs hybridised across the beta-globin gene clusters. Other methods include amplification refractory mutation system (ARMS), reversed dot blot hybridisation (RDBH), and more recently, pyrosequencing in carrier screening and prenatal diagnosis will be described in this review. In prenatal diagnosis, invasive methods of obtaining fetal cells such as amniocentesis and chorionic villus sampling are

* Corresponding author: Dr Sherry Ho Sze Yee, Molecular Diagnosis Centre, Department of Laboratory Medicine, National University Hospital, 5 Lower Kent Ridge Road, Singapore 119074, Tel: 67724294; Fax: 67724407, Email: sherry_sy_ho@nuhs.edu.sg.

necessary. These methods carry up to 1% risk of miscarriage and are unacceptable to some couples. Cell-free fetal DNA from maternal plasma offers an alternative source of fetal genetic material for noninvasive prenatal diagnosis. However, the presence of high levels of maternal DNA impedes the use of conventional methods in detecting mutations in the fetus. Developments including the use of next generation sequencing (NGS) to identify fetal alleles for the detection of beta-thalassaemia mutations amongst a high background maternal alleles will be discussed.

Introduction

Haemoglobinopathies are the most common monogenic disorder worldwide. Amongst the haemoglobinopathies, mutations affecting the beta-globin gene (HBB) lead to the most diverse genetic heterogeneity and phenotypic severity causing beta-thalassaemia. To date, there are more than 800 variants in HBB out of which more than 280 cause beta-thalassaemia with varying genotypes and phenotypes (http://globin.bx.psu.edu/hbvar). HBB, together with the alpha-globin gene (HBA) code for the beta- and alpha- globin chains respectively. In a normal adult haemoglobin, there are two alpha-globin chains (α_2) and two beta-globin chains (β_2) forming a tetramer ($\alpha_2\beta_2$). Mutations in the beta-globin gene will either prevent or decrease the production of beta-globin chains, leading to an imbalance of alpha- and beta-globin chain synthesis. The excess alpha-globin chains cannot form soluble tetramers and instead precipitate and aggregate in erythroid precursors, leading to ineffective erythropoiesis (Weatherall 2001; Khandros et al., 2012; Ribeil et al., 2013). Patients suffer from anaemia which in turn causes extensive proliferation of the spleen and non-functional bone marrow, leading to extensive skeletal deformities, growth retardation and splenomegaly (Cao and Galanello 2010).

Beta-thalassaemias are classified mainly into beta-thalassaemia major (or Cooley's anaemia), beta-thalassaemia minor (or beta-thalassaemia trait), and thalassaemia intermedia. The two genetic defects that produce beta-thalassaemias are (i) nondeletional, where single base substitution or small deletions or insertions occur near or upstream of the beta-globin gene, usually in the promoter regions; (ii) deletional, where larger deletions occur involving the beta-globin gene. The severity of clinical phenotypes for homozygous or compound heterozygous beta-thalassaemia varies. Patients with beta-thalassaemia major inherit two β^0 thalassaemia alleles (homozygous or compound heterozygous states) which result in complete absence of HbA ($\alpha_2\beta_2$). This leads to severe microcytic, hypochromic anaemia that is fatal if left untreated. Conventional therapies consist of splenectomy if enlarged spleen is present, regular blood transfusions which in turn require iron chelation to treat iron overload caused by blood transfusions, and in selected cases, bone marrow transplantation of human leukocyte antigen (HLA)-matched haematopoietic stem cells (Al-Salem 2014; Goss et al., 2014; Fisher et al., 2013; La Nasa et al., 2013). The use of fetal haemoglobin (HbF) inducer drugs including hydroxyurea, histone deacetylase (HDAC) inhibitor agents and new immunomodulator drugs such as pomalidomide, lenalidomide and thalidomide to reduce alpha-globin chain production in erythroid progenitors for improving the alpha:beta chain imbalance was recently introduced (Fard et al., 2013; Musallam et al., 2013). Human gene therapy studies to cure beta-thalassaemia had also been conducted with promising results (Breda et al., 2012; Cavazzana-Calvo et al., 2010; Miccio et al., 2011; Samakoglu et al.,

2006). In recent years, gene therapy together with HbF inducer drugs was proposed as a novel alternative therapeutic approach (Breda et al., 2013; Chandrakasan and Malik 2014; Fucharoen et al., 2013).

In beta-thalassaemia minor, individuals inherit a single beta-thalassaemia allele, whether β^0 or β^+. As only one beta-globin allele is affected with the mutation, most patients with beta-thalassaemia minor are phenotypically 'silent'. Although beta-thalassaemia minor patients are clinically asymptomatic with no or mild anaemia with characteristic hypochromic microcytic red blood cells, elevated levels of HbA2 ($\alpha_2\delta_2$) and variable increases of HbF ($\alpha_2\gamma_2$), screening is important to identify and prevent high-risk marriages and pregnancies (Hashemizadeh and Noori 2013). Patients with beta-thalassaemia intermedia inherit two beta-thalassaemia alleles. Their condition ranges from slightly less severe than transfusion-dependence to asymptomatic, and tend to present later in life with mild anaemia. Occasional blood transfusion may be required depending on the severity of the condition, and cardiac deaths due to renal and cardiac causes are common (Matta et al., 2013). Molecular diagnosis of beta-thalassaemia mutations are therefore important for establishing proper treatment, disease prognosis, as well as family planning. Most variants in the beta-globin gene cluster include single nucleotide polymorphisms (SNPs) and small insertions deletions (INDELs). DNA sequencing is the current gold standard for detecting SNPs and INDELs in beta-thalassaemia. Minisequencing, amplification refractory mutation system (ARMS), reversed dot blot hybridisation (RDBH), arrayed primer extension (APEX), flow-through hybridisation and pyrosequencing are common alternative methods to detect beta-thalassaemia mutations. To detect large deletions, gap-PCR, multiplex ligation-dependent probe amplification (MLPA), array comparative genomic hybridisation (array-CGH), and real-time PCR had been reported and being routinely used in clinical diagnostic laboratories. This review paper will discuss the principles of some of these methods that are routinely used for screening and genotyping.

In prenatal diagnosis, fetal cells are obtained via invasive procedures such as amniocentesis and chorionic villus sampling. In addition to the attendant risk of fetal loss, the invasive nature of the procedures can cause considerable anxiety and stress to the couple. In recent years, next generation sequencing (NGS) technologies had enabled the analysis of cell-free fetal DNA in the maternal plasma, thus allowing noninvasive prenatal testing of common chromosomal aneuploidies. Single gene disorders such as beta-thalassaemia can also be detected noninvasively using the same technologies, which will be described in this review.

Common Molecular Diagnostic Methods for Genetic Screening of Beta-thalassaemia Mutations

DNA Sequencing

DNA sequencing is the process used to determine the nucleotide order of a given DNA fragment, known as the DNA sequence. The target DNA is denatured and annealed to an oligonucleotide primer, which is then extended by DNA polymerase using a mixture of deoxynucleotide triphosphates (normal dNTPs) and chain-terminating dideoxynucleotide triphosphates (ddNTPs). ddNTPs lack the 3'-OH group to which the next dNTP of the growing DNA chain is added. Without the 3'-OH group, nucleotides can no longer be added and the DNA polymerase dissociates and falls off. The resulting newly synthesised DNA chains will be a mixture of different lengths. Dye terminator sequencing technique, which is a cheaper and faster alternative to the chain termination method (Sanger sequencing) is now commonly used in diagnostic laboratories. In dye terminator sequencing, each ddNTP (ddG, ddA, ddT or ddC) is labeled with a different fluorescent dye, which fluoresces at a different wavelength that is activated and captured by an automated genetic analyser. This labeling of each dideoxynucleotide chain-terminators with a separate fluorescent dye enables visualisation of the DNA sequence by the genetic analyser. As the majority of beta-thalassaemia mutations are point mutations including single nucleotide substitutions and small insertions and deletions, DNA sequencing is the most common direct method of detecting beta-thalassaemia mutations. In our laboratory, beta-thalassaemia mutations including the common IVS-II-654 (C>T), Codons 41/42 (-TCTT), Hb Malay/ Cd19 (T>C), Codons 8/9 (+G), Hb S(A>T), CAP+1 (A>C), and Codons 71/72(+A) are targeted by DNA sequencing. Gap-PCR amplifies an intact beta-globin gene fragment and/or a 619 bp deletion junction fragment (NG_000007.3:g.71609_72227del619) with the use of a common forward primer and two reverse primers (Wang et al., 2003). In the presence or absence of a 619 bp deletion, an amplicon of 1671 or 1457 bp will be detected on gel electrophoresis respectively. Therefore, the presence of both amplicons would indicate that a sample is heterozygous for the 619 bp deletion. The bands are then excised, purified using the QIAquick Gel Extraction Kit (Qiagen, GmbH, Hilden, Germany), and cycle sequenced using the BigDye Terminator v3.1 Cycle Sequencing Kit (Applied Biosystems, ThermoFisher Scientific, Waltham, Massachusetts, USA) before capillary chemistry separation using the ABI3130xl Genetic Analyzer (Applied Biosystems) according to the manufacturers' recommendations. Data analysis to detect mutations is performed using SeqScape® Software v3.0 (Applied Biosystems). DNA sequencing is suitable for detecting point mutations, small deletions and insertions, as well as to confirm or to characterise rare or new Hb variants. However, for deletional mutations involving large regions such as HBB:c.-74_31del, with a 105 bp deletion, or a 619 bp deletion in NG_000007.3:g.71609_72227del619, direct DNA sequencing is not the optimal method of detection.

Amplification Refractory Mutation System (ARMS)

ARMS is a simple method to detect any known mutation involving single base changes or small deletions. It was first described by Newton et al. (1989) and developed to detect common beta-thalassaemia mutations found in all main ethnic groups (Meena et al., 2013; Miri-Moghaddam et al., 2013; Newton et al., 1989; Sahoo, Biswal, and Dixit 2014). Sequence-specific PCR primers were designed to amplify DNA only when the target al.lele is present. Therefore, the presence or absence of a PCR product is equivalent to the presence or absence of the target al.lele (Little 2001). With its direct detection of amplified products by gel electrophoresis, common beta-thalassaemia mutations can be detected rapidly with high accuracy (Tan et al., 1994). Combine-ARMS (c-ARMS) and multiplex-ARMS (MARMS) were an extension of ARMS that were developed to detect multiple beta-thalassaemia mutations within a single PCR reaction. This reduces the assay turnaround time and improves cost-effectiveness for molecular diagnosis of common beta-thalassaemia mutations (Hassan et al., 2013; Tan et al., 2001).

Multiplex Ligation-Dependent Probe Amplification (MLPA)

MLPA is designed to detect deletions or duplications using quantitative amplification of multiple probe pairs that are hybridized across the alpha- and beta- globin gene clusters and neighbouring regions. Universal tags are hybridised to each ligated primer set, which differ in length among each other, before amplification using a labeled universal PCR primer. The resulting amplicons differ in length and are separated by an automated fragment analyser which detects each amplicon by quantifying the fluorescence of each probe. The decrease or increase in signals as compared to a normal reference is indicative of the deletions or duplications respectively, across the locus analyzed. MLPA is usually used as a supplementary method to gap-PCR when studying known or unknown rearrangements (Harteveld 2013). There are two types of commercial MLPA kits for each of the alpha- and beta- globin gene clusters. The kit from MRC-Holland bv (Amsterdam, The Netherlands, www.mlpa.com) utilise cloned cosmid probes, which are restricted to the alpha- and beta-gene cluster and to the regulatory elements (respectively, P140B2 and P102B). The kit from LGTC (Leiden Genome Technology Center, Leiden, The Netherlands, www.LGTC.nl) makes use of oligonucleotide probes designed over a larger region allowing the detection of both smaller and more extensive deletions involving the alpha- and beta- globin gene cluster and neighbouring regions (respectively HBA- and HBB- MLPA kit; Leiden Genome Technology Center, Leiden, The Netherlands).

Reversed Dot Blot Hybridisation (RDBH)

RDBH is a technique for hybridising amplified DNA to short allele-specific oligonucleotide (ASO) probes bound on a nylon membrane for radioactive, chemical or enzymatic detection. The hybridisation conditions can be adjusted so that a single base pair mismatch can be discriminated using multiple pairs of mutant and normal ASO probes. RDBH was subsequently developed for detection of genes with a high mutation spectrum such as beta-thalassaemia (Saiki et al., 1988; Saiki et al., 1985). Multiplex allele specific diagnostic assay (MASDA) enables characterisation of a variety of mutations in the same locus, which is useful for beta-thalassaemia screening. Today, RDBHs are most often arrayed so that the normal oligonucleotide probes sit on a line adjacent to each other, while variant probes are not on the same line. This permits rapid interpretation of heterozygotes where one normal and one variant allele are indicated. However, where two mutations are close to each other and fall within the sequence of the ASO such as HbA, HbS and HbC, a different pattern is obtained (Gold 2003).

Pyrosequencing

Pyrosequencing is a real-time sequencing-by-synthesis method that enables rapid (SNPs analysis of short DNA sequences. In pyrosequencing, the annealing of a dispensed nucleotide with the template during synthesis will cause the release of a pyrophosphate which is converted to fluorescence emission through a series of enzymatic reactions. The fluorescence emission is measured to determine the amounts of synthesised nucleotide molecules, hence, determining the sequence of the template. Timbs et al. (2012) described the use of pyrosequencing in the prenatal diagnosis of 12 common nondeletional alpha- and beta- globin gene mutations in the UK population (Timbs et al., 2012). Recently, we developed a pyrosequencing-based panel targeting 27 most common nondeletional and deletional beta-thalassemia mutations in Singapore, and was able to achieve 100% sensitivity (lower 95% CI, 97.8%) and 100% specificity (lower 95% CI, 92.4%) (Ho et al., 2013).

Noninvasive Prenatal Testing for Beta-thalassaemia

Prenatal diagnosis is an essential part of obstetric practice, and genetic diagnosis is currently offered to women at risk of carrying a fetus with an aneuploidy, either predicted by a high risk Down's syndrome screening result or due to fetal abnormalities seen on a scan (Nicolaides 2004), or to couples who are known to be carriers of a particular single gene disorder. Prenatal diagnosis of fetal genetic status or aneuploidy depends on the use of invasive diagnostic tests to collect a sample of the baby's genetic material. Amniocentesis (taking fluid from around the baby) and chorion villus sampling (CVS) (taking a small sample from the placenta) carry a small but significant risk of miscarriage of around 1% (Tabor and Alfirevic 2010). Additionally, these techniques cannot be performed until after 11 weeks of gestation, which may give rise to increased parental anxiety, particularly if the parents are known carriers of a disorder or have a previously affected child (Alfirevic, Sundberg, and Brigham 2003).

Because of the risk to the fetus, a major goal in prenatal diagnosis has been to develop methods to carry out the tests noninvasively using a maternal blood sample. Initial studies focused on diagnosis from fetal cells, but this has proven to be technically challenging due to the fact that these cells are very difficult to isolate (Bianchi 2010). Additionally, many types of fetal cells persist in the mother's body for years after the pregnancy, and so are not pregnancy-specific (Rust and Bianchi 2009). The discovery that circulating cell-free fetal DNA (cffDNA) exists in maternal plasma has laid the groundwork for the development of noninvasive methods for safer prenatal diagnosis (Lo et al., 1997). Noninvasive prenatal testing (NIPT) using (cffDNA), originating from the placenta (Alberry et al., 2009), provides an alternative means of prenatal diagnosis that does not carry a risk of miscarriage. Cell-free fetal DNA circulates alongside cell-free maternal DNA in maternal plasma from as early as 5 weeks gestation (Birch et al., 2005), constitutes around 10% of the total cell-free DNA (cfDNA) (Lun, Chiu, et al., 2008), and is made up of small fragments with an average length of 143 bp, 23 bp less than maternal DNA, which has an average length of 166 bp (Lo et al., 2010). Of great significance for prenatal diagnosis is the fact that cffDNA is rapidly cleared from maternal circulation with a very short half-life of sixteen minutes, and thus, is usually undetectable two hours after birth (Lo et al., 1999).

NIPT is already available for some indications such as fetal sex determination using Y chromosome sequences in women at risk of X-linked disorders (Finning and Chitty 2008) and the testing of Rhesus D (RhD) negative women at risk of haemolytic disease of the fetus and newborn (HDFN) (van der Schoot, Hahn, and Chitty 2008). Sensitivity and specificity are close to 100% (Devaney et al., 2011; Zhu et al., 2014), and these tests are relatively straightforward, since a sequence unique to the fetus is being detected. The use of NIPT for Down's syndrome diagnosis was first reported in 2008 (Chiu et al., 2008; Fan et al., 2008) and a huge number of large-scale validity studies had been conducted to evaluate testing based on massively parallel sequencing (Chiu et al., 2011; Palomaki et al., 2011; Bianchi et al., 2012; Dan et al., 2012). Targeted approaches to aneuploidy testing are also being developed (Sparks et al., 2012; Zimmermann et al., 2012) providing a more cost-effective route to aneuploidy testing. NIPT tests for Down's syndrome are now available commercially in some countries and more widespread clinical implementation is underway (Chitty et al., 2012). NIPT for aneuploidy is not considered fully diagnostic as the small but significant rate of false-positives means that an invasive test is still required to confirm a screen-positive result (Benn et al., 2012; Grati et al., 2014; Benn et al., 2013).

One of the disadvantages of the high maternal background is that it is very difficult to distinguish maternal from fetal alleles. Initial studies were confined to detection of paternally inherited or sporadic disorders, identifying mutations absent from the mother's DNA, but contributed to the cfDNA by the fetus. A number of paternally inherited disorders have been examined (Lench et al., 2013) using techniques including PCR (Meaney and Norbury 2009), quantitative fluorescence-PCR (QF-PCR) (Gonzalez-Gonzalez et al., 2008; Gonzalez-Gonzalez, Trujillo, Rodriguez de Alba, Garcia-Hoyos, et al., 2003; Gonzalez-Gonzalez, Trujillo, Rodriguez de Alba, and Ramos 2003), quantitative real-time PCR (qPCR) (Au et al., 2011), coamplification at lower denaturation temperature-PCR (COLD-PCR) (Galbiati et al., 2011), and Snapshot sequencing (Bustamante-Aragones, Vallespin, et al., 2008). Sporadic disorders are similarly amenable to testing (Chitty et al., 2011; Saito et al., 2000; Li et al., 2004; Chitty et al., 2013)

Noninvasive prenatal diagnosis (NIPD) for autosomal recessive or maternally transmitted autosomal dominant disorders is more complicated. First attempts involved the exclusion of the paternal mutation in autosomal recessive conditions where the parents were carriers of different mutations. If a paternally identified allele can be detected, there is a 50% risk that the fetus will inherit the disorder, and therefore invasive testing would be recommended. Alternatively, in the absence of a paternal allele, the fetus would be a carrier at worst, and invasive testing would not be necessary. A number of publications had demonstrated that paternal exclusion is readily achieved (Chiu, Lau, Cheung, et al., 2002; Bustamante-Aragones, Gallego-Merlo, et al., 2008; Bustamante-Aragones, Perez-Cerda, et al., 2008; Ho et al., 2010; Papasavva et al., 2006; Papasavva et al., 2013). However, in the 50% of cases where the fetus has inherited the paternal allele, an invasive test is still required. Therefore the ultimate goal of future research is to remove the requirement for any invasive testing regardless of the parental mutations.

NIPT for Exclusion of Paternally Inherited Beta-thalassaemia Mutations

Due to the fact that the thalassaemias are the most common single gene disorders worldwide, many groups are focussing their efforts on developing NIPD for these conditions. More than 280 mutations had been identified for beta-thalassaemia, and the distribution of these varies by geographical area (Henderson et al., 2009). There had been a number of publications describing exclusion of the paternal mutation, which will remove the need for an invasive test in 50% of high-risk pregnancies.

The first report of noninvasive prenatal testing for beta-thalassaemia used allele specific PCR primers and a fluorescent probe to detect paternal inheritance of the Codons 41/42 (-TCTT) mutant allele using qPCR (Chiu, Lau, Leung, et al., 2002). Of eight cases tested, the mutation was excluded in two and detected in the remaining six. Real-time allele-specific PCR (RT-ASPCR) was used by Tungwiwat et al., to determine paternal inheritance in 60 plasma samples (Tungwiwat et al., 2006). In all cases, this simple method using standard PCR protocols provided a correct result.

Ding et al. used a single allele base extension reaction (SABER) followed by mass spectrometry (MS) to exclude paternal inheritance of the four most common Southeast Asian beta-thalassaemia mutations (Ding et al., 2004). This method was found to be more sensitive than standard base extension, since only the mutant allele was being analysed, and in fact was successful in all 11 cases tested. Additionally they used haplotype analysis to determine informative paternal SNPs in a further case where both parents were carriers of the Codons 41/42 (-TCTT) mutation. SABER detected the paternal allele. The main drawback to this approach is that haplotyping is not always possible, since the father is not always known or available for typing. Furthermore, DNA is required from grandparents who may live a great distance away or already deceased. Another study indicated that size fractionation prior to the SABER reaction may improve the signal detection by MS, but this was only carried out in one sample. One of the main disadvantages to the SABER-MS technique is that it is expensive, and requires sophisticated equipment not available to all laboratories, particularly those in developing countries.

Size selection was also used to isolate fetal DNA, followed by PCR using primers containing a peptide-nucleic-acid (PNA) clamp to suppress amplification of the wild type maternal allele. Allele-specific PCR was then performed to detect the paternal allele, which showed a high sensitivity and specificity for the detection of four beta-thalassaemia mutations (Li et al., 2005). Advantages to this approach include the fact that it is cheap, and relatively simple to perform. However, extensive handling of the samples is required, with consequent potential for sample contamination during the size selection procedure. Galbiati et al. proposed using a PNA clamp PCR strategy coupled with use of a microelectronic chip containing fluorescent-labeled probes specific for wild type and mutant alleles (Galbiati et al., 2008), achieving correct classifications in 41/41 samples. They also successfully classified 27/28 of these samples using Sanger sequencing and 4/4 using pyrosequencing. Despite these successes, they concluded that establishing the optimal PNA concentration for each target is time-consuming, and so the technique may not be applicable to high-throughput scenarios or in cases where a large number of mutations need to be screened.

COLD-PCR has been shown to be effective at diagnosing mutations in the beta-globin gene (HBB) that are causative for beta-thalassaemia (Galbiati et al., 2011). This technique makes use of the fact that there are melting temperature differences between mutant and wild type sequences, and uses a critical denaturation temperature lower than the melting temperature to specifically amplify the mutant alleles (Li et al., 2008). Thirty-five samples were Sanger sequenced following COLD-PCR, and the inheritance status of the paternal allele was correctly diagnosed in all cases. Similar to the PNA clamp approach, extensive optimisation is needed for each primer set. A high resolution melting (HRM) technique was used to detect a number of paternal thalassaemia mutations from 32 pregnancies at risk of beta-thalassaemia, as well as from 57 pregnancies at risk of sickle cell anaemia (HbS mutation) (Yenilmez, Tuli, and Evruke 2013).

Papasavva et al. had been developing SNP-based approaches for detection of beta-thalassaemia in the Cypriot population (Papasavva et al., 2006; Papasavva et al., 2013; Papasavva et al., 2008). In their preliminary studies, 11 informative SNPs linked to the beta-thalassaemia locus with a high degree of heterozygosity in the Cypriot population were assessed. Arrayed Primer Extension (APEX) was carried out on a microarray chip (known as a thalassochip) consisting of oligonucleotide probes specific for informative SNPs and common Mediterranean mutations on a solid support (Papasavva et al., 2008). They were able to correctly determine inheritance of the mutant paternal allele in six out of seven cases, but highlighted the need for a large number of SNPs to be screened to obtain at least 2-3 informative ones for accurate classification. Of the 34 families that were initially tested, 11 had one informative SNP or fewer, and so the test could not be used in these patients. More recently, next generation sequencing (NGS) was used to sequence four SNPs located in the beta-thalassaemia locus in ten plasma samples where parental haplotypes were known (Papasavva et al., 2013). Six sites could not be used, since the mother was heterozygous for these SNPs. Of the 34 examined SNPs, 27 cases were concordant with CVS results. Thus, eight cfDNA samples were correctly classified using SNPs correlating with previously identified paternal haplotype. It was concluded that more than four SNPs and more replicates should be used to develop a reliable assay using this methodology.

Pyrophosphorolysis-activated polymerisation (PAP) was used to detect paternally-inherited alleles based on twelve informative SNPs within the beta-globin gene cluster (Phylipsen et al., 2012). PAP makes use of oligonucleotides with a blocked 3' end that can be removed to allow extension when annealed to a specific sequence. A variant within 16 nucleotides of the 3' end will prevent binding, and therefore a specific sequence can be detected using a primer specific for that SNP. Dilution of plasma DNA confirmed that the assay was sensitive down to 3% for a particular SNP. Detection of paternally-inherited SNPs was shown in plasma from 13 couples, and a proof-of-principle NIPD was carried out in one additional case where a previous unaffected child was available for association of the SNP with the wild type paternal HbS (sickle cell) allele; it was found that the fetus had inherited the SNP associated with the normal paternal allele, and this was confirmed by CVS. This method is low cost and a single amplicon can be used to test a number of mutations. However, a major limitation is that a previous child or another family member is required for linkage of the SNP to the mutant allele. There is a recombination hotspot between the beta- and delta- globin genes, and so if an informative SNP is not available within the beta-globin gene itself, two SNPs should be used, one on either side of the hotspot.

Excluding inheritance of paternal mutations allows us to avoid an invasive procedure in fifty percent of pregnancies; more complicated techniques are required to determine maternal inheritance, since it is impossible to differentiate the maternal from the fetal alleles.

Techniques for Determining Inheritance of Maternal Alleles

A quantitative approach to NIPD where both parents carry the same mutation known as Relative Mutation Dosage (RMD) was developed for beta-thalassaemia and haemoglobin E (HbE) mutations using digital PCR (dPCR) (Lun, Tsui, et al., 2008). Template DNA is diluted to an average concentration of less than one molecule per well, and thousands of replicates of a PCR reaction are analysed using digital PCR (Vogelstein and Kinzler 1999). Because most positive wells contain one or fewer molecules, counting allows quantification of the initial number of molecules in the DNA sample. Primers and probes specific for the mutant and wild type alleles were designed, and 12 panel digital PCR arrays (Dube, Qin, and Ramakrishnan 2008) were used to run thousands of duplex PCR reactions for each sample. If a woman is heterozygous for a particular allele and the fetus is also a heterozygote, it is expected that there will be an allelic balance between the wild type and mutant alleles; if the fetus is homozygous for either the mutant or the wild type allele there will be an over-representation of the respective allele. A statistical test known as sequential probability ratio testing (SPRT) can be used to assess whether the counts from the digital PCR are balanced or whether there is an imbalance for the over-represented allele. Using RMD, Lun et al. looked at two different beta-thalassaemia mutations in ten patients and were able to correctly classify five of these (Lun, Tsui, et al., 2008). This technique is dependent upon accurate quantification of fetal fraction, since the degree of over-representation will be greater when there is a higher fetal component to the plasma DNA. This can be easily determined in male fetuses using Y chromosome sequences, but in cases where there is a female fetus we rely on detection of paternally inherited SNPs or insertion/deletion (indel) polymorphisms (Barrett et al., 2012). In cases where the fetal fraction is relatively low, and the degree of over-representation is smaller, the number of counts required for an accurate classification will increase (Lun, Tsui, et al., 2008), and therefore more digital PCR chips per sample are required. With the advent of droplet digital PCR technology (Hindson et al., 2011) it may be possible to do RMD more accurately, since a single reaction can produce 20,000 counts. However, this technology has not yet been extensively validated clinically. In addition, digital PCR requires a separate probe for each wild type and each mutant allele making this approach expensive, particularly in the case of beta-thalassaemia, where there are more than 280 potential mutations.

A more high-throughput method that can be used for screening all known mutations is NGS. Using NGS it was shown that the entire fetal genome is represented in maternal plasma (Lo et al., 2010). In a sample from a woman whose partner carried the Codons 41/42 (-TCTT) deletion it was possible to directly detect that the paternal deletion had been inherited. Relative Haplotype Dosage (RHDO) was then used to assess whether, having inherited a paternal Codons 41/42 (-TCTT) mutation, the fetus had also inherited the maternal -28A>G mutation. A SNP Array covering 900,000 SNPs was used to identify the SNPs on maternal and paternal genomic DNA, and SNPs were classified into different categories, the category with the father being homozygous and the mother being heterozygous for a particular SNP being chosen for determining inheritance. The maternal mutation was found to be on HapII; RHDO showed that there was an over-representation of HapI, indicating that the fetus had inherited the maternal wild-type allele, and was therefore only a carrier of beta-thalassaemia.

To overcome the problems of expense associated with whole genome sequencing followed by RHDO, it was shown that a targeted approach in which only the region of interest is captured can be implemented (Lam et al., 2012). Using over 54,000 biotinylated probes for in-solution capture, the HBB gene as well as SNPs within a 288 kb region were captured and sequenced. Two samples were examined, first of all with respect to inheritance of the paternal mutation. In the first family, the fetus had inherited the Codons 41/42 (-TCTT) mutation from the father, but in family 2, the paternal CD17(A>T) had not been inherited. Using RHDO it was then shown that in family 1 the maternal -28A>T mutation had not been inherited, whereas in family 2 the Codons 41/42 (-TCTT) maternal mutation had been inherited; therefore both fetuses were carriers of beta-thalassameia. This method still requires extensive work to haplotype the parents using digital PCR, but does not require DNA from the grandparents. Using newer techniques it may be possible to carry out the haplotyping in a simpler fashion. 93.8% of the probes included in the hybridisation were targeted to chromosomes 7, 13, 18, 21 and X, suggesting that using this method a single gene disorder can be screened at the same time as an aneuploidy.

Psychosocial Aspects to NIPT for Thalassaemia

For implementation of noninvasive testing into clinical practice it is essential that social and ethical issues are taken into consideration. There is a growing body of work demonstrating that women have positive attitudes to the introduction of noninvasive tests for both aneuploidies and single gene disorders (Lewis et al., 2012; Lewis, Silcock, and Chitty 2013; Lewis, Hill, and Chitty 2014; Hill et al., 2012; Kooij, Tymstra, and Berg 2009; Tischler et al., 2011; Yotsumoto et al., 2012; Friel, Czerwinski, and Singletary 2013; Verweij et al., 2013). Understandably, women tend to focus on the advantages and disadvantages to the individual, prioritising safety to the fetus, improvements to decision making, management of pregnancy, and preparation for birth of an affected child (Skirton and Patch 2013), whereas health professionals indicated concerns that noninvasive testing may lead to change in attitude to the fetus and to the disabled. Recently, two studies conducted in the UK have looked at the attitudes of women (Lewis, Hill, and Chitty 2014) and health professionals (Hill et al., 2013) to the introduction of NIPD for thalassaemia as well as two other common autosomal recessive conditions, cystic fibrosis (CF) and sickle cell disease. Views of NIPD were extremely positive and demonstrate that carriers of thalassaemia would value a safe test that was available early in pregnancy. This work showed that uptake of prenatal testing was likely to increase, as women who have previously declined invasive testing expressed interest in having NIPD; for example, women who have conceived through the use of assisted reproductive technology, or for women of advanced maternal age, there is often a particular reluctance to risk harming the precious fetus, and so they would be more amenable to testing with NIPD.

One of the major concerns regarding aneuploidy for NIPT has been the idea that testing could become routinized, and therefore women may not be aware of the implications of consenting to the test. It is possible that this could also apply to testing for single gene disorders. One scenario presented by Deans et al. (Deans et al., 2013) is of a woman who was unaware that she is a carrier of a haemoglobinopathy until she was pregnant. Whilst still processing this information, she was offered NIPT for her current pregnancy and accepted the test as 'just another blood test" without full consideration. She did not realised the implications of a positive result for continuation of her pregnancy. Another possibility is that the woman's partner may decline carrier screening. Although she has the right to continue with noninvasive testing of the fetus if she is identified as a positive carrier, her partner also has a right not to know his own result (Gilbar, 2007). This moral dilemma will also exist if an invasive test is carried out, but it is possible that the ease with which the noninvasive test can be performed will prevent the couple from discussing the options fully. These two situations highlighted the fact that, as with NIPT for aneuploidy, comprehensive genetic counselling should be given before offering NIPD to a couple at risk of a single gene disorder.

Conclusion

Molecular diagnosis of beta-thalassaemia mutations has evolved with the advent of new technologies throughout the decades. The wide variety of mutations consisting of short insertions, deletions, single base pair substitutions, large insertions and deletions, and duplications allow many different platforms to be tested for diagnosis. New test developments have reduced the assay turnaround time and improve cost-effectiveness in genetic screening, which are important for prenatal diagnosis. With the progress in technologies for NIPT using cffDNA from the maternal plasma, we envisioned that amniocentesis or CVS to detect beta-thalassaemia mutations in the fetus will become a thing of the past.

Table 1. Methods used for NIPD

Testing Method	Mutations Examined	Number of Cases	Outcomes Correct	Reference
Allele-specific qPCR	CD41/42(-CTTT)	8	8/8	(Chiu, Lau, Leung, et al., 2002)
Allele-specific qPCR	HbE CD41/42(-CTTT) Cd17(A>T)	39 12 9	39/39 12/12 9/9	(Tungwiwat et al., 2006)
HRM analysis	Cap +22(G>A) IVSI-1(G>A) IVSI05(G>A) IVSI-6(T>C) IVSI-110(G>A) CD8(-AA) CD9/10(+T) CD15(G>A) CD39(C>T) IVSII-1(G>A) IVSII-745(C>G)	32	32/32	(Yenilmez, Tuli, and Evruke 2013)
SABER-MS	CD41/42 (-CTTT) IVS2 654(C>T) nt -28A>G CD17(A>T) M&F CD41/42	6 3 1 1 1	6/6 3/3 1/1 1/1 1/1	(Ding et al., 2004)
Size selection & PNA clamp followed by allele-specific qPCR	IVSI-1(G>A) IVSI-6(T>C) IVSI-110(G>A) CD39(C>T)	7 4 5 16	6/7 4/4 5/5 13/16 (2 inc., 1 excluded)	(Li et al., 2005)

Testing Method	Mutations Examined	Number of Cases	Outcomes Correct	Reference
PNA clamp followed by microchip analysis using fluorescent probes	IVSI-110(G>A) CD39(C>T) IVSI-6(T>C) Lepore Boston IVSII-745(C>G) IVSI-1(G>A)	14 8 7 4 3 3	14/14 8/8 7/7 4/4 3/3 3/3	(Galbiati et al., 2008)
APEX	rs10837631A>T	7	6/7 (1FN)	(Papasavva et al., 2008)
Targeted NGS	rs3834466 rs968857 rs10768683 rs7480526	9 10 8 7	6/9 (2FN and 1FP) 7/10 (2FP and 1 FN) 7/8 (1FP) 7/7	(Papasavva et al., 2013)
PAP	HbS	1	1/1	(Phylipsen et al., 2012)
COLD-PCR	IVSI-110(G>A) CD39(C>T)	14 21	14/14 21/21	(Galbiati et al., 2011)
Relative Mutation Dosage using dPCR	CD41/42(-CTTT) HbE (G>A)	5 5	3/5 (1FN and 1 inc.) 2/5 (3 inc)	(Lun, Tsui, et al., 2008)
MPS	F: CD41/42(-CTTT), M: -28(A>T)	1	1/1	(Lo et al., 2010)
In solution target capture followed by MPS	F: CD41/42(-CTTT), M: -28A>T F: CD17(A>T), M: CD41/42 (-CTTT)	1 1	1/1 1/1	(Lam et al., 2012)

M- Mother's mutation, F – Father's mutation, FN – false negative, FP – false positive, Inc. - inconclusive

References

Al-Salem, A. H. (2014). Splenectomy for Children With Thalassemia: Total or Partial Splenectomy, Open or Laparoscopic Splenectomy. *J Pediatr Hematol Oncol*.

Alberry, M. S., Maddocks, D. G., Hadi, M. A., Metawi, H., Hunt, L. P., Abdel-Fattah, S. A., Avent, N. D. & Soothill, P. W. (2009). Quantification of cell free fetal DNA in maternal plasma in normal pregnancies and in pregnancies with placental dysfunction. *Am J Obstet Gynecol*, *200*, 98 e1-6.

Alfirevic, Z., Sundberg, K. & Brigham, S. (2003). Amniocentesis and chorionic villus sampling for prenatal diagnosis. *Cochrane Database Syst Rev*, CD003252.

Au, P. K., Kwok, Y. K., Leung, K. Y., Tang, L. Y., Tang, M. H. & Lau, E. T. (2011). Detection of the S252W mutation in fibroblast growth factor receptor 2 (FGFR2) in fetal DNA from maternal plasma in a pregnancy affected by Apert syndrome. *Prenat Diagn*, *31*, 218-20.

Barrett, A. N., McDonnell, T. C., Chan, K. C. & Chitty, L. S. (2012). Digital PCR Analysis of Maternal Plasma for Noninvasive Detection of Sickle Cell Anemia. *Clin Chem*.

Benn, P., Borell, A., Chiu, R., Cuckle, H., Dugoff, L., Faas, B., Gross, S., Johnson, J., Maymon, R., Norton, M., et al. (2013). Position statement from the Aneuploidy

Screening Committee on behalf of the Board of the International Society for Prenatal Diagnosis. *Prenat Diagn*, *33*, 622-9.

Benn, P., Borrell, A., Cuckle, H., Dugoff, L., Gross, S., Johnson, JA., Maymon, R., Odibo, A., Schielen, P., Spencer, K., et al. (2012). Prenatal Detection of Down Syndrome using Massively Parallel Sequencing (MPS): a rapid response statement from a committee on behalf of the Board of the International Society for Prenatal Diagnosis, 24 October 2011. *Prenat Diagn*, *32*, 1-2.

Bianchi, D. W. (2010). From Michael to microarrays: 30 years of studying fetal cells and nucleic acids in maternal blood. *Prenat Diagn*, *30*, 622-3.

Bianchi, D. W., Platt, L. D., Goldberg, J. D., Abuhamad, A. Z., Sehnert, A. J. & Rava, R. P. (2012). Genome-wide fetal aneuploidy detection by maternal plasma DNA sequencing. Obstet *Gynecol*, *119*, 890-901.

Birch, L., English, C. A., O'Donoghue, K., Barigye, O., Fisk, N. M. & Keer, J. T. (2005). Accurate and robust quantification of circulating fetal and total DNA in maternal plasma from 5 to 41 weeks of gestation. *Clin Chem*, *51*, 312-20.

Breda, L., Casu, C., Gardenghi, S., Bianchi, N., Cartegni, L., Narla, M., Yazdanbakhsh, K., Musso, M., Manwani, D., Little, J., et al. (2012). Therapeutic hemoglobin levels after gene transfer in beta-thalassemia mice and in hematopoietic cells of beta-thalassemia and sickle cells disease patients. *PLoS One*, *7*, e32345.

Breda, L., Rivella, S., Zuccato, C. & Gambari, R. (2013). Combining gene therapy and fetal hemoglobin induction for treatment of beta-thalassemia. *Expert Rev Hematol*, *6*, 255-64.

Bustamante-Aragones, A., Gallego-Merlo, J., Trujillo-Tiebas, M. J., de, Alba, M. R., Gonzalez-Gonzalez, C., Glover, G., Diego-Alvarez, D., Ayuso, C. & Ramos, C. (2008). New strategy for the prenatal detection/exclusion of paternal cystic fibrosis mutations in maternal plasma. *J Cyst Fibros*, *7*, 505-10.

Bustamante-Aragones, A., Perez-Cerda, C., Perez, B., de, Alba, M. R., Ugarte, M. & Ramos, C. (2008). Prenatal diagnosis in maternal plasma of a fetal mutation causing propionic acidemia. *Mol Genet Metab*, *95*, 101-3.

Bustamante-Aragones, A., Vallespin, E., Rodriguez, de, Alba, M., Trujillo-Tiebas, M. J., Gonzalez-Gonzalez, C., Diego-Alvarez, D., Riveiro-Alvarez, R., Lorda-Sanchez, I., Ayuso, C. & Ramos, C. (2008). Early noninvasive prenatal detection of a fetal CRB1 mutation causing Leber congenital amaurosis. *Mol Vis*, *14*, 1388-94.

Cao, A. & Galanello, R. (2010). Beta-thalassemia. *Genet Med*, *12*, 61-76.

Cavazzana-Calvo, M., Payen, E., Negre, O., Wang, G., Hehir, K., Fusil, F., Down, J., Denaro, M., Brady, T., Westerman, K., et al. (2010). Transfusion independence and HMGA2 activation after gene therapy of human beta-thalassaemia. *Nature*, *467*, 318-22.

Chandrakasan, S & Malik, P. (2014). Gene Therapy for Hemoglobinopathies: The State of the Field and the Future. *Hematol Oncol Clin North Am*, *28*, 199-216.

Chitty, L. S., Griffin, D. R., Meaney, C., Barrett, A., Khalil, A., Pajkrt, E. & Cole, T. J. (2011). New aids for the non-invasive prenatal diagnosis of achondroplasia: dysmorphic features, charts of fetal size and molecular confirmation using cell-free fetal DNA in maternal plasma. *Ultrasound Obstet Gynecol*, *37*, 283-9.

Chitty, L. S., Hill, M., White, H., Wright, D. & Morris, S. (2012). Non-invasive prenatal testing for aneuploidy-ready for prime time? *Am J Obstet Gynecol*, *206*, 269-75.

Chitty, L. S., Khalil, A., Barrett, A. N., Pajkrt, E., Griffin, D. R. & Cole, T. J. (2013). Safe, accurate, prenatal diagnosis of thanatophoric dysplasia using ultrasound and free fetal DNA. *Prenat Diagn*, *33*, 416-23.

Chiu, R. W., Akolekar, R., Zheng, Y. W., Leung, T. Y., Sun, H., Chan, K. C., Lun, F. M., Go, A. T., Lau, E. T., To, W. W., et al. (2011). Non-invasive prenatal assessment of trisomy 21 by multiplexed maternal plasma DNA sequencing: large scale validity study. *BMJ*, *342*, c7401.

Chiu, R. W., Chan, K. C., Gao, Y., Lau, V. Y., Zheng, W., Leung, T. Y., Foo, C. H., Xie, B., Tsui, N. B., Lun, F. M., et al. (2008). Noninvasive prenatal diagnosis of fetal chromosomal aneuploidy by massively parallel genomic sequencing of DNA in maternal plasma. *Proc Natl Acad Sci U S A*, *105*, 20458-63.

Chiu, R. W., Lau, T. K., Cheung, P. T., Gong, Z. Q., Leung, T. N. & Lo, Y. M. (2002). Noninvasive prenatal exclusion of congenital adrenal hyperplasia by maternal plasma analysis: a feasibility study. *Clin Chem*, *48*, 778-80.

Chiu, R. W., Lau, T. K., Leung, T. N., Chow, K. C., Chui, D. H. & Lo, Y. M. (2002). Prenatal exclusion of beta thalassaemia major by examination of maternal plasma. *Lancet*, *360*, 998-1000.

Dan, S., Wang, W., Ren, J., Li, Y., Hu, H., Xu, Z., Lau, T. K., Xie, J., Zhao, W., Huang, H., et al. (2012). Clinical application of massively parallel sequencing-based prenatal noninvasive fetal trisomy test for trisomies 21 and 18 in 11,105 pregnancies with mixed risk factors. *Prenat Diagn*, *32*, 1225-32.

Deans, Z., Hill, M., Chitty, L. S. & Lewis, C. (2013). Non-invasive prenatal testing for single gene disorders: exploring the ethics. *Eur J Hum Genet*, *21*, 713-8.

Devaney, S. A., Palomaki, G. E., Scott, J. A. & Bianchi, D. W. (2011). Noninvasive fetal sex determination using cell-free fetal DNA: a systematic review and meta-analysis. *JAMA*, *306*, 627-36.

Ding, C., Chiu, R. W., Lau, T. K., Leung, T. N., Chan, L. C., Chan, A. Y., Charoenkwan, P., Ng, I. S., Law, H. Y., Ma, E. S., et al. (2004). MS analysis of single-nucleotide differences in circulating nucleic acids: Application to noninvasive prenatal diagnosis. *Proc Natl Acad Sci U S A*, *101*, 10762-7.

Dube, S., Qin, J. & Ramakrishnan, R. (2008). Mathematical analysis of copy number variation in a DNA sample using digital PCR on a nanofluidic device. *PLoS One*, *3*, e2876.

Fan, H. C., Blumenfeld, Y. J., Chitkara, U., Hudgins, L. & Quake, S. R. (2008). Noninvasive diagnosis of fetal aneuploidy by shotgun sequencing DNA from maternal blood. *Proc Natl Acad Sci U S A*, *105*, 16266-71.

Fard, A. D., Hosseini, S. A., Shahjahani, M., Salari, F. & Jaseb, K. (2013). Evaluation of Novel Fetal Hemoglobin Inducer Drugs in Treatment of beta-Hemoglobinopathy Disorders. *Int J Hematol Oncol Stem Cell Res*, *7*, 47-54.

Finning, K. M. & Chitty, L. S. (2008). Non-invasive fetal sex determination: impact on clinical practice. *Semin Fetal Neonatal Med*, *13*, 69-75.

Fisher, S. A., Brunskill, S. J., Doree, C., Gooding, S., Chowdhury, O. & Roberts, D. J. (2013). Desferrioxamine mesylate for managing transfusional iron overload in people with transfusion-dependent thalassaemia. *Cochrane Database Syst Rev*, *8*, CD004450.

Friel, L. A., Czerwinski, J. L. & Singletary, C. N. (2013). The Impact of Noninvasive Prenatal Testing on the Practice of Maternal-Fetal Medicine. *Am J Perinatol*.

Fucharoen, S., Inati, A., Siritanaratku, N., Thein, S. L., Wargin, W. C., Koussa, S., Taher, A., Chaneim, N., Boosalis, M., Berenson, R., et al. (2013). A randomized phase I/II trial of HQK-1001, an oral fetal globin gene inducer, in beta-thalassaemia intermedia and HbE/beta-thalassaemia. *Br J Haematol*, *161*, 587-93.

Galbiati, S., Brisci, A., Lalatta, F., Seia, M., Makrigiorgos, G. M., Ferrari, M. & Cremonesi, L. (2011). Full COLD-PCR protocol for noninvasive prenatal diagnosis of genetic diseases. *Clin Chem*, *57*, 136-8.

Galbiati, S., Foglieni, B., Travi, M., Curcio, C., Restagno, G., Sbaiz, L., Smid, M., Pasi, F., Ferrari, A., Ferrari, M., et al. (2008). Peptide-nucleic acid-mediated enriched polymerase chain reaction as a key point for non-invasive prenatal diagnosis of beta-thalassemia. *Haematologica*, *93*, 610-4.

Gilbar, R. (2007). Patient autonomy and relatives' right to know genetic information. *Med Law*, *26*, 677-97.

Gold, B. (2003). Origin and utility of the reverse dot-blot. *Expert Rev Mol Diagn*, *3*, 143-52.

Gonzalez-Gonzalez, M. C., Garcia-Hoyos, M., Trujillo-Tiebas, M. J., Bustamante, Aragones, A., Rodriguez de Alba, M., Diego Alvarez, D., Diaz-Recasens, J., Ayuso, C. & Ramos, C. (2008). Improvement in strategies for the non-invasive prenatal diagnosis of Huntington disease. *J Assist Reprod Genet*, *25*, 477-81.

Gonzalez-Gonzalez, M. C., Trujillo, M. J., Rodriguez de Alba, M., Garcia-Hoyos, M., Lorda-Sanchez, I., Diaz-Recasens, J., Ayuso, C. & Ramos, C. (2003). Huntington disease-unaffected fetus diagnosed from maternal plasma using QF-PCR. *Prenat Diagn*, *23*, 232-4.

Gonzalez-Gonzalez, M. C., Trujillo, M. J., Rodriguez de Alba, M. & Ramos, C. (2003). Early Huntington disease prenatal diagnosis by maternal semiquantitative fluorescent-PCR. *Neurology*, *60*, 1214-5.

Goss, C., Giardina, P., Degtyaryova, D., Kleinert, D., Sheth, S. & Cushing, M. (2014). Red blood cell transfusions for thalassemia: results of a survey assessing current practice and proposal of evidence-based guidelines. *Transfusion*.

Grati, F. R., Malvestiti, F., Ferreira, J. C., Bajaj, K., Gaetani, E., Agrati, C., Grimi, B., Dulcetti, F., Ruggeri, A. M., De, Toffol, S., et al. (2014). Fetoplacental mosaicism: potential implications for false-positive and false-negative noninvasive prenatal screening results. *Genet Med*.

Harteveld, C. L. (2013). State of the art and new developments in molecular diagnostics for hemoglobinopathies in multiethnic societies. *Int J Lab Hematol*.

Hashemizadeh, H. & Noori, R. (2013). Premarital Screening of Beta Thalassemia Minor in north-east of Iran. *Iran J Ped Hematol Oncol*, *3*, 210-5.

Hassan, S., Ahmad, R., Zakaria, Z., Zulkafli, Z. & Abdullah, W. Z. (2013). Detection of beta-globin Gene Mutations Among beta-thalassaemia Carriers and Patients in Malaysia: Application of Multiplex Amplification Refractory Mutation System-Polymerase Chain Reaction. *Malays J Med Sci*, *20*, 13-20.

Henderson, S., Timbs, A., McCarthy, J., Gallienne, A., Van, Mourik, M., Masters, G., May, A., Khalil, M. S., Schuh, A. & Old, J. (2009). Incidence of haemoglobinopathies in various populations - the impact of immigration. *Clin Biochem*, *42*, 1745-56.

Hill, M., Compton, C., Lewis, C., Skirton, H. & Chitty, L. S. (2012). Determination of foetal sex in pregnancies at risk of haemophilia: a qualitative study exploring the clinical practices and attitudes of health professionals in the United Kingdom. *Haemophilia*, *18*, 575-83.

Hill, M., Karunaratna, M., Lewis, C., Forya, F. & Chitty, L. S. (2013). Views and Preferences for the Implementation of Non-Invasive Prenatal Diagnosis for Single Gene Disorders from Health Professionals in the United Kingdom. *American Journal of Human Genetics*, Manuscript Accepted.

Hindson, B. J., Ness, K. D., Masquelier, D. A., Belgrader, P., Heredia, N. J., Makarewicz, A. J., Bright, I. J., Lucero, M. Y., Hiddessen, A. L., Legler, T. C., et al. (2011). High-throughput droplet digital PCR system for absolute quantitation of DNA copy number. *Anal Chem*, *83*, 8604-10.

Ho, S. S., Chong, S. S., Koay, E. S., Ponnusamy, S., Chiu, L., Chan, Y. H., Rauff, M., Baig, S., Chan, J., Su, L. L., et al. (2010). Noninvasive prenatal exclusion of haemoglobin Bart's using foetal DNA from maternal plasma. *Prenat Diagn*, *30*, 65-73.

Ho, S. S., Huan, P. T., Leow, G. H., Ching, L. K., Chiu, L., Law, H. Y. & Koay, E. S. (2013). Rapid prenatal diagnosis of common beta-thalassemia mutations in Southeast Asia using pyrosequencing. *Prenat Diagn*, *33*, 1017-22.

Khandros, E., Thom, C. S., D'Souza, J. & Weiss, M. J. (2012). Integrated protein quality-control pathways regulate free alpha-globin in murine beta-thalassemia. *Blood*, *119*, 5265-75.

Kooij, L., Tymstra, T. & Berg, P. (2009). The attitude of women toward current and future possibilities of diagnostic testing in maternal blood using fetal DNA. *Prenat Diagn*, *29*, 164-8.

La, Nasa, G., Caocci, G., Efficace, F., Dessi, C., Vacca, A., Piras, E., Sanna, M., Marcias, M., Littera, R., Carcassi, C., et al. (2013). Long-term health-related quality of life evaluated more than 20 years after hematopoietic stem cell transplantation for thalassemia. *Blood*, *122*, 2262-70.

Lam, K. W., Jiang, P., Liao, G. J., Chan, K. C., Leung, T. Y., Chiu, R. W. & Lo, Y. M. (2012). Noninvasive prenatal diagnosis of monogenic diseases by targeted massively parallel sequencing of maternal plasma: application to beta-thalassemia. *Clin Chem*, *58*, 1467-75.

Lench, N., Barrett, A., Fielding, S., McKay, F., Hill, M., Jenkins, L., White, H. & Chitty, L. S. (2013). The clinical implementation of non-invasive prenatal diagnosis for single-gene disorders: challenges and progress made. *Prenat Diagn*, *33*, 555-62.

Lewis, C., Hill, M. & Chitty, L. S. (2014). Non-invasive prenatal diagnosis for single gene disorders: experience of patients. *Clin Genet*, *85*, 336-42.

Lewis, C., Hill, M., Skirton, H. & Chitty, L. S. (2012). Fetal sex determination using cell-free fetal DNA: service users' experiences of and preferences for service delivery. *Prenat Diagn*, *32*, 735-41.

Lewis, C., Silcock, C. & Chitty, L. S. (2013). Non-invasive prenatal testing for Down's syndrome: pregnant women's views and likely uptake. *Public Health Genomics*, *16*, 223-32.

Li, J., Wang, L., Mamon, H., Kulke, M. H., Berbeco, R. & Makrigiorgos, G. M. (2008). Replacing PCR with COLD-PCR enriches variant DNA sequences and redefines the sensitivity of genetic testing. *Nat Med*, *14*, 579-84.

Li, Y., Di, Naro, E., Vitucci, A., Zimmermann, B., Holzgreve, W. & Hahn, S. (2005). Detection of paternally inherited fetal point mutations for beta-thalassemia using size-fractionated cell-free DNA in maternal plasma. *JAMA*, *293*, 843-9.

Li, Y., Holzgreve, W., Page-Christiaens, G. C., Gille, J. J. & Hahn, S. (2004). Improved prenatal detection of a fetal point mutation for achondroplasia by the use of size-fractionated circulatory DNA in maternal plasma--case report. *Prenat Diagn*, *24*, 896-8.

Little, S. (2001). Amplification-refractory mutation system (ARMS) analysis of point mutations. *Curr Protoc Hum Genet*, Chapter 9 Unit 9 8.

Lo, Y. M., Chan, K. C., Sun, H., Chen, E. Z., Jiang, P., Lun, F. M., Zheng, Y. W., Leung, T. Y., Lau, T. K., Cantor, C. R., et al. (2010). Maternal plasma DNA sequencing reveals the genome-wide genetic and mutational profile of the fetus. *Sci Transl Med*, *2*, 61ra91.

Lo, Y. M., Corbetta, N., Chamberlain, P. F., Rai, V., Sargent, I. L., Redman, C. W. & Wainscoat, J. S. (1997). Presence of fetal DNA in maternal plasma and serum. *Lancet*, *350*, 485-7.

Lo, Y. M., Zhang, J., Leung, T. N., Lau, T. K., Chang, A. M. & Hjelm, N. M. (1999). Rapid clearance of fetal DNA from maternal plasma. *Am J Hum Genet*, *64*, 218-24.

Lun, F. M., Chiu, R. W., Allen, Chan, K. C., Yeung, Leung, T., Kin, Lau, T. & Dennis Lo, Y. M. (2008). Microfluidics digital PCR reveals a higher than expected fraction of fetal DNA in maternal plasma. *Clin Chem*, *54*, 1664-72.

Lun, F. M., Tsui, N. B., Chan, K. C., Leung, T. Y., Lau, T. K., Charoenkwan, P., Chow, K. C., Lo, W. Y., Wanapirak, C., Sanguansermsri, T., et al. (2008). Noninvasive prenatal diagnosis of monogenic diseases by digital size selection and relative mutation dosage on DNA in maternal plasma. *Proc Natl Acad Sci U S A*, *105*, 19920-5.

Matta, B. N., Musallam, K. M., Maakaron, J. E., Koussa, S. & Taher, A. T. (2013). A killer revealed: 10-year experience with beta-thalassemia intermedia. *Hematology*.

Meaney, C. & Norbury, G. (2009). Noninvasive prenatal diagnosis of early onset primary dystonia I in maternal plasma. *Prenat Diagn*, *29*, 1218-21.

Meena, L. P., Kumar, K., Singh, V. K., Bharti, A., Rahman, S. K. & Tripathi, K. (2013). Study of Mutations in beta-Thalassemia Trait among Blood Donors in Eastern Uttar Pradesh. *J Clin Diagn Res*, *7*, 1394-6.

Miccio, A., Poletti, V., Tiboni, F., Rossi, C., Antonelli, A., Mavilio, F. & Ferrari, G. (2011). The GATA1-HS2 enhancer allows persistent and position-independent expression of a beta-globin transgene. *PLoS One*, *6*, e27955.

Miri-Moghaddam, E., Zadeh-Vakili, A., Nikravesh, A., Sistani, S. S. & Naroie-Nejad, M. (2013). Sistani population: a different spectrum of beta-thalassemia mutations from other ethnic groups of Iran. *Hemoglobin*, *37*, 138-47.

Musallam, K. M., Taher, A. T., Cappellini, M. D. & Sankaran, V. G. (2013). Clinical experience with fetal hemoglobin induction therapy in patients with beta-thalassemia. *Blood*, *121*, 2199-212; quiz 372.

Newton, C. R., Heptinstall, L. E., Summers, C., Super, M., Schwarz, M., Anwar, R., Graham, A., Smith, J. C. & Markham, A. F. (1989). Amplification refractory mutation system for prenatal diagnosis and carrier assessment in cystic fibrosis. *Lancet*, *2*, 1481-3.

Nicolaides, K. H. (2004). Nuchal translucency and other first-trimester sonographic markers of chromosomal abnormalities. *Am J Obstet Gynecol*, *191*, 45-67.

Palomaki, G. E., Kloza, E. M., Lambert-Messerlian, G. M., Haddow, J. E., Neveux, L. M., Ehrich, M., van den Boom, D., Bombard, A. T., Deciu, C., Grody, W. W., et al. (2011).

DNA sequencing of maternal plasma to detect Down syndrome: An international clinical validation. *Genetics in Medicine*, *13*, 913-20.

Papasavva, T., Kalakoutis, G., Kalikas, I., Neokli, E., Papacharalambous, S., Kyrri, A. & Kleanthous, M. (2006). Noninvasive prenatal diagnostic assay for the detection of beta-thalassemia. *Ann N Y Acad Sci*, *1075*, 148-53.

Papasavva, T., Kalikas, I., Kyrri, A. & Kleanthous, M. (2008). Arrayed primer extension for the noninvasive prenatal diagnosis of beta-thalassemia based on detection of single nucleotide polymorphisms. *Ann N Y Acad Sci*, *1137*, 302-8.

Papasavva, T., van Ijcken, W. F., Kockx, C. E., van den Hout, M. C., Kountouris, P., Kythreotis, L., Kalogirou, E., Grosveld, F. G. & Kleanthous, M. (2013). Next generation sequencing of SNPs for non-invasive prenatal diagnosis: challenges and feasibility as illustrated by an application to beta-thalassaemia. *Eur J Hum Genet*.

Phylipsen, M., Yamsri, S., Treffers, E. E., Jansen, D. T., Kanhai, W. A., Boon, E. M., Giordano, P. C., Fucharoen, S., Bakker, E. & Harteveld, C. L. (2012). Non-invasive prenatal diagnosis of beta-thalassemia and sickle-cell disease using pyrophosphorolysis-activated polymerization and melting curve analysis. *Prenat Diagn*, *32*, 578-87.

Ribeil, J. A., Arlet, J. B., Dussiot, M., Moura, I. C., Courtois, G. & Hermine, O. (2013). Ineffective erythropoiesis in beta -thalassemia. *ScientificWorldJournal*, 2013, 394295.

Rust, D. W. & Bianchi, D. W. (2009). Microchimerism in endocrine pathology. *Endocr Pathol*, *20*, 11-6.

Sahoo, S. S., Biswal, S. & Dixit, M. (2014). Distinctive mutation spectrum of the HBB gene in an urban eastern Indian population. *Hemoglobin*, *38*, 33-8.

Saiki, R. K., Chang, C. A., Levenson, C. H., Warren, T. C., Boehm, C. D., Kazazian, H. H. Jr. & Erlich, H. A. (1988). Diagnosis of sickle cell anemia and beta-thalassemia with enzymatically amplified DNA and nonradioactive allele-specific oligonucleotide probes. *N Engl J Med*, *319*, 537-41.

Saiki, R. K., Scharf, S., Faloona, F., Mullis, K. B., Horn, G. T., Erlich, H. A. & Arnheim, N. (1985). Enzymatic amplification of beta-globin genomic sequences and restriction site analysis for diagnosis of sickle cell anemia. *Science*, *230*, 1350-4.

Saito, H., Sekizawa, A., Morimoto, T., Suzuki, M. & Yanaihara, T. (2000). Prenatal DNA diagnosis of a single-gene disorder from maternal plasma. *Lancet*, *356*, 1170.

Samakoglu, S., Lisowski, L., Budak-Alpdogan, T., Usachenko, Y., Acuto, S., Di, Marzo, R., Maggio, A., Zhu, P., Tisdale, J. F., Riviere, I., et al. (2006). A genetic strategy to treat sickle cell anemia by coregulating globin transgene expression and RNA interference. *Nat Biotechnol*, *24*, 89-94.

Skirton, H. & Patch, C. (2013). Factors affecting the clinical use of non-invasive prenatal testing: a mixed methods systematic review. *Prenat Diagn*, *33*, 532-41.

Sparks, A. B., Struble, C. A., Wang, E. T., Song, K. & Oliphant, A. (2012). Noninvasive prenatal detection and selective analysis of cell-free DNA obtained from maternal blood: evaluation for trisomy 21 and trisomy 18. *Am J Obstet Gynecol*, *206*, 319 e1-9.

Tabor, A. & Alfirevic, Z. (2010). Update on procedure-related risks for prenatal diagnosis techniques. *Fetal Diagn Ther*, *27*, 1-7.

Tan, J. A., Tay, J. S., Lin, L. I., Kham, S. K., Chia, J. N., Chin, T. M., Aziz, N. B. & Wong, H. B. (1994). The amplification refractory mutation system (ARMS): a rapid and direct prenatal diagnostic technique for beta-thalassaemia in Singapore. *Prenat Diagn*, *14*, 1077-82.

Tan, K. L., Tan, J. A., Wong, Y. C., Wee, Y. C., Thong, M. K. & Yap, S. F. (2001). Combine-ARMS: a rapid and cost-effective protocol for molecular characterization of beta-thalassemia in Malaysia. *Genet Test*, *5*, 17-22.

Timbs, A. T., Rugless, M. J., Gallienne, A. E., Haywood, A. M., Henderson, S. J. & Old, J. M. (2012). Prenatal diagnosis of hemoglobinopathies by pyrosequencing: a more sensitive and rapid approach to fetal genotyping. *Hemoglobin*, *36*, 144-50.

Tischler, R., Hudgins, L., Blumenfeld, Y. J., Greely, H. T. & Ormond, K. E. (2011). Noninvasive prenatal diagnosis: pregnant women's interest and expected uptake. *Prenat Diagn*, *31*, 1292-9.

Tungwiwat, W., Fucharoen, S., Fucharoen, G., Ratanasiri, T. & Sanchaisuriya, K. (2006). Development and application of a real-time quantitative PCR for prenatal detection of fetal alpha(0).-thalassemia from maternal plasma. *Ann N Y Acad Sci*, *1075*, 103-7.

van der Schoot, C. E., Hahn, S. & Chitty, L. S. (2008). Non-invasive prenatal diagnosis and determination of fetal Rh status. *Semin Fetal Neonatal Med*, *13*, 63-8.

Verweij, E. J., Oepkes, D., de Vries, M., van den Akker, M. E., van den Akker, E. S. & de Boer, M. A. (2013). Non-invasive prenatal screening for trisomy 21: what women want and are willing to pay. *Patient Educ Couns*, *93*, 641-5.

Vogelstein, B. & Kinzler, K. W. (1999). Digital PCR. *Proc Natl Acad Sci U S A*, *96*, 9236-41.

Wang, W., Kham, S. K., Yeo, G. H., Quah, T. C. & Chong, S. S. (2003). Multiplex minisequencing screen for common Southeast Asian and Indian beta-thalassemia mutations. *Clin Chem*, *49*, 209-18.

Weatherall, D. J. (2001). Phenotype-genotype relationships in monogenic disease: lessons from the thalassaemias. *Nat Rev Genet*, *2*, 245-55.

Yenilmez, E. D., Tuli, A. & Evruke, I. C. (2013). Noninvasive prenatal diagnosis experience in the Cukurova Region of Southern Turkey: detecting paternal mutations of sickle cell anemia and beta-thalassemia in cell-free fetal DNA using high-resolution melting analysis. *Prenat Diagn*, *33*, 1054-62.

Yotsumoto, J., Sekizawa, A., Koide, K., Purwosunu, Y., Ichizuka, K., Matsuoka, R., Kawame, H. & Okai, T. (2012). Attitudes toward non-invasive prenatal diagnosis among pregnant women and health professionals in Japan. *Prenat Diagn*, *32*, 674-9.

Zhu, Y. J., Zheng, Y. R., Li, L., Zhou, H., Liao, X., Guo, J. X. & Yi, P. (2014). Diagnostic accuracy of non-invasive fetal RhD genotyping using cell-free fetal DNA: a meta analysis. *J Matern Fetal Neonatal Med.*

Zimmermann, B., Hill, M., Gemelos, G., Demko, Z., Banjevic, M., Baner, J., Ryan, A., Sigurjonsson, S., Chopra, N., Dodd, M., et al. (2012). Noninvasive prenatal aneuploidy testing of chromosomes 13, 18, 21, X, and Y, using targeted sequencing of polymorphic loci. *Prenat Diagn*, *32*, 1233-41.

In: Thalassemia
Editor: Makenzie Greene
ISBN: 978-1-63117-954-9

Chapter 8

Antioxidant Therapies for Thalassemia

Ruchaneekorn W. Kalpravidh and Suneerat Hatairaktham
Department of Biochemistry, Faculty of Medicine Siriraj Hospital,
Mahidol University, Bangkok, Thailand

Abstract

The cellular redox status in physiological condition is normally well-balanced between oxidant and antioxidant levels. Oxidative stress is defined as the disturbance state that the production of the oxidants is greater than the efficiency of the antioxidant system. In the pathogenesis of thalassemia, redox-active iron released from excess unpaired globin chains causes oxidative damage to the membrane of mature or immature red blood cells. This leads to increased premature removal of the affected red cells, ineffective erythropoiesis, chronic anemia, and finally, iron overload. Thus, patients with thalassemia have inevitably profound oxidative stress that triggers oxidation of intracellular biomolecules; causing tissue damage and then organ failure. Therefore, the antioxidant supplementation may be beneficial for the patients with thalassemia. This article briefly summarizes how oxidative stress raises and discusses several therapeutic strategies using antioxidant(s) to neutralize the oxidative burden in thalassemia; including direct scavenging of free radicals, detoxifying or removing oxidants, or boosting endogenous antioxidants. Several studies and clinical trials on the use of potential antioxidant agents such as pharmaceuticals, dietary compounds, and endogenous biomolecules in thalassemia have been reported. Some recent studies showed that various antioxidants when used in combination enhanced antioxidant capacity and decreased toxicity/side effects. Future research should address the optimization of combination strategies with the final goal to prevent hazardous complications and increase life expectancy of thalassemic patients. Moreover, it should focus on the investigation of the potential antioxidants for thalassemia which could be orally administered and readily absorbed, and highly bioavailable. Moreover, they should possess high antioxidative activities, have long half-life, do not interfere with other drugs, and are not toxic even at high concentrations.

1. Introduction

Thalassemia is a worldwide genetic anemia with approximately 300,000-400,000 infants annually born with the major form [1]. The excess of unpaired α- or β-globin chains related to the reduced or absent chain synthesis contributes to an oxidative environment in erythroid progenitor cells or mature red blood cells (RBCs). Toxic iron species liberated from the excess globin chains induce overproduction of reactive oxygen species (ROS) concurrent with rapid depletion of cellular antioxidants. The sequels of this redox imbalance are profound oxidative damage in RBC membrane components, ineffective erythropoiesis and extra hemolysis, and hemolytic anemia. To compensate the blood loss, patients with thalassemia often receive blood transfusions or significantly increase absorption of intestinal iron. Due to lack of removal system, uncontrolled accumulation of iron exacerbates oxidative stress throughout the body. Oxidative stress-induced complications are frequently observed in thalassemia patients and also responsible for the major cause of their mortality; especially iron-induced heart diseases [2]. Antioxidant administration has been used in various research thus far to neutralize the harmful effects of free radicals and attenuate oxidative damages to biological sites that result in decreasing the risks of pathological sequences arisen by iron-associated oxidative stress. This chapter briefly summarizes cause and consequences of oxidative stress implicated in thalassemia. Then, the strategies of antioxidants against oxidative stress are addressed, as well as the main results from the *in vitro*, *in vivo*, or clinical studies with antioxidants in thalassemia models are also reviewed.

2. Oxidative Stress in Thalassemia

Under physiological condition, cellular redox status is well-balanced between oxidant and antioxidant levels. “Oxidative stress” is defined as an imbalance state that the formation of harmful free radicals is greater than the ability of antioxidant defenses [3]. Many radicals are unstable and highly reactive to give or accept unpaired electron(s) from nearby biological molecules leading to malfunction or abnormality of physiological responses of such molecular systems. Moreover, various physiological processes including apoptosis, inflammation, and immunity are regulated by oxidation-reduction (redox) reactions. Thus, enhanced oxidative stress and disturbance of redox homeostasis contribute to the pathogenesis of many life-threatening diseases.

Thalassemia has been regarded as an oxidative stress disorder which the stress is mainly caused by secondary iron overload, an inevitably major consequence of chronic anemia (Figure 1). In order to evaluate the effective prevention or treatment of any disease, an understanding of the pathophysiology is essential. In thalassemia, the mutation(s) in globin gene(s) results in partial or complete deficiency of α- or β-globin synthesis. The unpaired chains are in excess and unstable; consequently, they are precipitated, denatured, and disintegrated releasing toxic iron species (e.g., hemicromes, inclusion bodies, Heinz bodies, free heme, free iron) into intraerythrocytic circumstance [4]. Transition metal especially iron is well known to be a powerful catalyst in the formation of hydroxyl radicals ($OH^{\bullet}$) via Fenton reaction as follows:

$$Fe^{2+} + H_2O_2 \longrightarrow Fe^{3+} + OH^{\bullet} + OH^{-}$$

Hydroxyl radicals are highly reactive ROS that cause devastating effects to virtually biological molecules including lipids, proteins, nucleic acids, and carbohydrates. The deleterious consequences include loss of membrane integrity by lipid peroxidation, mutagenesis by DNA lesions, and structural/functional changes of oxidized proteins and carbohydrates [5]. Compared to RBCs obtained from normal subjects, thalassemic RBCs contain significantly higher levels of ROS and oxidative products including malondialdehyde (MDA), F2-isoprostanes, carbonylated proteins, and DNA adducts; indicating oxidative stress state in thalassemia [6-9].

Once free radicals extensively oxidize protein and lipid components of red cell membrane, it leads to either phosphatidylserine (PS) exposure or clusterization of membrane proteins (e.g., band 3) expressed as a neoantigen on the surface of RBCs. Apoptosis and marrow/splenic phagocytosis triggering from PS-positive and neoantigen-expressed red cells result in ineffective erythropoiesis and extravascular hemolysis, respectively [4]. Moreover, oxidation of cytoskeletal proteins (e.g., band 4.1, spectrin, actin) destabilizes red cell membrane and leads to intravascular hemolysis when passing through capillaries. Chronic anemia in thalassemia is a combined outcome of ineffective erythropoiesis, intra-, and extravascular hemolysis [4].

Secondary iron overload in thalassemia is mainly caused by regular blood transfusions and significantly increased intestinal iron uptake. Frequent blood transfusions are the major supportive therapy for the patients with severe anemia. One mL of whole blood contains approximately 0.5 mg of iron [10]; therefore, there are approximately 225 mg of iron in one blood unit corresponding to 450 mL of whole blood. The patients with mild to moderate anemia also develop iron overload by increasing intestinal iron uptake for massive RBC production as an adaptive response to ineffective erythropoiesis. Absorption of dietary iron was increased 3-4 folds in patients with thalassemia intermedia, compared to that of the normal group [11].

Iron is an essential metal in the body with a tight regulation of systemic and cellular iron homeostasis. Since free iron is highly toxic; therefore, it normally binds tightly to appropriate ligands under physiological condition. In the circulation, iron mainly exists in the forms of transferrin bound iron, ferritin, hemoglobin-haptoglobin complex, or heme bound to hemopexin [12]. Once the concentration of iron in plasma exceeds the binding capacities of these ligands, excessive iron appears in the form of ferric (Fe^{3+}) loosely bound to any anionic ligands including proteins (e.g., albumin) or low-molecular weight molecules (e.g., citrate, acetate) termed as non-transferrin bound iron (NTBI). NTBI is greatly diverse in its structures and biological properties; however, most NTBI found in thalassemic sera has been identified as a ternary compound that ferric loosely binds to citrate and albumin [13]. Various research studies use the word "labile plasma iron (LPI)" to specifically describe the most redox-active form of plasma NTBI [10]. Unlike transferrin-bound iron, cellular uptake of NTBI and LPI is uncontrollable since it could not be regulated by the iron-regulatory element (IRE)/iron-regulatory protein (IRP) system. Liver, heart, and endocrine glands especially pancreatic beta cells are the main organs for iron deposition [10].

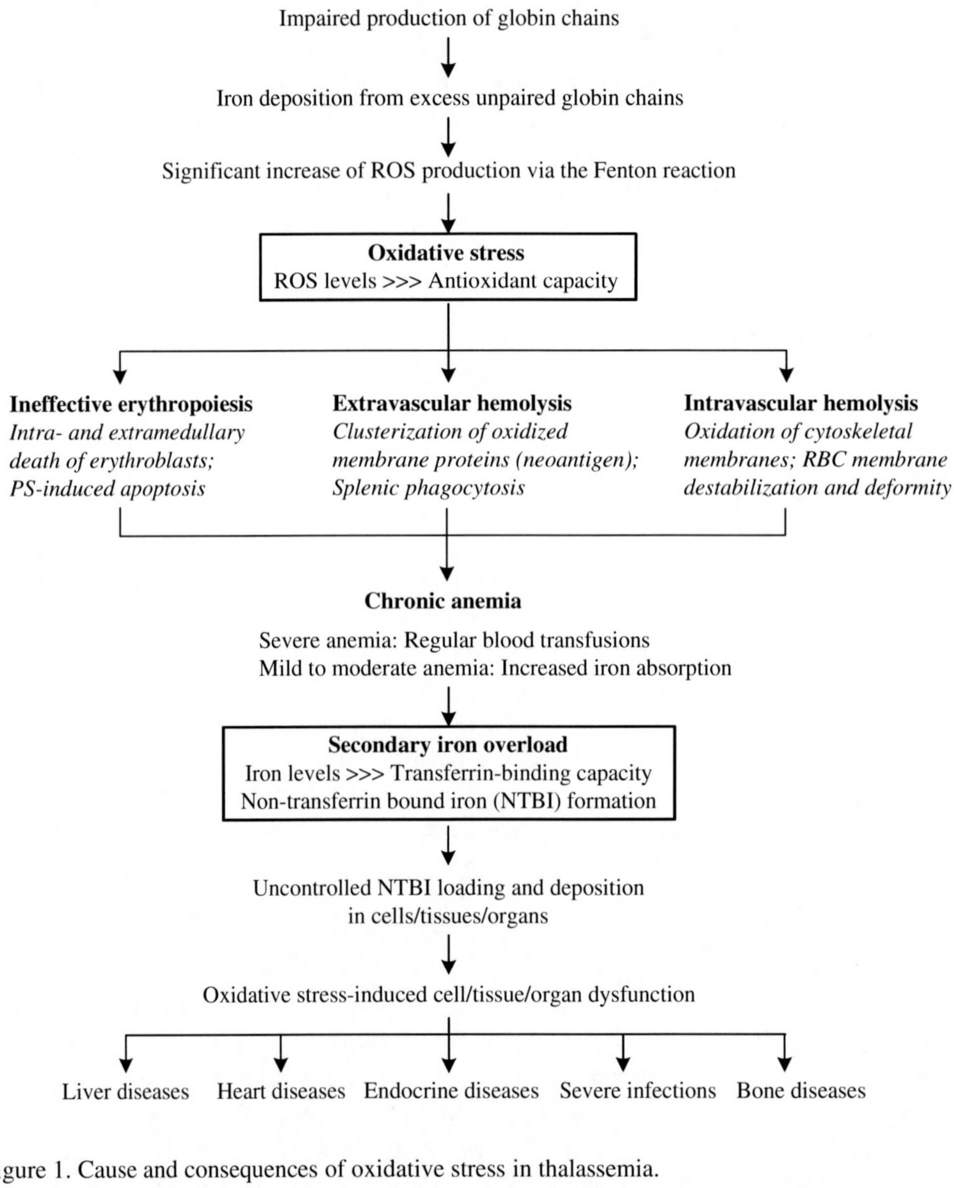

Figure 1. Cause and consequences of oxidative stress in thalassemia.

Most iron in cells is stored as ferritin and hemosiderin with a small amount of transient iron pool known as "labile iron pool (LIP)" presented in subcellular compartments to facilitate redox-sensitive biological processes [14]. Cellular LIP levels are dynamically changed as a net result of iron influx, iron chelation, ferritin synthesis, or ferritin degradation rates [15]. In iron overload, cellular LIP level is markedly increased with no active mechanisms for iron excretion generating a great amount of hydroxyl radicals followed by oxidative damage of biological molecules. Macromolecules with oxidative damage lose their efficiency or cellular functions leading to tissues/organs impairment followed by increasing the risk of oxidative stress-associated complications such as liver diseases (e.g., fibrosis/cirrhosis, hepatoma), heart diseases (e.g., heart failure), diabetes mellitus, bone diseases, severe infections, and endocrine disorders.

3. Antioxidant Defenses

Antioxidant is defined as any molecule that can prevent, inhibit, or repair the oxidative damage of biomolecules caused by free radicals. Human body contains systemic and cellular antioxidant defenses interacting as a network with different mechanisms due to vastly different half-life of radicals and their sites of oxidation. Hydroxyl radicals have very short half-life in nanoseconds with highest rate constants for oxidation, therefore, they rapidly oxidize biomolecules at the site of production; whereas peroxyl radicals ($ROO^{\bullet}$, generated from lipid peroxidation) are stable with the half-life in seconds and able to pass through membrane to cause oxidation at distant sites [16]. Cellular antioxidant defenses are varied widely by tissue types. Liver, heart, and pancreatic beta-cells are the tissues at high risk of oxidation because they contain a large number of mitochondria resulting in high steady-state rates in superoxide and hydrogen peroxide generation. Under iron overload, pancreatic beta-cells are the most sensitive tissue to oxidative damage due to relatively poor antioxidant defenses and high iron uptake compared with other cell types [17].

The strategies against oxidative stress can be divided into three levels: prevention, interception, and repair [16]. At prevention level, antioxidants minimize the generation of ROS by metal chelation (e.g., metal-binding proteins, chelating drugs), detoxification of potential oxidants (e.g., glutathione-S-transferase), and modification of target molecules to increase their resistance to oxidation (e.g., modified low-density lipoproteins by dehydro-L-ascorbic acid [18]). Once free radicals are formed, antioxidants intercept their deleterious effects by direct scavenging (e.g., vitamin C, glutathione, thiol-containing compounds, polyphenolic compounds), chain breaking (e.g., vitamin E, plant polyphenols), and converting to nonradical products (e.g., antioxidant enzymes). As capacities of preventive and interceptive antioxidants are insufficient and oxidation reaction has occurred, damaged biomolecules are repaired by several enzymes involved in DNA repair system, proteolysis of oxidized protein, and oxidized phospholipid turnover.

According to their originated sources, antioxidants can be divided into 2 main types: endogenous and exogenous antioxidants [19].

(1) Endogenous Antioxidant Defenses

Endogenous antioxidants are produced in the body to maintain proper redox status which is critical for normal cellular functions. They can be divided into enzymatic and non-enzymatic antioxidants.

Enzymatic Antioxidants

The major enzymatic antioxidants including superoxide dismutase (SOD), catalase (CAT), glutathione peroxidase (GPx), glutathione reductase (GR), peroxiredoxin (Prx), and thioredoxin reductase (TR) are the front-line defense to catalyze the detoxification reactions of toxic radical intermediates generating during oxygen reduction in aerobic respiration (Table 1). Enzymatic antioxidants possess transition metals including copper, zinc, selenium, iron, and manganese at the active sites acting as cofactors to donate or accept electron(s) to substrates.

Table 1. Enzymatic antioxidant defenses

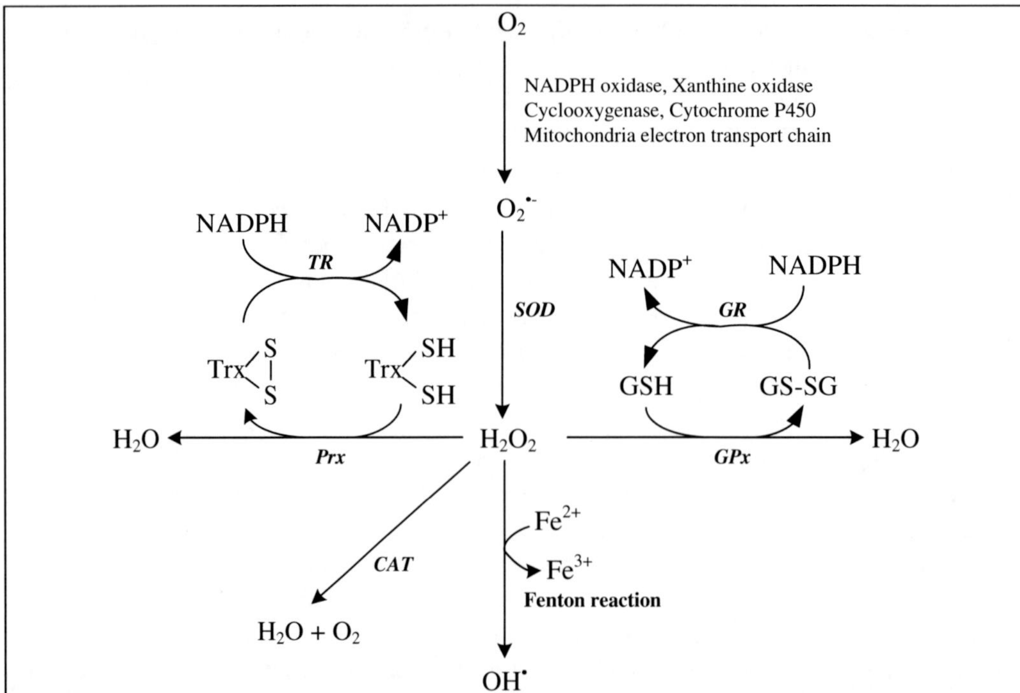

Enzymatic antioxidants	Location	Defense mechanisms
Superoxide dismutase (SOD)	biological fluids (plasma, milk), cellular compartments (cytosol, mitochondria), extracellular space	catalyzes the dismutation of $O_2^{\bullet-}$ to H_2O_2 $2\,O_2^{\bullet-} + 2\,H^+ \xrightarrow{SOD} H_2O_2 + O_2$
Catalase (CAT)	cellular compartments (peroxisomes)	catalyzes the conversion of H_2O_2 to H_2O $2\,H_2O_2 + 2\,H^+ \xrightarrow{CAT} 2\,H_2O + O_2$
Glutathione peroxidase (GPx)	plasma, cellular compartments (cytosol, mitochondria)	catalyzes the reduction of peroxides $H_2O_2 + 2\,GSH \xrightarrow{GPx} 2\,H_2O + GSSG$ $ROOH + 2\,GSH \xrightarrow{GPx} H_2O + GSSG + ROH$
Glutathione reductase (GR)	cellular compartments (cytosol, mitochondria)	regenerates GSH from GSSG $GSSG + NADPH + H^+ \xrightarrow{GR} 2\,GSH + NADP^+$
Peroxiredoxin (Prx)	cellular compartments (cytosol, nucleus, mitochondria, membrane, golgi)	catalyzes the reduction of peroxides $H_2O_2 + Trx\text{-}(SH)_2 \xrightarrow{Prx} 2\,H_2O + Trx\text{-}S_2$ $ROOH + Trx\text{-}(SH)_2 \xrightarrow{Prx} H_2O + Trx\text{-}S_2 + ROH$
Thioredoxin reductase (TR)	cellular compartments (cytosol, nucleus)	regenerates $Trx\text{-}(SH)_2$ from $Trx\text{-}S_2$ $Trx\text{-}S_2 + NADPH + H^+ \xrightarrow{TR} Trx\text{-}(SH)_2 + NADP^+$

In mammalian cells, superoxide anions are converted to H_2O_2 by the reaction catalyzed by SOD. H_2O_2 can be further converted to water by the reactions catalyzed by CAT (in peroxisome), GPx with electrons transferred from glutathione (GSH), and Prx utilizing electrons from thioredoxin (Trx-$(SH)_2$). GR and TR play essential roles in cellular antioxidant system by reversing glutathione disulfide (GSSG) and thioredoxin disulfide (Trx-S_2), the oxidized forms of GSH and Trx-$(SH)_2$ respectively, to their reduced forms for maintaining sufficient antioxidant capacity. Glutathione-S-transferase (GST) is the detoxifying enzyme that conjugates GSH to peroxides and other oxidative metabolites for excretion out of body.

Non-Enzymatic Antioxidants

Most non-enzymatic antioxidants produced in the body are metal-binding proteins, thiol-containing peptides/proteins, or other low-molecular weight compounds. One strategy to prevent ROS formation is to minimize free metal ions. Endogenous iron-binding proteins including transferrin, lactotransferrin, ferritin, hemopexin, and haptoglobin function as antioxidants by sequestering iron so that iron is not available for catalyzing the formation of hydroxyl radicals (Fenton reaction).

Thiol-containing peptides/proteins act as powerful antioxidants through several mechanisms such as participating in thiol/disulfide redox buffer system, chelating metal, quenching radicals, using as substrates for both redox and conjugation reactions (e.g., glutathione), and facilitating reduction of disulfide bonds in proteins (e.g., thioredoxin) [20]. Antioxidative activity of thiol compounds is derived from the sulfur atom of cysteine that is readily to donate electron [21]. Among these, a tripeptide glutathione (GSH, γ-glutamylcystenylglycine) is the most important thiol compound localized in all cell compartments and biological fluids. GSH serves multiple functions such as detoxifying xenobiotics; maintaining cellular redox balance and thiol proteins by thiol-disulfide exchange; participating in antioxidant defenses (e.g., radical scavenging, GPx-catalyzed reaction); providing endogenous reservoir for cysteine; and modulating various biological processes (e.g., immunity, cell cycle, apoptosis) [22]. Moreover, GSH can regenerate vitamin C from its oxidized form, dehydroascorbate [23]. Another major thiol antioxidant is thioredoxin (Trx) ubiquitously expressed in mammalian cells with oxidoreductase activity. Trx contains two sulfhydryl groups in its reduced form which are converted to a disulfide bond when it is oxidized in thiol-disulfide exchange reactions with various proteins.

Other small molecules exhibit antioxidant activities such as Coenzyme Q_{10} (CoQ_{10}, ubiquinone/ubiquinol), bilirubin, and uric acid. CoQ_{10} is an endogenous hydrophobic antioxidant consisting of a quinone group attached to 10 units of highly hydrophobic isoprenoids. CoQ_{10} is found in eukaryotic cell membrane, mitochondria, and circulating lipoproteins. It is an effective free radical scavenger by donating 2 electrons to lipid peroxyl radicals during the initiation and propagation steps of lipid peroxidation with efficiency equivalent to or higher than vitamin E [23]. Furthermore, CoQ_{10} is the main antioxidant to inhibit hydroxyl radical production in low-density lipoprotein and also regenerate α-tocopherol from α-tocopheroxyl radical [24]. Bilirubin is a product of heme degradation and can act as an antioxidant because it scavenges peroxyl radicals with high efficiency relative to vitamin E [25]. Uric acid is a product from purine base degradation which exerts antioxidative effects by radical scavenging, iron chelating, and stabilizing vitamin C from oxidation reactions in biological fluids [26]. Major non-enzymatic endogenous antioxidants in human are summarized in Table 2.

Table 2. Major non-enzymatic endogenous antioxidants in human

Non-enzymatic antioxidants	Location	Defense mechanisms
Glutathione	plasma, cellular compartments (cytosol, mitochondria)	scavenges free radicals; as a substrate for both redox and conjugation reactions
Thioredoxin	plasma, cellular compartments (cytosol, nucleus)	scavenges free radicals; catalyzes thiol-disulfide exchange reactions
Transferrin/Lactoferrin	plasma/ biological fluids	binds to ferric iron and transfers to tissues
Ferritin	cellular compartments (cytosol), plasma	binds to ferric iron; intracellular storage form of iron
Hemopexin/Haptoglobin	plasma	binds to free heme/hemoglobin released during intravascular hemolysis and transfers to spleen for iron recycling
Coenzyme Q_{10}	plasma lipoproteins, cellular compartments (membrane, mitochondria)	scavenges free radicals, breaks chain reaction
Bilirubin	plasma	scavenges free radicals
Uric acid	plasma	scavenges free radicals, binds to ferric iron

(2) Exogenous Antioxidant Defenses

Under oxidative stress, endogenous antioxidants may be insufficient and other antioxidants from exogenous sources are required to maintain redox balance in cells. Exogenous antioxidants are provided mainly from diet (e.g., fruits, vegetables, grains, beverages). Moreover, some drugs have antioxidant properties such as chelating agents or thiol-replenishing drugs. Diet-derived compounds and drugs with antioxidant properties that have been studied in thalassemia will be described below.

Antioxidant capacity can be evaluated by measuring either total antioxidant capacity expressed as trolox equivalents or determining levels of individual antioxidants/markers of oxidative damage in cells/biological fluids [27]. Previous studies have been indicated that patients with thalassemia have decreased antioxidant capacity as well as increased oxidant levels. Significantly decreased total antioxidant capacity and levels of antioxidants (vitamin E, vitamin C, vitamin A, β-carotene, and lycopene) accompanied with significantly elevated levels of ROS and oxidative products (e.g., MDA, F2-isoprostanes, carbonylated proteins, DNA adducts) were observed in sera and RBCs of the patients [6-9, 28-30]. The alteration of redox state toward oxidative stress leads to the upregulation of several antioxidants and detoxifying enzymes. Thalassemic patients, as compared to normal subjects, showed significant increases of antioxidant enzyme activities (e.g., SOD, GPx, GST, GR), decreased levels of GSH and increased levels of its oxidized form (GSSG) resulting in lower GSH/GSSG ratio [7, 31, 32]. Therefore, the supplementation of exogenous antioxidants has been investigated over decades and should be beneficial to patients with thalassemia to restore the balance of oxidants and antioxidants.

4. Dietary Antioxidants in Thalassemia

Diet contains many compounds that possess antioxidant activities contributing to beneficial health effects in human. Antioxidant compounds from diet that have been used to treat thalassemia are described as follows:

4.1. Vitamin E

Vitamin E is the main hydrophobic antioxidant that inhibits lipid peroxidation in cells or plasma lipoproteins. The structure of vitamin E is a chromanol ring with a hydroxyl group which is responsible for chain-breaking activity. Although natural vitamin E consists of four tocopherols and four tocotrienols, α-tocopherol is the most abundant isomer in diet and the human body with the highest biological activity [33]. α-tocopherol (vit E-OH) inhibits the propagation step of lipid peroxidation in cell membranes by providing hydrogen and electron on the hydroxyl group to lipid peroxyl radical ($LOO^{\bullet}$) to yield α-tocopheroxyl radical (vit E-$O^{\bullet}$) and a relatively stable lipid hydroperoxide (LOOH) terminating the radical chain reaction. α-tocopheroxyl radical can be regenerated to its reduced form by various reducing agents including vitamin C, retinol, CoQ_{10}, and GSH [34]. If the oxidation between α-tocopheroxyl radical and $LOO^{\bullet}$ still continues, the reaction provides LOOH and an irreversible α-tocopheryl quinone which is mainly secreted into the bile and eventually, eliminated in the feces.

Vitamin E treatment decreases oxidative stress in RBCs and white blood cells (WBCs) in thalassemic patients. In a study performed by Pfeifer et al. [35], patients with thalassemia intermedia supplemented with vitamin E (400 IU daily dose) for three months significantly decreased ROS in RBCs and WBCs, declined serum thiobarbituric reactive substances (TBARS); and increased GSH levels. Although vitamin E did not affect hemoglobin concentrations in this study, reticulocyte counts were significantly decreased at the end of treatment. After completion of the treatment for 3 months, levels of all analyzed parameters tended to basal values. The similar results were also supported by a study of Tesoriere and colleague [36] which showed an improvement of oxidative stress biomarkers in plasma, low-density lipoproteins and RBCs in β-thalassemia intermedia patients after 9-month supplementation with 600 mg/day vitamin E.

Besides the decrease of oxidative stress in blood cells, platelet functions were also improved. A double-blinded, placebo-controlled crossover study had been established to treat β-thalassemia/Hb E patients (nine splenectomized (SP) and 16 non-splenectomized (NS)) with 525 IU daily dose of vitamin E for three months [37]. At baseline, the SP group showed higher levels of serum ferritin, plasma TBARS, and platelet reactivity than the NS, while both groups had low levels of plasma vitamin E. After 3 months of treatment, all patients had a significant increase in plasma vitamin E and reduction in plasma TBARS with unchanged serum ferritin. Vitamin E also decreased platelet reactivity of the SP patients close to normal values. Therefore, vitamin E treatment may delay hypercoagulable state and reduce thromboembolic events in SP thalassemic patients.

Vitamin E also improves RBCs membrane fluidity of thalassemic patients. Using spin labeling techniques, values indicating RBCs membrane fluidity of the SP β-thalassemia/Hb E patients were significantly higher than that of the NS and normal subjects. Administration of 350 mg/day vitamin E for one month significantly lowered erythrocyte membrane fluidity, whereas the increased levels were reported in the placebo group [38]. A study by Das et al. showed the protective effect of vitamin E (10 mg/kg/day for four weeks) on thalassemic erythrocyte membranes by decreased levels of degraded membrane proteins compared to the untreated ones [39].

Vitamin C plays an indirect role to regenerate α-tocopherol from α-tocopheroxyl radical, co-administration of vitamin E and C has benefits more than vitamin E alone. Twenty young patients with β-thalassemia major who had low baseline levels of plasma vitamin C and E were treated with both vitamins for three months [40]. There were significant increases of plasma vitamin C, E, and GSH levels at the end of treatment, while total antioxidant status and MDA levels did not show the differences during the study.

Most studies on vitamin E monotherapy in thalassemia have not shown an improvement in hematological parameters especially hemoglobin (Hb) concentration. Significant increase of Hb concentration had been explored when vitamin E used in combination with other vitamins. A prospective study was performed in 39 young β-thalassemia major patients with low initial serum vitamin levels [41]. They were administered with combined vitamins (E, C, and A) for one year as compared to the controls who were 21 young patients with normal initial serum vitamin levels. Patients treated with the combined vitamins improved their redox balance as shown by significantly increased levels of GSH, Hb concentration, GR activities paralleled by continuous decline in MDA, ferritin, serum transaminase, SOD activity levels during the therapy. A significant improvement of hepatic fibrosis determined by hepatic transient elastography did not show in this study, whereas liver iron concentrations using magnetic resonance imaging R2* were significantly decreased.

4.2. Plant Polyphenols

Plant polyphenols contribute to human health benefits with the consumption of fruits, vegetables, cereals or even beverages. Recently, over 8000 types of polyphenols have been identified in various plant species as secondary metabolites contributing to color, flavor, and odor of plants. They also possess powerful antioxidant activities to scavenge free radicals or chelate redox-active metals through their chemical structures. However, the major limitation of these phenolic compounds is poor bioavailability owing to their hydrophobic ring structures. This results in inadequate concentration to exert *in vivo* antioxidant effect.

Curcuminoids

Curcuminoids are polyphenolic compounds extracted from rhizomes of turmeric (*Curcuma longa* Linn); which consist mainly of ~77% curcumin, ~17% demethoxycurcumin, ~3% bisdemethoxycurcumin [42]. Curcuminoids exhibit antioxidant activities by several mechanisms including free radicals scavenging via β-diketone and hydroxyl/methoxyl groups; increasing GSH synthesis via upregulation of the transcription factor Nrf2; and iron chelating via β-diketone moieties (a bidentate ligand, ligand:iron ratio = 3:1) [43-45]. Low bioavailability of curcuminoids were reported that at 1 hour after orally given at a single dose of two grams to normal volunteers, undetectable or extremely low levels (0.006±0.005 μg/mL) of curcuminoids in human sera were observed [46].

Oxidative stress and iron overload in thalassemic patients were improved by administration of curcuminoids at 500 mg/day for 12 months as seen by significantly increased GSH and decreased MDA levels concomitant with reduced activities of SOD and GPx antioxidant enzymes in RBCs [7]. Moreover, the levels of serum NTBI were also significantly decreased. Further plasma proteomics study using two-dimensional fluorescence difference gel electrophoresis indicated significantly decreased intensities of 2 groups of proteins in thalassemic plasma, coagulation factors and proteins in iron homeostasis, as compared to the normal controls [47]. Curcuminoids treatment was able to increase plasma contents as well as reduce oxidative damage of such proteins detected by carbonyl immunoblotting. Another study using a mouse model of iron-overloaded β-thalassemia intermedia, treatment with curcuminoids (200 mg/kg/day) for four months successfully decreased concentrations of plasma NTBI, MDA, cardiac iron burden, and also improved cardiac functions (cardiac autonomic activity) measured by heart rate variability (HRV) analysis [48].

Catechins

Catechins are flavonol extracted from leaves of tea (*Camellia sinensis*) comprising of 48-55% (-)-epigallocatechin-3-gallate (EGCG), 9-12% (-)-epigallocatechin (EGC), 9-12% (-)-epicatechin gallate (ECG), and 5-7% (-)-epicatechin (EC) [49]. Multiple hydroxyl groups, *O*-dihydroxyphenol, and gallate group contribute to the antioxidant properties of catechins either free radical scavenging or iron chelating [50]. Moreover, tea catechins are able to suppress the expressions of pro-oxidant enzymes (e.g., inducible nitric oxide synthase, xanthine oxidase) and activate the expressions of antioxidant enzymes (SOD, catalase, and GPx) [49]. Very few studies have been performed so far using catechins in iron-overloaded or thalassemic models. Intervention thalassemic RBCs and plasma with green tea extract for 1 hour before incubating with iron significantly decreased levels of intracellular ROS and plasma NTBI [51]. Similar results have been reported in iron-overloaded rats [52], and in thalassemic mice [53]. To evaluate the efficiency of tissue iron removal, β-thalassemia intermedia mice with iron overload were fed Fe-diet together with green tea extract (300 mg/kg daily) compared to that with deferiprone (50 mg/kg daily) or deionized water (placebo) for eight weeks [53]. After completion of the treatment, the liver iron concentration in the green tea-treated and deferiprone-treated groups were significantly decreased about 1.615±0.895 and 1.355±0.999 μg Fe/mg protein, respectively; whereas, the placebo increased approximately 22 folds liver iron content.

Resveratol

Resveratol (3,5,4'-trihydroxy-stilbene) is the principle stilbene mainly found in various plants including grape skins, tea, apples, berries, peanuts, and Japanese knotweed (*polygonum cuspidatum*). Fibach et al. demonstrated beneficial effects of resveratrol on K562 cells, normal and β-thalassemic blood cells [54]. Resveratol showed a dose-dependent manner in alleviation of oxidative stress shown by decreased levels of ROS in RBCs, platelets, and WBCs accompanied with increased GSH levels and lipid peroxidase activities. Moreover, the inhibition of cell growth and induction of erythroid differentiation in K562 cells were also achieved by resveratrol treatment. Another interesting effect of resveratrol is the ability to enhance transcriptional activities of γ- and β-globin promoters. Similar to hydroxyurea and butyrate which are clinically used as Hb F inducer, resveratrol increased cellular Hb F content varied from 1.27 to 5.78 folds compared to the untreated in different genotypes of β-thalassemia. These dual effects of resveratrol were also revealed in a murine model of β-thalassemia [55]. Therefore, resveratrol may be considered as a potentially therapeutic intervention to ameliorate oxidative stress and anemia in patients with β-hemoglobinopathies.

Silymarin

Silymarin is a natural flavonolignan complex extracted from milk thistle (*Silybum marianum* L. Gaertn). The complex comprises of silybin, silychristin, and silydianin; which have been regarded as hepatoprotective agents by their powerful antioxidant, iron-chelating, and immunomodulatory properties. Antioxidative effects of silymarin in *in vitro* and *in vivo* studies were involved in its ability for radical scavenging (superoxide anion and hydroxyl radicals), increased GSH bioavailability, anti-lipoperoxidation, and raised expressions/activities of antioxidant enzymes (SOD, GPx, and GR) [56]. In 2006, Alidoost et al. collected peripheral blood mononuclear cells (PBMCs) from 28 each of β-thalassemia major patients and healthy subjects [57]. After incubating the cells with silymarin (5-20 μg/mL), a significantly increased intracellular GSH and depressed PBMCs proliferation were reported in thalassemic samples. Unfortunately, most recent research on silymarin in thalassemia emphasizes its role as an iron chelator rather than an effective antioxidant as shown in clinical trials using silymarin in combination with desferrioxamine [58, 59].

Besides antioxidants described earlier, only a few dietary antioxidants have been reported in thalassemic models including indicaxanthin derived from beet [60] and fermented papaya [61].

5. Pharmaceutical Antioxidants in Thalassemia

Some pharmaceutical agents show antioxidant effects that may associate to their pharmacological activity. Such synthetic antioxidants that have been studied in thalassemia are listed as follows:

5.1. Thiol-replenishing Drug

The maintenance of redox homeostasis is crucial for the functioning of various biological processes. The thiol-disulfide system is the major intracellular and extracellular redox buffer in mammals. Therefore, it would be beneficial to increase thiol concentrations under oxidative stress state.

In mammalian cells, the thiol-disulfide buffer usually refers to the GSH/GSSG pair since it is the most abundant redox couple in all cell types and biological fluids with strong electron-donating via thiol group of cysteine residue [62]. Exogenous thiols may be supplied as cysteine-donating compounds (a rate-limiting substrate) such as N-acetyl-L-cysteine (NAC) and its derivatives. N-acetylcysteine amide (AD4), the amide form of NAC with more hydrophobicity and better membrane diffusion, was studied *in vitro* and *in vivo* effects on thalassemic model [63]. RBCs, platelets, and polymorphonuclear (PMN) leukocytes obtained from thalassemic patients treated with AD4 showed significantly increased GSH and declined ROS levels with higher efficiency than NAC. In the murine model of β-thalassemia, intra-peritoneal injection of 150 mg/kg AD4 significantly reduced ROS and raised GSH levels. Nacystelyn (NAL), the lysine salt of NAC, was developed with 2-fold increase of intracellular GSH levels and providing neutral solution instead of acidic pH when NAC is solubilized [64]. Glutathione monoethyl and diethyl esters may be efficiently used to increase cellular GSH pools as they are rapidly transported into cells and then hydrolyzed to GSH [65]. Unfortunately, no any studies using such compounds in thalassemic model have been established so far.

Inhibition of GSH efflux mechanism results in restoration of cellular GSH. Muanprasat and colleague studied the GSH efflux in β-thalassemia/Hb E erythrocytes via cystic fibrosis transmembrane conductance regulator (CFTR) and multidrug resistance-associated protein (MRP) [66]. Treatment with GlyH-101 (CFTR inhibitor) and MK571 (MRP1 inhibitor) reduced H_2O_2-induced ROS generation by 80% and 50%, respectively. Combined treatment with both inhibitors completely inhibited ROS formation. H_2O_2-induced glutathione efflux was decreased by 87% and 66% after treatment with GlyH-101 and MK571, respectively. Therefore, pharmacological inhibitor of glutathione efflux may alleviate oxidative stress and premature destruction of thalassemic erythrocytes. However, further studies of safety should be performed since these drugs may produce side effects and may be not suitable for long-term use.

5.2. Iron Chelators

Iron chelators mobilize excess iron in tissues or biological fluids to form stable complexes that can be eliminated from the body in feces and/or urine. Typically, the goal of chelation therapy is to correct iron imbalance keeping iron levels within safety threshold and to reduce extensive accumulation of iron in vital organs. These reduce iron-related complications and improve survival as well as quality of life in iron-overloaded patients. Since 2004, more than 100 articles about iron-chelation therapy in thalassemic patients have been published on PubMed database. Almost all of these used high-doses of chelating drugs to remove iron deposited in organs/circulation in transfused-dependent thalassemic patients. Only a few studies aimed to maintain iron burden by low-dose chelating drugs used in transfused-independent patients.

Among three clinically used iron chelators, only deferasirox (DFX) has been used to maintain negative iron balance in non-transfusion-dependent thalassemia (NTDT) patients. The standard dose of DFX is 20-40 mg/kg/day for patients with liver iron overload (liver iron concentration (LIC) > 7 mg Fe/g dry weight) [67]. The THALASSA project is the first clinical trial to study the efficacy of DFX in NTDT patients with iron overload. One-year phase 2 trial of the project showed the effectiveness and safety of DFX at the dose 5 and 10 mg/kg/day to reduce liver iron overload in NTDT patients [68]. In 2013, the results of one-year THALASSA extension reported progressively decreased LIC with mean change -7.14 mg Fe/g dry weight at mean DFX dose 9.8 ± 3.6 mg/kg/day. From initial 166 patients enrolled, 64 (38.6%) and 24 (14.5%) patients achieved the goal of LIC <5 and <3 mg Fe/g dry weight, respectively [69]. Unfortunately, there were no measurements indicating oxidative status performed in this clinical trial.

5.3. Erythropoietin

Recombinant human erythropoietin (rHuEPO) is a drug used to treat anemia in patients with hemolytic anemia, on hemodialysis, or on chemotherapy. Thirteen-week treatment of rHuEPO (at escalating dose from 500 to 950 U/kg, 3 times/week) increased hemoglobin levels in β-thalassemic patients from 7.1±0.1 to 9.3±0.1 g/dL without changes in biomarkers indicating oxidative stress, iron-loading, and other hematological parameters [70]. The antioxidative properties of rHuEPO were shown in an *in vitro* study done by Amer et al. [71]. RBCs obtained from 11 thalassemic patients were under oxidative stress with increased ROS and decreased GSH levels compared to their normal counterparts. Incubating these RBCs with 1 U/mL EPO for two hours significantly decreased intracellular ROS by 1.5- to 2-fold and increased GSH by 1.25-fold compared to that of the untreated. Moreover, decreased percentages of PS-exposed RBCs were also reported resulting in decreased relative percentages of hemolyzed and phagocytized cells. However, the concentration of EPO that exert antioxidative activity is far higher than its physiological concentration and EPO cost is more expensive than other potential antioxidants. These make EPO not appropriate used as an antioxidative drug only.

5.4. Coenzyme Q_{10}

Synthetic CoQ_{10} is used as a medicine to prevent or alleviate various pathological conditions including heart and blood vessel problems, migraine, Huntington's disease, Parkinson's disease, and HIV/AIDS. So far, there has been only one clinical trial using CoQ_{10} in thalassemia. Kalpravidh et al. studied the antioxidant effect of CoQ_{10} in 12 β-thalassemia/Hb E patients [72]. Patients had extremely low levels of plasma CoQ_{10} at baseline and the levels significantly increased after supplementation at 100 mg daily dose for six months (baseline 0.28±0.13 μg/mL VS. month 6 0.50±0.15 μg/mL). The results also showed a significant improvement of oxidative stress as declined MDA levels and decreased activities of CAT and GPx.

6. Future Research of Antioxidants in Thalassemia

Although antioxidant therapies in thalassemia have been investigated over four decades, data limitation is still the main obstacle to consider as a treatment in practice. Further research studies are needed and some of these are summarized as follows:

(1) Combination strategies of antioxidants in thalassemia should be examined. Some antioxidants act synergistically when taken in combination and enhance antioxidant efficacy greater than the individually used.
(2) Recently, there are attempts to explore novel compounds with promising antioxidant potency such as large scale screenings of edible plant extracts with superoxide or hydroxyl radicals scavenging potential [73, 74]. Some of them may be potential and suitable for treatment oxidative stress in thalassemia. Appropriate antioxidants should be orally administered and readily absorbed, inexpensive, possess high antioxidative activities, have a long half-life, do not interfere with other drugs, and are not toxic even at high concentrations.
(3) Various antioxidants have low bioavailability that may be responsible for poor responses in patients. Possible reasons include poor absorption, increased metabolism, inactivity/low activity of antioxidants or their metabolites under physiological/pathological conditions, or rapid elimination out of body. The actual rationale behind these should be clarified, and pharmacodynamic/pharmacokinetic studies are encouraged to perform. Moreover, several techniques to date have been developed to improve bioavailability including liposome encapsulation, adjuvant, and emulsifying system. The experiments should be carefully designed to prevent pro-oxidant effect of such substances at inappropriate dose.
(4) From the literature review, many of published articles were studied in *in vitro* models and only a few were further performed in *in vivo*. The *in vivo* studies, either in animal models or patients with thalassemia, should be established.
(5) Experimental results are widely varied among studies. Numerous factors contributing these great variations include criteria for subject recruitment, dose and supplementation schedule, time of treatment, differential endpoints, sources and extraction procedures of dietary antioxidants. Therefore, therapeutic efficacy and adverse effects observed in one trial may not be directly compared to another trial. Normalization methods for comparative analysis should be considered to find the best regime for thalassemic patients.
(6) Safety implications of natural or synthetic antioxidants in either short-term or long-term treatment period need clarification.

Conclusion

Patients with thalassemia are under oxidative stress induced by secondary iron overload; mainly caused by chronic hemolysis, regular blood transfusions, and significantly increased intestinal absorption of iron. The generation of redox-active labile iron pool promotes the uncontrolled production of hydroxyl radicals leading to oxidative damages of intra- and extracellular biological molecules. However, a number of endogenous and exogenous antioxidant defenses counteract ROS and neutralize deleterious effects resulting in depletion of such antioxidants. Antioxidant supplementation from exogenous sources should increase antioxidant capacity in thalassemic patients. The studies using various antioxidants on thalassemic models as monotherapy or in combination regime are reviewed. Unfortunately, no any mono- or combined therapies have been completely neutralized harmful effects of iron-induced ROS in thalassemia so far. To date, scientific information is still limited with high variation of results. More research is required to find the best regime and some recommendations based on current knowledge are suggested in this chapter.

References

[1] De Franceschi, L; Bertoldi, M; Matte, A; Santos Franco, S; Pantaleo, A; Ferru, E, et al. Oxidative stress and beta-thalassemic erythroid cells behind the molecular defect. *Oxid. Med. Cell Longev.*, 2013; doi: 10.1155/2013/985210.

[2] Borgna-Pignatti, C; Rugolotto, S; De Stefano, P; Zhao, H; Cappellini, MD; Del Vecchio, GC, et al. Survival and complications in patients with thalassemia major treated with transfusion and deferoxamine. *Haematologica*, 2004; 89, 1187-93.

[3] Betteridge, DJ. What is oxidative stress? *Metabolism*, 2000; 49, 3-8.

[4] Rund, D; Rachmilewitz, E. Beta-thalassemia. *N. Engl. J. Med.*, 2005; 353, 1135-46.

[5] Halliwell, B; Gutteridge, JMC. Free Radicals in Biology and Medicine. New York: Oxford University Press Inc.; 1998.

[6] Amer, J; Goldfarb, A; Fibach, E. Flow cytometric analysis of the oxidative status of normal and thalassemic red blood cells. *Cytometry A*, 2004; 60, 73-80.

[7] Kalpravidh, RW; Siritanaratkul, N; Insain, P; Charoensakdi, R; Panichkul, N; Hatairaktham, S, et al. Improvement in oxidative stress and antioxidant parameters in beta-thalassemia/Hb E patients treated with curcuminoids. *Clin. Biochem.*, 2010; 43, 424-9.

[8] Trombetta, D; Gangemi, S; Saija, A; Minciullo, PL; Cimino, F; Cristani, M, et al. Increased protein carbonyl groups in the serum of patients affected by thalassemia major. *Ann. Hematol.*, 2006; 85, 520-2.

[9] Meerang, M; Nair, J; Sirankapracha, P; Thephinlap, C; Srichairatanakool, S; Arab, K, et al. Accumulation of lipid peroxidation-derived DNA lesions in iron-overloaded thalassemic mouse livers: comparison with levels in the lymphocytes of thalassemia patients. *Int. J. Cancer*, 2009; 125, 759-66.

[10] Kohgo, Y; Ikuta, K; Ohtake, T; Torimoto, Y; Kato, J. Body iron metabolism and pathophysiology of iron overload. *Int. J. Hematol.*, 2008; 88, 7-15.

[11] Fiorelli, G; Fargion, S; Piperno, A; Battafarano, N; Cappellini, MD. Iron metabolism in thalassemia intermedia. *Haematologica*, 1990; 75 Suppl 5, 89-95.

[12] Brissot, P; Ropert, M; Le Lan, C; Loreal, O. Non-transferrin bound iron: a key role in iron overload and iron toxicity. *Biochim. Biophys. Acta*, 2012; 1820, 403-10.

[13] Evans, RW; Rafique, R; Zarea, A; Rapisarda, C; Cammack, R; Evans, PJ, et al. Nature of non-transferrin-bound iron: studies on iron citrate complexes and thalassemic sera. *J. Biol. Inorg. Chem.*, 2008; 13, 57-74.

[14] Patel, M; Ramavataram, DV. Non Transferrin Bound Iron: Nature, Manifestations and Analytical Approaches for Estimation. *Indian J. Clin. Biochem.*, 2012; 27, 322-32.

[15] Kakhlon, O; Cabantchik, ZI. The labile iron pool: characterization, measurement, and participation in cellular processes(1). *Free Radic. Biol. Med.*, 2002; 33, 1037-46.

[16] Sies, H. Strategies of antioxidant defense. *Eur. J. Biochem.*, 1993; 215, 213-9.

[17] Eaton, JW; Qian, M. Molecular bases of cellular iron toxicity. *Free Radic. Biol. Med.*, 2002; 32, 833-40.

[18] Retsky, KL; Freeman, MW; Frei, B. Ascorbic acid oxidation product(s) protect human low density lipoprotein against atherogenic modification. Anti- rather than prooxidant activity of vitamin C in the presence of transition metal ions. *J. Biol. Chem.*, 1993; 268, 1304-9.

[19] Pham-Huy, LA; He, H; Pham-Huy, C. Free radicals, antioxidants in disease and health. *Int. J. Biomed. Sci.*, 2008; 4, 89-96.

[20] Deneke, SM. Thiol-based antioxidants. *Curr. Top Cell Regul.*, 2000; 36, 151-80.

[21] Rahman, K. Studies on free radicals, antioxidants, and co-factors. *Clin. Interv. Aging*, 2007; 2, 219-36.

[22] Lu, SC. Glutathione synthesis. *Biochim. Biophys. Acta*, 2013; 1830, 3143-53.

[23] Young, IS; Woodside, JV. Antioxidants in health and disease. *J. Clin. Pathol.*, 2001; 54, 176-86.

[24] Thomas, SR; Neuzil, J; Stocker, R. Cosupplementation with coenzyme Q prevents the prooxidant effect of alpha-tocopherol and increases the resistance of LDL to transition metal-dependent oxidation initiation. *Arterioscler. Thromb. Vasc. Biol.*, 1996; 16, 687-96.

[25] Stocker, R; Yamamoto, Y; McDonagh, AF; Glazer, AN; Ames, BN. Bilirubin is an antioxidant of possible physiological importance. *Science*, 1987; 235, 1043-6.

[26] Sevanian, A; Davies, KJ; Hochstein, P. Serum urate as an antioxidant for ascorbic acid. *Am. J. Clin. Nutr.*, 1991; 54, 1129S-34S.

[27] Young, IS. Measurement of total antioxidant capacity. *J. Clin. Pathol.*, 2001; 54, 339.

[28] Behera, S; Dixit, S; Bulliyya, G; Kar, SK. Fat-Soluble Antioxidant Vitamins, Iron Overload and Chronic Malnutrition in beta-Thalassemia Major. *Indian J. Pediatr.*, 2013; doi: 10.1007/s12098-013-1162-0.

[29] Livrea, MA; Tesoriere, L; Pintaudi, AM; Calabrese, A; Maggio, A; Freisleben, HJ, et al. Oxidative stress and antioxidant status in beta-thalassemia major: iron overload and depletion of lipid-soluble antioxidants. *Blood*, 1996; 88, 3608-14.

[30] Awadallah, S; Al Arrayed, K; Bahareth, E; Saeed, Z. Total antioxidant capacity and ischemia modified albumin in beta thalassemia. *Clin. Lab.*, 2013; 59, 687-91.

[31] Kalpravidh, RW; Tangjaidee, T; Hatairaktham, S; Charoensakdi, R; Panichkul, N; Siritanaratkul, N, et al. Glutathione redox system in beta -thalassemia/Hb E patients. *The Scientific World Journal*, 2013; doi: 10.1155/2013/543973.

[32] Kukongviriyapan, V; Somparn, N; Senggunprai, L; Prawan, A; Kukongviriyapan, U; Jetsrisuparb, A. Endothelial dysfunction and oxidant status in pediatric patients with hemoglobin E-beta thalassemia. *Pediatr. Cardiol.*, 2008; 29, 130-5.

[33] Herrera, E; Barbas, C. Vitamin E: action, metabolism and perspectives. *J. Physiol. Biochem.*, 2001; 57, 43-56.

[34] Traber, MG; Stevens, JF. Vitamins C and E: Beneficial effects from a mechanistic perspective. *Free Radic. Biol. Med.*, 2011; 51, 1000-13.

[35] Pfeifer, WP; Degasperi, GR; Almeida, MT; Vercesi, AE; Costa, FF; Saad, ST. Vitamin E supplementation reduces oxidative stress in beta thalassaemia intermedia. *Acta Haematol.,* 2008; 120, 225-31.

[36] Tesoriere, L; D'Arpa, D; Butera, D; Allegra, M; Renda, D; Maggio, A, et al. Oral supplements of vitamin E improve measures of oxidative stress in plasma and reduce oxidative damage to LDL and erythrocytes in beta-thalassemia intermedia patients. *Free Radic. Res.*, 2001; 34, 529-40.

[37] Unchern, S; Laoharuangpanya, N; Phumala, N; Sipankapracha, P; Pootrakul, P; Fucharoen, S, et al. The effects of vitamin E on platelet activity in beta-thalassaemia patients. *Br. J. Haematol.*, 2003; 123, 738-44.

[38] Sutipornpalangkul, W; Morales, NP; Unchern, S; Sanvarinda, Y; Chantharaksri, U; Fucharoen, S. Vitamin E supplement improves erythrocyte membrane fluidity of thalassemia: an ESR spin labeling study. *J. Med. Assoc. Thai*, 2012; 95, 29-36.

[39] Das, N; Das Chowdhury, T; Chattopadhyay, A; Datta, AG. Attenuation of oxidative stress-induced changes in thalassemic erythrocytes by vitamin E. *Pol. J. Pharmacol.*, 2004; 56, 85-96.

[40] Dissayabutra, T; Tosukhowong, P; Seksan, P. The benefits of vitamin C and vitamin E in children with beta-thalassemia with high oxidative stress. *J. Med. Assoc. Thai*, 2005; 88 Suppl 4, S317-21.

[41] Elalfy, MS; Adly, AA; Attia, AA; Ibrahim, FA; Mohammed, AS; Sayed, AM. Effect of antioxidant therapy on hepatic fibrosis and liver iron concentrations in beta-thalassemia major patients. *Hemoglobin*, 2013; 37, 257-76.

[42] Goel, A; Kunnumakkara, AB; Aggarwal, BB. Curcumin as "Curecumin": from kitchen to clinic. *Biochem. Pharmacol.*, 2008; 75, 787-809.

[43] Ak, T; Gulcin, I. Antioxidant and radical scavenging properties of curcumin. *Chem. Biol. Interact.*, 2008; 174, 27-37.

[44] Lee, JS; Surh, YJ. Nrf2 as a novel molecular target for chemoprevention. *Cancer Lett.*, 2005; 224, 171-84.

[45] Jiao, Y; Wilkinson, Jt; Di, X; Wang, W; Hatcher, H; Kock, ND, et al. Curcumin, a cancer chemopreventive and chemotherapeutic agent, is a biologically active iron chelator. *Blood*, 2009; 113, 462-9.

[46] Shoba, G; Joy, D; Joseph, T; Majeed, M; Rajendran, R; Srinivas, PS. Influence of piperine on the pharmacokinetics of curcumin in animals and human volunteers. *Planta Med.*, 1998; 64, 353-6.

[47] Weeraphan, C; Srisomsap, C; Chokchaichamnankit, D; Subhasitanont, P; Hatairaktham, S; Charoensakdi, R, et al. Role of curcuminoids in ameliorating oxidative modification in beta-thalassemia/Hb E plasma proteome. *J. Nutr. Biochem.*, 2013; 24, 578-85.

[48] Thephinlap, C; Phisalaphong, C; Lailerd, N; Chattipakorn, N; Winichagoon, P; Vadolas, J, et al. Reversal of cardiac iron loading and dysfunction in thalassemic mice by curcuminoids. *Med. Chem.*, 2011; 7, 62-9.

[49] Babu, PV; Liu, D. Green tea catechins and cardiovascular health: an update. *Curr. Med. Chem.*, 2008; 15, 1840-50.

[50] Cabrera, C; Artacho, R; Gimenez, R. Beneficial effects of green tea--a review. *J. Am. Coll. Nutr.*, 2006; 25, 79-99.

[51] Thephinlap, C; Ounjaijean, S; Khansuwan, U; Fucharoen, S; Porter, JB; Srichairatanakool, S. Epigallocatechin-3-gallate and epicatechin-3-gallate from green

tea decrease plasma non-transferrin bound iron and erythrocyte oxidative stress. *Med. Chem.*, 2007; 3, 289-96.

[52] Ounjaijean, S; Thephinlap, C; Khansuwan, U; Phisalapong, C; Fucharoen, S; Porter, JB, et al. Effect of green tea on iron status and oxidative stress in iron-loaded rats. *Med. Chem.*, 2008; 4, 365-70.

[53] Saewong, T; Ounjaijean, S; Mundee, Y; Pattanapanyasat, K; Fucharoen, S; Porter, JB, et al. Effects of green tea on iron accumulation and oxidative stress in livers of iron-challenged thalassemic mice. *Med. Chem.*, 2010; 6, 57-64.

[54] Fibach, E; Prus, E; Bianchi, N; Zuccato, C; Breveglieri, G; Salvatori, F, et al. Resveratrol: Antioxidant activity and induction of fetal hemoglobin in erythroid cells from normal donors and beta-thalassemia patients. *Int. J. Mol. Med.*, 2012; 29, 974-82.

[55] Franco, SS; De Falco, L; Ghaffari, S; Brugnara, C; Sinclair, DA; Matte, A, et al. Resveratrol accelerates erythroid maturation by activation of FoxO3 and ameliorates anemia in beta-thalassemic mice. *Haematologica*, 2014; 99, 267-75.

[56] Agarwal, R; Agarwal, C; Ichikawa, H; Singh, RP; Aggarwal, BB. Anticancer potential of silymarin: from bench to bed side. *Anticancer Res.*, 2006; 26, 4457-98.

[57] Alidoost, F; Gharagozloo, M; Bagherpour, B; Jafarian, A; Sajjadi, SE; Hourfar, H, et al. Effects of silymarin on the proliferation and glutathione levels of peripheral blood mononuclear cells from beta-thalassemia major patients. *Int. Immunopharmacol.*, 2006; 6, 1305-10.

[58] Gharagozloo, M; Moayedi, B; Zakerinia, M; Hamidi, M; Karimi, M; Maracy, M, et al. Combined therapy of silymarin and desferrioxamine in patients with beta-thalassemia major: a randomized double-blind clinical trial. *Fundam. Clin. Pharmacol.*, 2009; 23, 359-65.

[59] Moayedi, B; Gharagozloo, M; Esmaeil, N; Maracy, MR; Hoorfar, H; Jalaeikar, M. A randomized double-blind, placebo-controlled study of therapeutic effects of silymarin in beta-thalassemia major patients receiving desferrioxamine. *Eur. J. Haematol.*, 2013; 90, 202-9.

[60] Tesoriere, L; Allegra, M; Butera, D; Gentile, C; Livrea, MA. Cytoprotective effects of the antioxidant phytochemical indicaxanthin in beta-thalassemia red blood cells. *Free Radic. Res.*, 2006; 40, 753-61.

[61] Fibach, E; Tan, ES; Jamuar, S; Ng, I; Amer, J; Rachmilewitz, EA. Amelioration of oxidative stress in red blood cells from patients with beta-thalassemia major and intermedia and E-beta-thalassemia following administration of a fermented papaya preparation. *Phytother. Res.*, 2010; 24, 1334-8.

[62] Wu, G; Fang, YZ; Yang, S; Lupton, JR; Turner, ND. Glutathione metabolism and its implications for health. *J. Nutr.*, 2004; 134, 489-92.

[63] Amer, J; Atlas, D; Fibach, E. N-acetylcysteine amide (AD4) attenuates oxidative stress in beta-thalassemia blood cells. *Biochim. Biophys. Acta*, 2008; 1780, 249-55.

[64] Gillissen, A; Jaworska, M; Orth, M; Coffiner, M; Maes, P; App, EM, et al. Nacystelyn, a novel lysine salt of N-acetylcysteine, to augment cellular antioxidant defence in vitro. *Respir. Med.*, 1997; 91, 159-68.

[65] Levy, EJ; Anderson, ME; Meister, A. Transport of glutathione diethyl ester into human cells. *Proc. Natl. Acad. Sci. U. S. A.*, 1993; 90, 9171-5.

[66] Muanprasat, C; Wongborisuth, C; Pathomthongtaweechai, N; Satitsri, S; Hongeng, S. Protection against oxidative stress in beta thalassemia/hemoglobin E erythrocytes by

inhibitors of glutathione efflux transporters. *PLoS One*, 2013; doi: 10.1371/journal.pone.0055685.

[67] Wood, JC; Kang, BP; Thompson, A; Giardina, P; Harmatz, P; Glynos, T, et al. The effect of deferasirox on cardiac iron in thalassemia major: impact of total body iron stores. *Blood*, 2010; 116, 537-43.

[68] Taher, AT; Porter, J; Viprakasit, V; Kattamis, A; Chuncharunee, S; Sutcharitchan, P, et al. Deferasirox reduces iron overload significantly in nontransfusion-dependent thalassemia: 1-year results from a prospective, randomized, double-blind, placebo-controlled study. *Blood*, 2012; 120, 970-7.

[69] Taher, AT; Porter, JB; Viprakasit, V; Kattamis, A; Chuncharunee, S; Sutcharitchan, P, et al. Deferasirox effectively reduces iron overload in non-transfusion-dependent thalassemia (NTDT) patients: 1-year extension results from the THALASSA study. *Ann. Hematol.*, 2013; 92, 1485-93.

[70] Rachmilewitz, EA; Aker, M; Perry, D; Dover, G. Sustained increase in haemoglobin and RBC following long-term administration of recombinant human erythropoietin to patients with homozygous beta-thalassaemia. *Br. J. Haematol.*, 1995; 90, 341-5.

[71] Amer, J; Dana, M; Fibach, E. The antioxidant effect of erythropoietin on thalassemic blood cells. *Anemia*, 2010; doi: 10.1155/2010/978710.

[72] Kalpravidh, RW; Wichit, A; Siritanaratkul, N; Fucharoen, S. Effect of coenzyme Q10 as an antioxidant in beta-thalassemia/Hb E patients. *Biofactors*, 2005; 25, 225-34.

[73] Saito, K; Kohno, M; Yoshizaki, F; Niwano, Y. Extensive screening for edible herbal extracts with potent scavenging activity against superoxide anions. *Plant Foods Hum. Nutr.*, 2008; 63, 65-70.

[74] Niwano, Y; Saito, K; Yoshizaki, F; Kohno, M; Ozawa, T. Extensive screening for herbal extracts with potent antioxidant properties. *J. Clin. Biochem. Nutr.*, 2011; 48, 78-84.

In: Thalassemia
Editor: Makenzie Greene

ISBN: 978-1-63117-954-9

Chapter 9

Calcifications in Thalassemia: An Important Complication

Somsri Wiwanitkit[1] and Viroj Wiwanitkit[2]
[1]Wiwanitkit House, Bangkhae, Bangkok Thailand
[2]Visiting Professor, Hainan Medical University, China;
Visiting professor,
Faculty of Medicine, University of Nis, Serbia; Adjunct professor,
Joseph Ayobabalola University, Nigeria

Abstract

Thalassemia is an important congenital hematological disorder. This congenital disorder result in hemoglobin defect and causes several signs and symptoms. This problem can be seen around the world and is still an important public health threat in several countries. There are many complications of thalassemia and those complications can be the causes of death. In the present short article, the authors will present and discuss on an important complication, calcification. The calcification is an important but usually forgotten complication. The calcified tissue can be seen in many organs and become the problem.

Keywords: Thalassemia, calcification

Introduction

Thalassemia is an important congenital hematological disorder. This congenital disorder result in hemoglobin defect and causes several signs and symptoms. The examples of signs and symptoms include pale, organomegaly and growth retardation [1 – 3]. Due to the defective, the patients usually have short life span. This problem can be seen around the world and is still an important public health threat in several countries (such as Thailand, Laos, etc) [4]. There are many complications of thalassemia and those complications can be the causes of death. It should be mentioned that most thalassemic patient died of complications of disease. In the present short article, the authors will present and discuss on an important complication, calcification. The calcification is an important but usually forgotten complication. The calcified tissue can be seen in many organs and become the problem.

How Can Calcification Occurs in Thalassemic Patients?

The first question to be discussed is on the pathogenesis of calcification in thalassemia. First, it should be mentioned that the abnormal calcification is usually pathology. The cause is usually relating to the aberration of calcium metabolism within the patient's body. In fact, the control of calcium in human body is based on the two important hormone, calcitonin and parathromone. The calcitonin reduce the blood calcium and stimulate the accumulation in tissue whereas parathromone has the counteraction. The balancing between the two hormone is the key point for calcium homeostasis in human. The two main endocrine glands, thyroid and parathyroid gland that secrete both hormones become the vital organ that control the regulation of calcium dynamics in human body [5].

In thalassemia, the abnormality of the parathyroid gland can be seen and this is mentioned as the cause of calcification. The endocrine disturbance is closely relating to the bone defect that is common in the patients with thalassemia. In thalassemic patients, there are many problems on bone system. Voskaridou and Terpos Noted that "the pathogenesis of bone loss in thalassemia is multifactorial. The delay in sexual maturation, the presence of diabetes and hypothyroidism, the parathyroid gland dysfunction, the accelerated hemopoiesis with progressive marrow expansion, the direct iron toxicity on osteoblasts, the iron chelators, the deficiency of growth hormone or insulin growth factors, all have been identified as major causes of osteoporosis in thalassemia [6]." Parathyroid malfunction is the main problem that affect the calcium metabolism and this result in further observed abnormal calcification [7].

Abnormal Calcification in Internal Organs in Thalassemic Patients

A. Brain Calcification

Brain calcification is a common king of internal organ calcification that can be seen in thalassemic patients. Karimi et al. noted that most cases were firstly observed at adolescent age [8 - 9].The calcification can be seen at any sites of brain [8]. However, the common affected site includes basal ganglia, and frontoparietal areas of the brain [10]. Karimi et al. noted that "no relationship was observed between the degree of cerebral calcification and the severity of hypoparathyroidism at diagnosis [8]. Mahmoodi et al. noted that "prompt treatment with oral calcium supplements and an active form of vitamin D can prevent hypoparathyroidism and its neurologic complications [11]. Finally, it should be noted that not only hypoparathyroidism but also other rare underlying disorders can causes intracranial calcification in thalassemic patients. The good example is the intracranial calcification in the patient with thalassemia as a secondary problem to nephrogenic diabetes insipidus [12].

B. Liver Calcification

The liver calcification can also be seen in the thalassemic patients. The underlying parathyroidism is accepted as the cause of liver calcification [13]. The problem can be seen early in fetal life [14].

C. Heart Calcification

Heart calcification is another internal calcification that can be seen in thalassemia. It is relating to another pathological condition, pseudoxanthomaelasticum-like diffuse elastic tissue defect [15]. The problem of calcification usually attacks heart valve [15].

Conclusion

In thalassemia, the calcification is an important but usually forgotten complication. The calcified tissue can be seen in many organs and become the problem in clinical practice. General practitioner has to aware and properly manage.

References

[1] Festa RS. Modern management of thalassemia. *Pediatr Ann.* 1985 Sep;14(9):597-600, 602-3, 606.

[2] Fondu P. Thalassemia in 1985. *Rev. Med. Brux.* 1985 Apr;6(4):281-5.

[3] Huisman TH. A short review of human gamma-globin gene anomalies.*ActaHaematol.* 1987;78(2-3):80-4.

[4] Fucharoen S, Winichagoon P. Haemoglobinopathies in Southeast Asia. *Indian J. Med. Res.* 2011 Oct;134:498-506.

[5] Kleeman CR, Massry SG, Coburn JW. The clinical physiology of calcium homeostasis, parathyroid hormone, and calcitonin. II. *Calif. Med.* 1971 Apr;114(4):19-30.

[6] Voskaridou E, Terpos E. Pathogenesis and management of osteoporosis in thalassemia. *Pediatr Endocrinol Rev.* 2008 Oct;6. Suppl 1:86-93.

[7] Galanello R, Origa R. Beta-thalassemia. *Orphanet. J. Rare Dis.* 2010 May 21;5:11. doi: 10.1186/1750-1172-5-11.

[8] Karimi M, Habibzadeh F, De Sanctis V. Hypoparathyroidism with extensive intracerebral calcification in patients with beta-thalassemia major. *J. Pediatr. Endocrinol. Metab.* 2003 Jul-Aug;16(6):883-6.

[9] Verma S, Saxena AK, Marwaha RK.Intracranial calcification in beta-thalassemia major. *Indian Pediatr.* 2007 Nov;44(11):856-8.

[10] Karimi M, Rasekhi AR, Rasekh M, Nabavizadeh SA, Assadsangabi R, Amirhakimi GH. Hypoparathyroidism and intracerebral calcification in patients with beta-thalassemia major. *Eur. J. Radiol.* 2009 Jun;70(3):481-4.

[11] Mahmoodi M, De Sanctis V, Karimi M. Diffuse intracerebral calcification in a beta-thalassaemia major patient with hypoparathyroidism: a case report. *Pediatr. Endocrinol. Rev.* 2011 Mar;8. Suppl 2:331-3.
[12] Dimple J, Alka J, Mona G, Atul D. Nephrogenic diabetes insipidus with intracranial calcification in a child with thalassemia minor. *Arab. J. Nephrol. Transplant.* 2013 Sep;6(3):185-7.
[13] Saki F, Bordbar MR, Imanieh MH, Karimi M. Diffuse hepatic calcifications in a transfusion-dependent patient with Beta-thalassemia: A case report. *Iran J. Med. Sci.* 2013 Sep;38(3):271-4.
[14] Buxton PJ, Maheswaran P, Dewbury KC, Moore IE. Neonatal hepatic calcification in subcapsularhaematoma with hydropsfetalis. *Br. J. Radiol.* 1991 Nov;64(767):1058-60.
[15] Farmakis D, Polonifi A, Deftereos S, Tsironi M, Papaioannou I, Aessopos A.Aortic valve replacement in a patient with thalassemia intermedia. *Ann. Thorac. Surg*. 2006 Feb;81(2):737-9.

In: Thalassemia
Editor: Makenzie Greene
ISBN: 978-1-63117-954-9

Chapter 10

Multi-Target Therapeutic Modalities for β-Hemoglobinopathies

*Eitan Fibach**

Department of Hematology, Hadassah, Hebrew University Medical Center, Jerusalem, Israel

Abstract

The primary defects in the β-hemoglobinopathies: β-thalassemia and sickle cell anemia (SCA), are quantitative and qualitative abnormalities in hemoglobin (Hb), respectively, leading to chronic anemia. To cure, these primary defects should be corrected. This can be accomplished by two therapeutic modalities: Hematopoietic stem cell transplantation [1] and gene therapy [2, 3]. However neither is currently applicable to most patients with these diseases because of technical difficulties, the costs involved, and a lack of the highly sophisticated medical care necessary to provide these therapies in developing countries where the diseases are most prevalent. In addition to chronic anemia, which is treated by blood transfusion, other associated pathologies cause morbidity and mortality. Among these are: Ineffective erythropoiesis – the abortive attempt of the body to overcome the state of anemia [4]; iron overload (IO) – the result of repeated blood transfusions and increased iron uptake [5], and oxidative stress – due to the instability of the Hb and iron-mediated generation of cytotoxic free radicals [6].Advances in the treatment of the chronic anemia and its accompanying IO significantly prolong the life-span of most patients, but with older age come additional pathologies associated with the underlying disease and its treatment modalities.

Treatment modalities are usually target-specific. Sometimes, such as in the case of malignancy, to achieve maximal efficacy a combination of drugs is used. For the β-hemoglobinopathies, each modality aims to treat one aspect of the disease: Blood transfusion for the chronic anemia, iron chelation for IO and anti-oxidants for oxidative stress. But usually drugs have more than one target. In most cases, their “side effects” on “secondary” targets are deleterious, causing therapy-associated symptoms. But

* Corresponding author: Eitan Fibach, Department of Hematology, Hadassah – Hebrew University Medical Center, Ein-Kerem, Jerusalem 91120, Israel. Fax: 972-2-6423067; E-mail address: Fibach@yahoo.com.

sometimes the effects, either direct or indirect on "secondary" targets are beneficial, synergizing with the primary effect to optimize the therapeutic influence..

Many drugs used for treating β-hemoglobinopathies have a pleiotropic effect, and as such they are associated with a variety of effects, both beneficial and deleterious. Among the beneficial effects are: (A) Stimulation of erythropoiesis, aimed at ameliorating the state of anemia. (B) Specific stimulation of fetal Hb production, thereby decreasing the relative concentration of β^S-globin chains (leading to sickling in SCA), or the excess of α-globin chains – the main cause of the short life-span of RBC in β-thalassemia. (C) Reducing IO – by iron chelation, increasing iron utilization or decreasing iron uptake. (D) Amelioration of oxidative stress – by directly scavenging free radicals in erythroid and non-erythroid cells, as well as in the extracellular milieu, or by its indirect effect on iron. These effects may influence the proliferation and maturation of erythroid precursors in the bone marrow as well as the senescence and removal of RBC from the peripheral blood, and also reduce cytotoxicity to other cells in vital organs.

The following is a review of such modalities and a discussion of their potential application for treatment of β-hemoglobinopathies. I believe that on the basis of the data summarized in this review, the time has come to define, by studying *in vitro* and *in vivo* models, as well as by controlled clinical trials, the multi-target effects of drugs for the treatment of patients with various forms of these diseases.

Keywords: Thalassemia, sickle cell anemia, erythrocytes, oxidative stress, antioxidants, iron overload, fetal hemoglobin

Quantitative and Qualitative Abnormalities of HbA and Their Amelioration by HbF

The β-hemoglobinopathies are hereditary hemolytic anemias due to mutations in the β-globin cluster. The β-globin polypeptide chains together with the α-globin chains constitute the major Hb species – adult Hb (HbA, $\alpha_2\beta_2$). In β-thalassemia, the mutations decrease (β^+-thalassemia) or abolish (β^o-thalassemia) synthesis of the β-globin chains [7]. In addition to the low presence of HbA, or its absence, the thalassemic RBC contain an excess of α-globin chains – the main cause for their membrane damage and short survival (see below). In SCA, a specific mutation causes a structural change in the β-globin (β^S), leading to production of sickle Hb (HbS, $\alpha_2\ \beta^S{}_2$). This abnormal Hb polymerizes under the deoxygenating conditions present in small capillaries, resulting in morphological and functional changes in RBC (sickling). During most of fetal life, the γ-globin genes, rather than the β-globin genes, are transcribed, and the major Hb is fetal Hb (HbF, $\alpha_2\gamma_2$). Postnatally, the γ-globin genes are almost completely switched off while the β-globin genes are turned on and thus, normally, HbF is replaced by HbA. Thus, abnormalities in HbA such as in β-hemoglobinopathies, do not affect the fetus or the newborn; their pathological consequences start at early childhood.

Epidemiological studies showed that patients with β-hemoglobinopathies who co-inherited additional mutations that allowed γ-globin gene expression in adults (hereditary persistence of fetal Hb) had less severe clinical courses [8, 9]. This was subsequently shown to be due to the ability of the γ-globin chains to bind to and thus reduce the excess of α-globin chains in β-thalassemia and of β^S-globin and HbS in SCA [10]. It has been therefore proposed that reactivation of the γ-globin genes could provide an effective treatment strategy [11].

Desimone et al., first in baboons [12] and then in patients [13], demonstrated the ability of the nucleoside analogue 5-azacytidine (5-Aza) to stimulate γ-globin gene expression and HbF production. Following these studies, more than 75 various chemical agents have been shown to share a similar activity. Currently, the only clinically approved drug is hydroxyurea (HU) [14].

Oxidative Stress

Although the primary lesions in β-hemoglobinopathies are mutations in the β-globin gene, the damage to the RBC and other cells is mediated in part by oxidative stress [15, 16]. The oxidative status in cells is maintained by the equilibrium between oxidants, such as reactive oxygen species (ROS) and nitrogen species, which are balanced by antioxidants, such as reduced glutathione (GSH). When this equilibrium is tilted by an increase in oxidants and/or a decrease in antioxidants – oxidative stress ensues. The redox status of cells and the presence of ROS are important for normal functioning of all cells. However, excess ROS, through their interaction with various cell constituents, such as proteins, DNA and lipids, are deleterious [17].

It has been shown that in β-hemoglobinopathies RBC are under oxidative stress [18]. Using flow cytometry methodology, we have demonstrated increased generation of ROS with a concurrent decreased content of GSH, in thalassemic RBC compared with that in normal RBC at basal level, as well as following an oxidative insult such as treatment of the cells with hydrogen peroxide [19, 20]. These effects were associated with membrane changes, including lipid peroxidation, and externalization of phosphatidylserine – a marker of cell senescence [21]. The changes in the RBC membranes resulted in increased susceptibility to hemolysis and to phagocytosis by macrophages [22]. Oxidative stress was also found in the polymorphonuclears [19] and platelets [23] of these patients, explaining, in part, their propensity for recurrent infections and thromboembolic complications [24].

The main contributor to oxidative stress in the β-hemoglobinopathies is the instability of various Hb species. In β-thalassemia, the excess α-globin chains form homotetramers that are unstable and dissociate into monomers which, following a change in their tertiary structure, are oxidized to hemichromes [25]. In SCA, HbS becomes unstable following repeated cycles of sickling and unsickling. In both diseases the outcome of these processes is the release of iron and proteins, which precipitate in the cytosol and in the plasma membrane. The chain of events has deleterious effects mainly on the membrane lipids and proteins, including oxidation of membrane protein band 4.1 and a decrease in the spectrin/band3 ratio [26].

Treatment of oxidative stress is based on the finding that in thalassemia and SCA, as well as in other hemolytic anemias, hydrophilic and hydrophobic antioxidants are depleted because of the increased need to neutralize the oxidative stress [27]. Since vitamin E is frequently deficient in β-thalassemia patients, its supplementation was studied extensively [28]. The results showed that in heterozygous patients, a high dose of oral vitamin E decreased lipid peroxidation in RBC and increased their survival [29]. Other studies showed an improvement in the plasma antioxidant/oxidant balance, in the oxidation of low density lipoproteins and in the impaired osmotic fragility of RBC [30]. Most of these studies, however, failed to find a significant improvement in clinical parameters, i.e., Hb concentration and transfusion requirement.

Iron-Overload (IO)

Another contributor to oxidative stress is iron overload (IO), which is a major complication in thalassemia patients and to some extent also in SCA, affecting both morbidity and mortality, mainly in older patients [5]. The major cause of IO is blood transfusions, commonly used in severe cases of these diseases. Blood transfusion introduces iron (in the form of Hb in the transfused RBC) beyond its disposal capacity by the body. Another cause of IO, which exists even in non-transfused patients [31], is increased iron uptake from the gastrointestinal tract. Iron homeostasis is mediated by hepcidin which inhibits iron transport across the gut mucosa, thereby preventing excess iron absorption, and out of macrophages (where iron is stored), thus lowering its mobilization. Hepcidin functions by binding to the iron export channel ferroportin, which is located on the cell surface, leading to its intracellular degradation. Hepcidin binding to ferroportin in the gut enterocytes and in the reticuloendothelial macrophages reduces iron uptake and mobilization.

The production of hepcidin is regulated by multiple factors, including iron and cytokines such as Il-6. In thalassemia, hepcidin production is reduced. leading to increased iron absorption and mobilization. The main cause of low hepcidin levels in thalassemia is believed to be augmented erythropoiesis, where the body attempts, ineffectively, to overcome the state of anemia. The mechanism was suggested to involve increased synthesis of the growth differentiation factor 15 (GDF15) [32].

Iron is transported in the circulation bound to transferrin and is taken up by cells through a transferrin receptor [33]. Inside the cells, most of the iron is bound, in a redox-inactive form, to various components such as Hb, heme and cytochrome C, whereas the excess is stored in ferritin [34]. When serum iron exceeds the binding capacity of transferrin, it is present in the form of non-transferrin-bound iron [35]. This form of iron enters cells through transferrin-independent pathways to form the labile iron pool (LIP) [36, 37], which was suggested to be a transitory intermediate between the cellular iron pools [38]. LIP is redox active and participates, through the Fenton and Haber-Weiss reactions, in the generation of ROS which, when present in excess, are cytotoxic as discussed above. It is postulated that this is the main reason for morbidity and mortality due to IO in major organs [39] such as the heart, liver and endocrine glands.

IO is treated by limiting the frequency of blood transfusions and by iron chelation. Three chelators are currently in clinical practice. The most widely used is deferoxiamine. Although its side effects are minimal, compliance is often problematic since this drug is taken parenterally through a portable infusion pump on a daily basis. Two oral chelators have been developed – deferiprone and deferasirox; their application improved compliance and the quality of life [40]. Interestingly, co-adminstration of deferiprone and deferoxiamine to thalassemic patients resulted in iron excretion rates much higher than of deferoxiamine alone [41]. The term "shuttle effect" was coined to imply that the combination of a weak chelator, with efficient cell penetration with a strong chelator with poor cell penetration, may have a synergistic effect through iron shuttling between the two drugs.

This mechanism was confirmed in an animal study [42]. By removing intra and extra-cellular iron species which generate ROS, iron chelators act as antioxidants [43]. The anti-oxidant effect of treatment with deferasirox was also demonstrated in multi-transfused patients with myelodysplastic syndrome in which amelioration of oxidative stress parameters was achieved after three months [44].

HbF and Oxidative Stress

After many years of intensive research, the mechanism of drug-mediated HbF induction remains elusive. Traditionally, most HbF-inducing agents have been viewed as affecting γ-globin gene expression by altering local promoter chromatin structure or by changing the kinetics of erythroid differentiation (cytotoxic agents). Recently, the key effect of most HbF-inducing agents has been attributed to the activation of cell stress signaling. Free radicals are important mediators of several cell signaling pathways [45]. Witt et al. showed that induction of erythroid differentiation and Hb production in K562 cells by butyrate was associated with increased p38 MAPK phosphorylation and that pharmacologic inhibition of p38 activity prevented this action [46]. Inhibition of this pathway also repressed the inducing potential of the histone deacetylase (HDAC) inhibitors apicidin and valproic acid [47, 48]. ROS are one of the signals for p38 MAPK phosphorylation. Pace et al. [49] provided further evidence that HDAC inhibitors not only cause histone hyperacetylation, but also lead to production of ROS which in turn, cause p38 MAPK phosphorylation and downstream activation of the cAMP response element binding protein (CREBP) and activating transcription factor 2 (ATF2), which are transcriptional activator proteins.

Evidence in support of this model includes the ability of inhibitors of ROS generation to decrease HbF induction, demonstration of p38 phosphorylation in response to HbF-inducing agents and inhibition of induction by an inhibitor of p38 activity, the ability of constitutively active forms of MKK3 and MKK6 (upstream activators of p38 MAPK) to independently increase γ-globin gene expression and the finding that CREB and ATF2 bind an element in the γ^G-globin upstream promoter following HDAC inhibitor treatment. Thalidomide, another HbF inducer in K562 cells, has also been shown to induce generation of ROS which, in turn, cause p38 MAPK phosphorylation and globally increase histone H4 acetylation. Pharmacologic inhibition of ROS generation or p38 MAPK activation reduced its effect on HbF [50]. Other experiments have shown that inhibition of p38 MAPK activation prevents HU induced γ-globin gene expression in K562 cells [51].

Other agents have been shown to induce γ-globin by activating antioxidative systems such as the nuclear factor erythroid–related factor 2/antioxidant response element (NRF2/ARE) pathway. NRF2 is a primary transcriptional activator of a large battery of genes involved in cellular responses to oxidants and electrophiles [52]. Macari et al. [53] found that several activators of this pathway increased γ-globin mRNA at nontoxic doses in K562 cells. Tert-butylhydroquinone, the most active of these compounds, increased cellular levels and nuclear translocation of NRF2 and binding of NRF2 to the γ-globin promoter. siRNA knock-down of NRF2 inhibited the γ-globin induction. Experiments in human primary erythroid cells showed NRF2 binding to the γ-globin promoter, increased γ-globin mRNA and HbF, and suppressed β-globin mRNA and HbA, resulting in a greater proportion of HbF.

We have studied agents, angelicin [54] and resveratrol [55, 56], that have been shown to induce cell signaling through the same pathway [57, 58]. Resveratrol, a 3, 5, 4′-trihydroxystilbene, is a natural phytoalexin present in red wine and other constituents of the human diet [59]. This polyphenol has a wide range of biological properties (e.g., [60]) and was implicated in chemoprevention, which may explain the low incidence of breast and prostate cancers among vegetarians and Orientals, respectively [61]. Resveratrol is a radical scavenger that prevents many heart disorders by inhibiting lipoprotein oxidation and platelet aggregation (e.g., [62]). This molecule was associated with the low incidence of ischaemic heart disease observed in the French population, a phenomenon called the 'French Paradox' [59]. The latter was attributed to the presence of resveratrol in wine and to a moderate consumption of red wine.

We have studied its effect in K562 cells and in normal and thalassemic human primary erythroid cultures [11]. We found that it decreased oxidative stress parameters and induced HbF at sub-toxic concentrations. This dual effect of resveratrol suggests its therapeutic potential in patients with β-hemoglobinopathies.

Hemin

Hemin is another drug that relates HbF stimulation to the oxidative status of erythroid cells. Hemin is the chloride form of heme – an iron-containing protoporphyrin which is included in Hb and several other molecules as a prostatic group. An excess of heme has been suggested, via iron-mediated generation of free radicals, to be toxic to cells (e.g., [63]). Heme, however, is not necessarily cytotoxic to all cells [64]. Exogenously supplied hemin is readily taken up by cultured erythroid cells [65] and its iron is incorporated into Hb or stored in ferritin [66]. Following the addition of succinylacetone, a potent inhibitor of heme synthesis, exogenously supplied hemin could replace intracellularly synthesized heme and be incorporated into *de novo* formed Hb [66].

Several groups reported that hemin supplementation to cultures promotes the growth of normal erythroid precursors, (e.g., [67]). We previously showed, in a two-phase liquid culture, that hemin promotes erythropoiesis of normal and thalassemic precursors, as well as precursors from children with Diamond-Blackfan anemia – a congenital pure red-cell anemia due to a block in erythroid precursors [68]. This effect was noted both in the presence [69] and absence [70] of holo-transferrin, the iron-transporting protein.

Hemin is a well-known inducer of erythroid differentiation, including hemoglobinization, of human (K562) [71] and murine (MEL) [72, 73] leukemia cell lines. We found that hemin stimulates HbF production in primary cultures of human, normal and thalassemic, erythroid cells [69] as well. The growth promoting and HbF stimulating effects in primary cells were particularly prominent during the early stages of maturation.

Based on these findings, we suggested that the exogenously supplied heme accelerates hemoglobinization when iron-uptake and heme synthesis are limited. Moreover, since HbF is mostly produced when Hb production is initiated [74-76], accelerating hemoglobinization at these stages favors mainly HbF. Additional studies have indicated that the effect of hemin on globin gene expression in primary erythroid cultures involves also transcriptional and posttranscriptional regulation [77].

However, heme participates in many metabolic pathways, including the regulation of transcription through inhibition of DNA binding of the repressor, Bach1 [78], or globin translation through inhibition of substrate phosphorylation by the repressor, erythroid-specific eukaryotic initiation factor 2α kinase (eIF2α kinase) [79]. In erythroid cells it also stabilizes the globin chains by forming Hb [80].

Hemin was also shown to use the Nrf2 pathway, e.g., induction of thioredoxin [81]. In K562 cells, hemin was found to induce γ-globin expression and to cause Nrf2 binding to the γ-globin promoter [53]. Knockdown of Nrf2 by treating the cells with siRNA prior to exposure to hemin attenuated induction of γ-globin.

The use of hemin as a therapeutic modality for patients with β-hemoglobinization [82] may be based on its multi-target effects: stimulation of Hb, particularly HbF, production and stimulation of the cellular antioxidant systems. Its potential effect on IO should, however, be considered.

Erythropoietin

Also erythropoietin (Epo), the major regulator of erythropoiesis, is a multi-target agent. This hormone is produced and released by the kidneys in response to hypoxia. By binding to a surface receptor (EpoR), it stimulates proliferation and inhibits apoptosis of erythroid progenitors and precursors in the bone marrow [83, 84]. The clinically-approved recombinant human Epo preparations include epoetin-α, epoetin-β, and the long-acting darbepoetin-α, all effective stimulators of erythropoiesis. They are widely used for the treatment of chronic anemia of different etiologies, e.g., in patients undergoing chemotherapy [85] or hemodialysis [86], as well as in patients with myelodysplastic syndrome [87].

In spite of the state of chronic anemia, the level of serum Epo in thalassemia, and to some extent in SCA, is low relative to the degree of anemia [88, 89], probably due to its increased utilization. Several studies demonstrated clinical improvement in these patients following treatment with Epo [90-95]. For example, darbepoetin-α was shown to substantially increase Hb levels in patients with HbE–β-thalassemia [96]. The therapeutic effect is mainly related to stimulation of erythropoiesis, thus, ameliorating ineffective erythro-poiesis and anemia. It should be noted, however, that Epo stimulates both pathological and less pathological HbF-containing, RBC.

Nevertheless, Epo is a pleiotropic cytokine, and as such its administration in patients with β-hemoglobinopathies can be associated with a variety of beneficial and deleterious effects.

In addition to its effect on total Hb by increasing the production of RBC, Epo treatment can specifically stimulate HbF. Based primarily on studying cultures of human erythroid precursors, we [97] suggested that this effect depends on changes in the Epo stimulus due to the drop in the abundance of EpoR during the maturation process of these cells [98] and the changes in Epo level following Epo treatment of anemic patients [99]. Attempts to increase HbF *in vivo*, either by Epo alone or in combination with HU, produced contradictory results [90, 95, 100-104]. This could be caused by the different timing, dose and frequency of Epo administration.

Several studies suggested that Epo reduces oxidative stress: Starvation of rats, which reduces endogenous Epo production, was found to increase lipid peroxidation in the RBC membrane, whereas administration of Epo reversed the effect [105]. An improved antioxidant status was also found following Epo treatment of newborn rabbits. This could be due to utilization of excess iron for developing erythroid precursors, as discussed above, thus making it unavailable for ROS generation [106].

The antioxidant effect of Epo treatment was first suggested for patients with chronic renal failure on dialysis. The RBC in these patients are under oxidative stress, resulting in externalization of phosphatidylserine, a marker of senescence, which tags RBC for elimination by phagocytosis [107, 108]. Epo treatment of these patients resulted in reduced lipid peroxidation concomitant with an increase in superoxide dismutase, catalase, and other antioxidant activities [109-113, 114]. It also caused, within 4 hours, a decrease in the number of RBC exhibiting surface phosphatidylserine [21, 115, 116]. Thus, although the main effect of Epo is related to stimulation of erythropoiesis and improvement in the anemia, as discussed above, it was suggested that in these patients the Epo effect may also be associated with prolongation of the life span of mature RBC [117].

We investigated the effect of Epo on the oxidative status of normal and β-thalassemic RBC and platelets [97]. When human blood samples were incubated with Epo, ROS levels were decreased and GSH levels were concurrently increased in RBC and platelets from both normal and thalassemic donors compared with those in untreated cells. The *in vivo* effect of Epo on oxidative stress was studied in heterozygous ($Hbb^{th3/+}$) β-thalassemic mice. Two hours after i.p. injection of Epo (5,000 U/kg), the ROS and lipid peroxides of their RBC were significantly reduced with a concomitant increase in GSH levels compared with those in control mice [97].

Although in our *in vitro* studies the effects on oxidative stress required Epo concentrations far above normal serum levels, continuous, cumulative sub-threshold effects, which could not be detected by the methodology used, at physiological Epo concentrations are possible. Epo is obviously not a practical anti-oxidant drug as it is less potent and much more expensive than other anti-oxidants and, in addition, has to be administrated by injection. However, its protective effect as an antioxidant on RBC and platelet survival should be taken into account when Epo is used therapeutically.

Epo is also known to have a protective effect in non hematopoietic cells, such as cardiomyocytes [118]. Thus, a significant improvement was demonstrated in patients with stroke, who were treated with Epo within 8 hours of the onset of neurological symptoms [119]. The mechanism of Epo-induced protection in non-erythroid cells was reported to involve a number of signaling pathways, including the Jak-2/STAT [120], a crucial pathway of its erythropoietic effect [121]. However, the mechanism of the Epo effect on non-erythroid cells probably differs from that on erythropoiesis: Whereas the latter requires the continuous presence of Epo, a brief exposure is sufficient for neuroprotection [122]. Consequently, desialylated Epo, which has a high affinity for EpoR but a short life-span (and therefore a reduced erythropoietic effect), is neuroprotective [123]. Carbamylated Epo, another Epo analog, which does not bind to EpoR and lacks erythropoietic activity, also confers neuroprotection and cardioprotection [124]. It was suggested that the protective effect of this Epo analog is mediated through a hetero-receptor complex consisting of EpoR and a β-receptor subunit (CD131), a signal-transducing subunit shared by receptors to several cytokines [125].

The protective effect of Epo on non-erythroid cells may have a significant beneficial effect also in thalassemia. The main causes of morbidity and mortality in older thalassemia patients are associated with damage to cells of vital organs due to IO-mediated oxidative stress. If Epo can directly alleviate the stress of these cells, in addition to improving the chronic anemia, it may contribute significantly to amelioration of a variety of the disease's symptoms.

The effect of Epo on malignancy is also of therapeutic importance, since as the life expectancy of thalassemic patients increases, the likelihood of developing malignancies grows as well [126]. In recent years, several studies have reported the association of thalassemia with malignancies, mainly in the liver and in the hematopoietic system (e.g., [127]). A possible link between these two diseases could be IO, which has been reported to be associated with various malignancies, including in the liver and in the hematopoietic system [128, 129]. I*n vitro* studies related IO and malignant transformation, mainly through the generation of ROS [130], which can initiate the generation of a neoplastic clone through genetic or epigenetic alterations.

Anemia is an independent prognostic factor in patients with cancer [131]. The pathophysiology of malignancy-related anemia can be related to the anemia of chronic disease, nutritional deficiencies, bleeding, hemolysis, bone marrow involvement with malignant cells, and chemoradiotherapy. A direct relationship has been reported between acute anemia and intratumoral hypoxia [132], although the effect of chronic anemia is more difficult to interpret [133]. There is also evidence that anemia might be associated with a reduced response to radiotherapy [134], chemotherapy [135], and surgery [136].

The use of Epo in malignancies focuses on its anemia-correcting effect. It reduces blood transfusion requirements, improves both the quality of life [137] and -survival [138]. In addition, Epo has been shown in animal models to restore radio- [139] and chemo-sensitivity [140]. Nevertheless, two randomized trials of the effect of Epo on progression-free survival reported negative results [141, 142]. The expression of EpoR on cancer cells [143] suggests that Epo treatment may exert direct effects on these cells, stimulating their proliferation, inhibiting their apoptosis and modulating their sensitivity to chemo-radiation therapy. Epo may also affect the tumor microenvironment: Epo or EpoR knockout embryos exhibited defects in angiogenesis. A recent study showed that Epo-EpoR signaling stimulates pathologic angiogenesis of diabetic retinopathy (37), however, its role in tumor angiogenesis, a process that is essential for tumor progression and metastasis, has not been established.

Epo may also have a therapeutic effect in malignancy. Epo treatment was reported to be associated with prolonged survival of multiple myeloma patients. This effect, which was supported by studies on murine myeloma models [144], is most probably not a direct one on the myeloma cells, but through stimulation of the immune system [145].

Administration of Epo is usually supplemented by iron. This may be crucial for anemia associated with iron-deficiency, where the iron supply is a limiting factor of erythropoiesis, but, it may not be required when the iron supply is abundant. We studied the effect of iron supplementation in patients with chronic renal failure on dialysis, where the kidneys fail to produce Epo, and consequently the patients suffer from anemia. These patients are treated by weekly injections of Epo, which is usually supplemented with IV iron. By using T2*MRI, we demonstrated iron deposition in the liver, spleen and pancreas. Discontinuation of iron supplementation for up to one year reduced IO (monitored by the decrease in serum ferritin and transferrin saturation levels), without interfering with the Hb-stimulating effect of Epo, indicating that under these conditions the stored iron could be mobilized for erythropoiesis. These results raise the question of the minimal iron supplementation required to support erythropoiesis during Epo treatment and suggest that in IO patients, such as in thalassemia, Epo may be given in order to increase the Hb level without iron supplementation. In fact, it is possible that such iron-free Epo treatment may reduce the consequences of IO by mobilizing iron not only from macrophages but also from parynchymal cells of vital organs (heart, liver) which are the main targets of IO damage.

Dietary Products As Iron-Chelating and Anti-Oxidant Agents

Many dietary products have the capacities to scavenge ROS as well as to chelate iron [146]. For example, Curcuminoids, a group of phenolic compounds derived from dried rhizomes of curcumin (*Curcuma longa Linn.*) also known as turmeric, a natural herb used as a food additive or traditional medicine for centuries. Curcumin extracts are non-toxic to animals or humans, even at high doses. Curcumin extracts are well known to possess antioxidant, anti-inflammatory, anticancer [147] as well as iron-chelator properties [148]. A variety of functional groups of curcuminoids is related to their biological properties. Although the mechanism of scavenging free oxygen radicals and chelating iron is not well understood, it has been proposed that the β-diketone group and the hydroxyl/ methoxy groups on the phenyl rings of curcuminoids participate in their antioxidant activity and iron chelating property [149, 15, 16]. Curcuminoids have been shown to reduce the oxidative stress in β-thalassemia/Hb E patients [150] and to synergize with deferiprone and desferrioxamine in iron chelation [151].

Fermented papaya preparation (FPP) is a product of the yeast fermentation of *Carica papaya Linn.* Studies in chronic and degenerative disease conditions have shown that it modulates various clinical aspects [for review see [152]]. The favorable effects in thalassemia include anti-oxidative and iron chelation activities [153, 154]. *In vitro* and *in vivo* (in patients and experimental animals) studies revealed that FPP ameliorates multiple parameters of oxidative stress in RBC, granulocytes and platelets [153].

As for the chelation activity, it has been shown that FPP protects against damage to DNA (induction of single and double strand breaks) and proteins (albumin) caused by combined treatment with ferric nitrilotriacetate and hydrogen peroxide, suggesting that the antioxidant properties of FPP are related to both hydroxyl scavenging as well as to iron chelating properties [155].

As LIP is the major culprit in iron-mediated cytotoxicity, we studied the ability of FPP to prevent (and revert) cellular accumulation of LIP [154]. Liver- and heart-derived cells, as well as RBC, were exposed to non-transferrin-bound iron in the form of ferrous ammonium sulfate in the presence or absence of FPP. The results showed that FPP decreased both LIP and ROS. Administering FPP per os to patients with thalassemia was found to be safe and effective in reducing their oxidative stress [153, 156]. The results suggest that this treatment may be preventive as well as therapeutic and that its the antioxidant mechanism of FPP may be related, at least in part, to its ability to chelate iron.

Conclusion

Therapeutic modalities may be multi-factorial and involve multiple targets. Some of them, with respect to treating patients with β-hemoglobinopathies, were discussed in this review. I believe that on the basis of the data, the time has come to define, by studying *in vitro* and *in vivo* models, as well as by controlled clinical trials, their effects and consider their use for the treatment of patients with various forms of these diseases.

References

[1] Bernaudin, F., Socie, G., Kuentz, M., Chevret, S., Duval, M., Bertrand, Y., Vannier, J. P., Yakouben, K., Thuret, I., Bordigoni, P., Fischer, A., Lutz, P., Stephan, J. L., Dhedin, N., Plouvier, E., Margueritte, G., Bories, D., Verlhac, S., Esperou, H., Coic, L., Vernant, J. P., Gluckman, E. Long-term results of related myeloablative stem-cell transplantation to cure sickle cell disease. *Blood*. 2007;110:2749-2756.

[2] Perumbeti, A., Malik, P. Therapy for beta-globinopathies: a brief review and determinants for successful and safe correction. *Ann. N. Y. Acad. Sci*. 2010;1202:36-44.

[3] Breda, L., Kleinert, D. A., Casu, C., Casula, L., Cartegni, L., Fibach, E., Mancini, I., Giardina, P. J., Gambari, R., Rivella, S. A preclinical approach for gene therapy of beta-thalassemia. *Ann. N. Y. Acad. Sci*. 2010;1202:134-140.

[4] Rivella, S. Ineffective erythropoiesis and thalassemias. *Curr. Opin. Hematol*. 2009;16: 187-194.

[5] Kohgo, Y., Ikuta, K., Ohtake, T., Torimoto, Y., Kato, J. Body iron metabolism and pathophysiology of iron overload. *Int. J. Hematol*. 2008;88:7-15.

[6] Fibach, E., Rachmilewitz, E. The role of oxidative stress in hemolytic anemia. *Curr. Mol. Med*. 2008;8:609-619.

[7] Rund, D., Rachmilewitz, E. Beta-thalassemia. *N. Engl. J. Med*. 2005;353:1135-1146.

[8] Edington, G. M., Lehmann, H. Expression of the sickle-cell gene in Africa. *Br. Med. J*. 1955;1:1308-1311.

[9] Conley, C. L., Weatherall, D. J., Richardson, S. N., Shepard, M. K., Charache, S. Hereditary persistence of fetal hemoglobin: a study of 79 affected persons in 15 Negro families in Baltimore. *Blood*. 1963;21:261-281.

[10] Nathan, D. G., Gunn, R. B. Thalassemia: the consequences of unbalanced hemoglobin synthesis. *Am. J. Med*. 1966;41:815-830.

[11] Papayannopoulou, T. H., Brice, M., Stamatoyannopoulos, G. Stimulation of fetal hemoglobin synthesis in bone marrow cultures from adult individuals. *Proc. Natl. Acad. Sci. US*. 1976;73:2033-2037.

[12] DeSimone, J., Heller, P., Hall, L., Zwiers, D. 5-Azacytidine stimulates fetal hemoglobin synthesis in anemic baboons. *Proc. Natl. Acad. Sci. US*.1982;79:4428-4431.

[13] Ley, T. J., DeSimone, J., Anagnou, N. P., Keller, G. H., Humphries, R. K., Turner, P. H., Young, N. S., Keller, P., Nienhuis, A. W. 5-azacytidine selectively increases gamma-globin synthesis in a patient with beta+ thalassemia. *N. Engl. J. Med*. 1982;307: 1469-1475.

[14] Ware, R. E., Aygun, B. Advances in the use of hydroxyurea. *Hematology Am. Soc. Hematol. Educ. Program*. 2009:62-69.
[15] Pavlova, L. E., Savov, V. M., Petkov, H. G., Charova, I. P. Oxidative stress in patients with beta-thalassemia major. *Prilozi*. 2007;28:145-154.
[16] Wood, K. C., Granger, D. N. Sickle cell disease: role of reactive oxygen and nitrogen metabolites. *Clin. Exp. Pharmacol. Physiol*. 2007;34:926-932.
[17] Fibach, E., Rachmilewitz, E. A. The role of antioxidants and iron chelators in the treatment of oxidative stress in thalassemia. *Ann. N. Y. Acad. Sci*. 2010;1202:10-16.
[18] Shinar, E., Rachmilewitz, E. A. Oxidative denaturation of red blood cells in thalassemia. *Semin. Hematol*. 1990;27:70-82.
[19] Amer, J., Fibach, E. Chronic oxidative stress reduces the respiratory burst response of neutrophils from beta-thalassaemia patients. *Br. J. Haematol*. 2005;129:435-441.
[20] Amer, J., Goldfarb, A., Fibach, E. Flow cytometric analysis of the oxidative status of normal and thalassemic red blood cells. *Cytometry A*. 2004;60:73-80.
[21] Lang, F., Lang, K. S., Lang, P. A., Huber, S. M., Wieder, T. Mechanisms and significance of eryptosis. *Antioxid. Redox Signal*. 2006;8:1183-1192.
[22] Amer, J., Atlas, D., Fibach, E. N-acetylcysteine amide (AD4) attenuates oxidative stress in beta-thalassemia blood cells. *Biochim. Biophys. Acta*. 2008;1780:249-255.
[23] Amer, J., Fibach, E. Oxidative status of platelets in normal and thalassemic blood. *Thromb. Haemost*. 2004;92:1052-1059.
[24] Eldor, A., Rachmilewitz, E. A. The hypercoagulable state in thalassemia. *Blood*. 2002; 99:36-43.
[25] Rachmilewitz, E. A., Harari, E. Intermediate hemichrome formation after oxidation of three unstable hemoglobins (Freiburg, Riverdale-Bronx and Koln). *Hamatol. Bluttransfus*. 1972;10:241-250.
[26] Advani, R., Sorenson, S., Shinar, E., Lande, W., Rachmilewitz, E., Schrier, S. L. Characterization and comparison of the red blood cell membrane damage in severe human alpha- and beta-thalassemia. *Blood*. 1992;79:1058-1063.
[27] Chan, A. C., Chow, C. K., Chiu, D. Interaction of antioxidants and their implication in genetic anemia. *Proc. Soc. Exp. Biol. Med*. 1999;222:274-282.
[28] Miniero, R., Canducci, E., Ghigo, D., Saracco, P., Vullo, C. Vitamin E in beta-thalassemia. *Acta Vitaminol. Enzymol*. 1982;4:21-25.
[29] Tesoriere, L., D'Arpa, D., Butera, D., Allegra, M., Renda, D., Maggio, A., Bongiorno, A., Livrea, M. A. Oral supplements of vitamin E improve measures of oxidative stress in plasma and reduce oxidative damage to LDL and erythrocytes in beta-thalassemia intermedia patients. *Free Radic. Res*. 2001;34:529-540.
[30] Kahane, I., Rachmilewitz, E. A. Alterations in the red blood cell membrane and the effect of vitamin E on osmotic fragility in beta-thalassemia major. *Isr. J. Med. Sci*. 1976; 12:11-15.
[31] Musallam, K. M., Rivella, S., Vichinsky, E., Rachmilewitz, E. A. Non-transfusion-dependent thalassemias. *Haematologica*. 2013;98:833-844.
[32] Tanno, T., Noel, P., Miller, J. L. Growth differentiation factor 15 in erythroid health and disease. *Curr. Opin. Hematol*. 2010;17:184-190.
[33] Wang, J., Pantopoulos, K. Regulation of cellular iron metabolism. *Biochem. J*. 2011; 434:365-381.

[34] Konijn, A. M., Meyron-Holtz, E. G., Fibach, E., Gelvan, D. Cellular ferritin uptake: a highly regulated pathway for iron assimilation in human erythroid precursor cells. *Adv. Exp. Med. Biol.* 1994;356:189-197.

[35] Breuer, W., Hershko, C., Cabantchik, Z. I. The importance of non-transferrin bound iron in disorders of iron metabolism. *Transfus. Sci.* 2000;23:185-192.

[36] Prus, E., Fibach, E. Flow cytometry measurement of the labile iron pool in human hematopoietic cells. *Cytometry A.* 2008;73:22-27.

[37] Prus, E., Fibach, E. The labile iron pool in human erythroid cells. *Br. J. Haematol.* 2008;142:301-307.

[38] Jacobs, A. Low molecular weight intracellular iron transport compounds. *Blood.* 1977; 50:433-439.

[39] Marsella, M., Pepe, A., Borgna-Pignatti, C. Better survival and less cardiac morbidity in female patients with thalassemia major: a review of the literature. *Ann. N. Y. Acad. Sci.* 2010;1202:129-133.

[40] Hoffbrand, A. V., Taher, A., Cappellini, M. D. How I treat transfusional iron overload. *Blood.* 2012;120:3657-3669.

[41] Grady, R., Giardina, P. () Iron chelation: rationale for combination therapy. In: D. Badman, Bergeron, R., Brittenham, G. (eds.) *Iron chelators: new development strategies*. Ponte Vedra, FL: Saratoga Group, 2000;293–310.

[42] Link, G., Konijn, A. M., Breuer, W., Cabantchik, Z. I., Hershko, C. Exploring the "iron shuttle" hypothesis in chelation therapy: effects of combined deferoxamine and deferiprone treatment in hypertransfused rats with labeled iron stores and in iron-loaded rat heart cells in culture. *J. Lab. Clin. Med.* 2001;138:130-138.

[43] Prus, E., Fibach, E. Effect of iron chelators on labile iron and oxidative status of thalassaemic erythroid cells. *Acta Haematol.* 2010;123:14-20.

[44] Ghoti, H., Fibach, E., Merkel, D., Perez-Avraham, G., Grisariu, S., Rachmilewitz, E. A. Changes in parameters of oxidative stress and free iron biomarkers during treatment with deferasirox in iron-overloaded patients with myelodysplastic syndromes. *Haematologica.* 2010; 95:1433-1434.

[45] Mabaera, R., West, R. J., Conine, S. J., Macari, E. R., Boyd, C. D., Engman, C. A., Lowrey, C. H. A cell stress signaling model of fetal hemoglobin induction: what doesn't kill red blood cells may make them stronger. *Exp. Hematol.* 2008;36:1057-1072.

[46] Witt, O., Sand, K., Pekrun, A. Butyrate-induced erythroid differentiation of human K562 leukemia cells involves inhibition of ERK and activation of p38 MAP kinase pathways. *Blood.* 2000;95:2391-2396.

[47] Witt, O., Monkemeyer, S., Ronndahl, G., Erdlenbruch, B., Reinhardt, D., Kanbach, K., Pekrun, A. Induction of fetal hemoglobin expression by the histone deacetylase inhibitor apicidin. *Blood.* 2003;101:2001-2007.

[48] Witt, O., Monkemeyer, S., Kanbach, K., Pekrun, A. Induction of fetal hemoglobin synthesis by valproate: modulation of MAP kinase pathways. *Am. J. Hematol.* 2002;71: 45-46.

[49] Pace, B. S., Qian, X. H., Sangerman, J., Ofori-Acquah, S. F., Baliga, B. S., Han, J., Critz, S. D. p38 MAP kinase activation mediates gamma-globin gene induction in erythroid progenitors. *Exp. Hematol.* 2003;31:1089-1096.

[50] Aerbajinai, W., Zhu, J., Gao, Z., Chin, K., Rodgers, G. P. Thalidomide induces gamma-globin gene expression through increased reactive oxygen species-mediated p38 MAPK

signaling and histone H4 acetylation in adult erythropoiesis. *Blood.* 2007;110:2864-2871.

[51] Park, J. I., Choi, H. S., Jeong, J. S., Han, J. Y., Kim, I. H. Involvement of p38 kinase in hydroxyurea-induced differentiation of K562 cells. *Cell Growth Differ.* 2001;12:481-486.

[52] Itoh, K., Chiba, T., Takahashi, S., Ishii, T., Igarashi, K., Katoh, Y., Oyake, T., Hayashi, N., Satoh, K., Hatayama, I., Yamamoto, M., Nabeshima, Y. An Nrf2/small Maf heterodimer mediates the induction of phase II detoxifying enzyme genes through anti-oxidant response elements. *Biochem. Biophys. Res. Commun.* 1997;236:313-322.

[53] Macari, E. R., Lowrey, C. H. Induction of human fetal hemoglobin via the NRF2 anti-oxidant response signaling pathway. *Blood.* 2011;117:5987-5997.

[54] Lampronti, I., Bianchi, N., Borgatti, M., Fibach, E., Prus, E., Gambari, R. Accumulation of gamma-globin mRNA in human erythroid cells treated with angelicin. *Eur. J. Haematol.* 2003;71:189-195.

[55] Fibach, E., Prus, E., Bianchi, N., Zuccato, C., Breveglieri, G., Salvatori, F., Finotti, A., Lipucci di Paola, M., Brognara, E., Lampronti, I., Borgatti, M., Gambari, R. Resveratrol: Antioxidant activity and induction of fetal hemoglobin in erythroid cells from normal donors and beta-thalassemia patients. *Int. J. Mol. Med.* 2012;29:974-982.

[56] Rodrigue, C. M., Arous, N., Bachir, D., Smith-Ravin, J., Romeo, P. H., Galacteros, F., Garel, M. C. Resveratrol, a natural dietary phytoalexin, possesses similar properties to hydroxyurea towards erythroid differentiation. *Br. J. Haematol.* 2001;113:500-507.

[57] Kode, A., Rajendrasozhan, S., Caito, S., Yang, S. R., Megson, I. L., Rahman, I. Resveratrol induces glutathione synthesis by activation of Nrf2 and protects against cigarette smoke-mediated oxidative stress in human lung epithelial cells. *Am. J. Physiol. Lung Cell Mol. Physiol.* 2008;294:L478-488.

[58] McMahon, M., Itoh, K., Yamamoto, M., Chanas, S. A., Henderson, C. J., McLellan, L. I., Wolf, C. R., Cavin, C., Hayes, J. D. The Cap'n'Collar basic leucine zipper transcription factor Nrf2 (NF-E2 p45-related factor 2) controls both constitutive and inducible expression of intestinal detoxification and glutathione biosynthetic enzymes. *Cancer Res.* 2001;61:3299-3307.

[59] Soleas, G. J., Diamandis, E. P., Goldberg, D. M. Resveratrol: a molecule whose time has come? And gone? *Clin. Biochem.* 1997;30:91-113.

[60] Pendurthi, U. R., Williams, J. T., Rao, L. V. Resveratrol, a polyphenolic compound found in wine, inhibits tissue factor expression in vascular cells: A possible mechanism for the cardiovascular benefits associated with moderate consumption of wine. *Arterioscler. Thromb. Vasc. Biol.* 1999;19:419-426.

[61] Jang, M., Cai, L., Udeani, G. O., Slowing, K. V., Thomas, C. F., Beecher, C. W., Fong, H. H., Farnsworth, N. R., Kinghorn, A. D., Mehta, R. G., Moon, R. C., Pezzuto, J. M. Cancer chemopreventive activity of resveratrol, a natural product derived from grapes. *Science.* 1997;275:218-220.

[62] Frankel, E. N., Waterhouse, A. L., Kinsella, J. E. Inhibition of human LDL oxidation by resveratrol. *Lancet.* 1993;341:1103-1104.

[63] Goldstein, L., Teng, Z. P., Zeserson, E., Patel, M., Regan, R. F. Hemin induces an iron-dependent, oxidative injury to human neuron-like cells. *J. Neurosci. Res.* 2003;73:113-121.

[64] Verger, C., Sassa, S., Kappas, A. Growth-promoting effects of iron- and cobalt- protoporphyrins on cultured embryonic cells. *J. Cell. Physiol.* 1983;116:135-141.

[65] Quigley, J. G., Yang, Z., Worthington, M. T., Phillips, J. D., Sabo, K. M., Sabath, D. E., Berg, C. L., Sassa, S., Wood, B. L., Abkowitz, J. L. Identification of a human heme exporter that is essential for erythropoiesis. *Cell.* 2004;118:757-766.

[66] Fibach, E., Konijn, A. M., Bauminger, R. E., Ofer, S., Rachmilewitz, E. A. Effect of extracellular hemin on hemoglobin and ferritin content of erythroleukemia cells. *J. Cell. Physiol.* 1987;130:460-465.

[67] Lu, L., Broxmeyer, H. E. The selective enhancing influence of hemin and products of human erythrocytes on colony formation by human multipotential (CFUGEMM) and erythroid (BFUE) progenitor cells in vitro. *Exp. Hematol.* 1983;11:721-729.

[68] Fibach, E., Aker, M. Hemin augments growth and hemoglobinization of erythroid precursors from patients with diamond-blackfan anemia. *Anemia*. 2012:940260.

[69] Fibach, E., Kollia, P., Schechter, A. N., Noguchi, C. T., Rodgers, G. P. Hemin-induced acceleration of hemoglobin production in immature cultured erythroid cells: preferential enhancement of fetal hemoglobin. *Blood.* 1995;85:2967-2974.

[70] Leimberg, J. M., Prus, E., Link, G., Fibach, E., Konijn, A. M. Iron-chelator complexes as iron sources for early developing human erythroid precursors. *Transl. Res.* 2008;151: 88-96.

[71] Rutherford, T. R., Clegg, J. B., Weatherall, D. J. K562 human leukaemic cells synthesise embryonic haemoglobin in response to haemin. *Nature*. 1979;280:164-165.

[72] Ross, J., Sautner, D. Induction of globin mRNA accumulation by hemin in cultured erythroleukemic cells. *Cell.* 1976;8:513-520.

[73] Nudel, U., Salmon, J., Fibach, E., Terada, M., Rifkind, R., Marks, P. A., Bank, A. Accumulation of alpha- and beta-globin messenger RNAs in mouse erythroleukemia cells. *Cell.* 1977;12:463-469.

[74] Papayannopoulou, T., Kalmantis, T., Stamatoyannopoulos, G. Cellular regulation of hemoglobin switching: evidence for inverse relationship between fetal hemoglobin synthesis and degree of maturity of human erythroid cells. *Proc. Natl. Acad. Sci. US.* 1979;76:6420-6424.

[75] Chui, D. H., Wong, S. C., Enkin, M. W., Patterson, M., Ives, R. A. Proportion of fetal hemoglobin synthesis decreases during erythroid cell maturation. *Proc. Natl. Acad. Sci. US.* 1980;77:2757-2761.

[76] Dalyot, N., Fibach, E., Rachmilewitz, E. A., Oppenheim, A. Adult and neonatal patterns of human globin gene expression are recapitulated in liquid cultures. *Exp. Hematol.* 1992;20:1141-1145.

[77] Kollia, P., Noguchi, C. T., Fibach, E., Loukopoulos, D., Schechter, A. N. Modulation of globin gene expression in cultured erythroid precursors derived from normal individuals: transcriptional and posttranscriptional regulation by hemin. *Proc. Assoc. Am. Physicians.* 1997;109:420-428.

[78] Tahara, T., Sun, J., Nakanishi, K., Yamamoto, M., Mori, H., Saito, T., Fujita, H., Igarashi, K., Taketani, S. Heme positively regulates the expression of beta-globin at the locus control region via the transcriptional factor Bach1 in erythroid cells. *J. Biol. Chem.* 2004;279:5480-5487.

[79] Tahara, S. M., Traugh, J. A., Sharp, S. B., Lundak, T. S., Safer, B., Merrick, W. C. Effect of hemin on site-specific phosphorylation of eukaryotic initiation factor 2. *Proc. Natl. Acad. Sci. US*. 1978;75:789-793.

[80] Iolascon, A., De Falco, L., Beaumont, C. Molecular basis of inherited microcytic anemia due to defects in iron acquisition or heme synthesis. *Haematologica*. 2009; 94: 395-408.

[81] Kim, Y. C., Masutani, H., Yamaguchi, Y., Itoh, K., Yamamoto, M., Yodoi, J. Hemin-induced activation of the thioredoxin gene by Nrf2. A differential regulation of the antioxidant responsive element by a switch of its binding factors. *J. Biol. Chem*. 2001; 276:18399-18406.

[82] Rund, D., Fibach, E., Goldfarb, A., Friedberg, A., Rachmilewitz, E. Heme arginate therapy for beta thalassemia: in vitro versus in vivo effects. *Acta Haematol*. 1998;100: 82-84.

[83] Krantz, S. B. Erythropoietin. *Blood*. 1991;77:419-434.

[84] Jelkmann, W. Erythropoietin: structure, control of production, and function. *Physiol. Rev*. 1992;72:449-489.

[85] Beutel, G., Ganser, A. Risks and benefits of erythropoiesis-stimulating agents in cancer management. *Semin. Hematol*. 2007;44:157-165.

[86] Eschbach, J. W. Anemia management in chronic kidney disease: role of factors affecting epoetin responsiveness. *J. Am. Soc. Nephrol*. 2002;13:1412-1414.

[87] Santini, V. Clinical use of erythropoietic stimulating agents in myelodysplastic syndromes. *Oncologist*. 2011;16 Suppl. 3:35-42.

[88] Manor, D., Fibach, E., Goldfarb, A., Rachmilewitz, E. A. Erythropoietin activity in the serum of beta thalassemic patients. *Scand. J. Haematol*. 1986;37:221-228.

[89] Dore, F., Bonfigli, S., Gaviano, E., Pardini, S., Cianciulli, P., Papa, G., Longinotti, M. Serum erythropoietin levels in thalassemia intermedia. *Ann. Hematol*. 1993;67:183-186.

[90] Goldberg, M. A., Brugnara, C., Dover, G. J., Schapira, L., Lacroix, L., Bunn, H. F. Hydroxyurea and erythropoietin therapy in sickle cell anemia. *Semin. Oncol*. 1992;19: 74-81.

[91] Olivieri, N. F., Freedman, M. H., Perrine, S. P., Dover, G. J., Sheridan, B., Essentine, D. L., Nagel, R. L. Trial of recombinant human erythropoietin: three patients with thalassemia intermedia. *Blood*. 1992;80:3258-3260.

[92] Rachmilewitz, E. A., Aker, M., Perry, D., Dover, G. Sustained increase in haemoglobin and RBC following long-term administration of recombinant human erythropoietin to patients with homozygous beta-thalassaemia. *Br. J. Haematol*. 1995;90:341-345.

[93] Rachmilewitz, E. A., Aker, M. The role of recombinant human erythropoietin in the treatment of thalassemia. *Ann. N. Y. Acad. Sci*. 1998;850:129-138.

[94] Kohli-Kumar, M., Marandi, H., Keller, M. A., Guertin, K., Hvizdala, E. Use of hydroxyurea and recombinant erythropoietin in management of homozygous beta0 thalassemia. *J. Pediatr. Hematol. Oncol*. 2002;24:777-778.

[95] Chaidos, A., Makis, A., Hatzimichael, E., Tsiara, S., Gouva, M., Tzouvara, E., Bourantas, K. L. Treatment of beta-thalassemia patients with recombinant human erythropoietin: effect on transfusion requirements and soluble adhesion molecules. *Acta Haematol*. 2004;111:189-195.

[96] Singer, S. T., Vichinsky, E. P., Sweeters, N., Rachmilewitz, E. Darbepoetin alfa for the treatment of anaemia in alpha- or beta- thalassaemia intermedia syndromes. *Br. J. Haematol*. 2011;154:281-284.

[97] Amer, J., Dana, M., Fibach, E. The antioxidant effect of erythropoietin on thalassemic blood cells. *Anemia*. 2010;2010:978710.

[98] Broudy, V. C., Lin, N., Brice, M., Nakamoto, B., Papayannopoulou, T. Erythropoietin receptor characteristics on primary human erythroid cells. *Blood*. 1991;77:2583-2590.

[99] Cho, S. H., Lim, H. S., Ghim, J. L., Choe, S., Kim, U. J., Jung, J. A., Bae, K. S. Pharmacokinetic, tolerability, and bioequivalence comparison of three different intravenous formulations of recombinant human erythropoietin in healthy Korean adult male volunteers: an open-label, randomized-sequence, three-treatment, three-way crossover study. *Clin. Ther*. 2009;31:1046-1053.

[100] Bourantas, K. L., Georgiou, I., Seferiadis, K. Fetal globin stimulation during a short-term trial of erythropoietin in HbS/beta-thalassemia patients. *Acta Haematol*. 1994;92: 79-82.

[101] Breymann, C., Fibach, E., Visca, E., Huettner, C., Huch, A., Huch, R. Induction of fetal hemoglobin synthesis with recombinant human erythropoietin in anemic patients with heterozygous beta-thalassemia during pregnancy. *J. Matern. Fetal. Med*. 1999;8:1-7.

[102] Little, J. A., McGowan, V. R., Kato, G. J., Partovi, K. S., Feld, J. J., Maric, I., Martyr, S., Taylor, J. Gt., Machado, R. F., Heller, T., Castro, O., Gladwin, M. T. Combination erythropoietin-hydroxyurea therapy in sickle cell disease: experience from the National Institutes of Health and a literature review. *Haematologica*. 2006;91:1076-1083.

[103] Rodgers, G. P., Dover, G. J., Uyesaka, N., Noguchi, C. T., Schechter, A. N., Nienhuis, A. W. Augmentation by erythropoietin of the fetal-hemoglobin response to hydroxyurea in sickle cell disease. *N. Engl. J. Med*. 1993;328:73-80.

[104] Saraf, S., Molokie, R., Gowhari, M., DO, Hassan, J., Gordeuk, V. Clinical Efficacy and Safety of Erythroid Stimulating Agents in Sickle Cell Disease. *Blood*. 2012;120: Abstract 3218.

[105] Biswas, T., Ghosal, J., Ganguly, C., Datta, A. G. Effect of erythropoietin on the interchange of cholesterol and phospholipid between erythrocyte membrane and plasma. *Biochem. Med. Metab. Biol*. 1986;35:120-124.

[106] Bany-Mohammed, F. M., Slivka, S., Hallman, M. Recombinant human erythropoietin: possible role as an antioxidant in premature rabbits. *Pediatr. Res*. 1996;40:381-387.

[107] Lang, K. S., Lang, P. A., Bauer, C., Duranton, C., Wieder, T., Huber, S. M., Lang, F. Mechanisms of suicidal erythrocyte death. *Cell. Physiol. Biochem*. 2005;15:195-202.

[108] Freikman, I., Ringel, I., Fibach, E. Oxidative stress-induced membrane shedding from RBCs is Ca flux-mediated and affects membrane lipid composition. *J. Membr. Biol*. 2011;240:73-82.

[109] Turi, S., Nemeth, I., Varga, I., Bodrogi, T., Matkovics, B. The effect of erythropoietin on the cellular defence mechanism of red blood cells in children with chronic renal failure. *Pediatr. Nephrol*. 1992;6:536-541.

[110] Rud'ko, I. A., Balashova, T. S., Pokrovskii, Iu. A., Ermolenko, V. M., Kubatiev, A. A. [The effect of human recombinant erythropoietin on the lipid peroxidation processes and antioxidant protection of the erythrocytes in patients with chronic kidney failure on hemodialysis]. *Gematol. Transfuziol*. 1993;38:24-26.

[111] Delmas-Beauvieux, M. C., Combe, C., Peuchant, E., Carbonneau, M. A., Dubourg, L., de Precigout, V., Aparicio, M., Clerc, M. Evaluation of red blood cell lipoperoxidation in hemodialysed patients during erythropoietin therapy supplemented or not with iron. *Nephron*. 1995;69:404-410.

[112] Cavdar, C., Camsari, T., Semin, I., Gonenc, S., Acikgoz, O. Lipid peroxidation and antioxidant activity in chronic haemodialysis patients treated with recombinant human erythropoietin. *Scand. J. Urol. Nephrol*. 1997;31:371-375.

[113] Sommerburg, O., Grune, T., Hampl, H., Riedel, E., van Kuijk, F. J., Ehrich, J. H., Siems, W. G. Does long-term treatment of renal anaemia with recombinant erythropoietin influence oxidative stress in haemodialysed patients? *Nephrol. Dial. Transplant*. 1998;13:2583-2587.

[114] Boran, M., Kucukaksu, C., Balk, M., Cetin, S. Red cell lipid peroxidation and antioxidant system in haemodialysed patients: influence of recombinant human erythropoietin (r-HuEPO) treatment. *Int. Urol. Nephrol*. 1998;30:507-512.

[115] Bonomini, M., Sirolli, V., Settefrati, N., Dottori, S., Di Liberato, L., Arduini, A. Increased erythrocyte phosphatidylserine exposure in chronic renal failure. *J. Am. Soc. Nephrol*. 1999;10:1982-1990.

[116] Myssina, S., Huber, S. M., Birka, C., Lang, P. A., Lang, K. S., Friedrich, B., Risler, T., Wieder, T., Lang, F. Inhibition of erythrocyte cation channels by erythropoietin. *J. Am. Soc. Nephrol*. 2003;14:2750-2757.

[117] Polenakovic, M., Sikole, A. Is erythropoietin a survival factor for red blood cells? *J. Am. Soc. Nephrol*. 1996;7:1178-1182.

[118] Joyeux-Faure, M. Cellular protection by erythropoietin: new therapeutic implications? *J. Pharmacol. Exp. Ther*. 2007;323:759-762.

[119] Ehrenreich, H., Hasselblatt, M., Dembowski, C., Cepek, L., Lewczuk, P., Stiefel, M., Rustenbeck, H. H., Breiter, N., Jacob, S., Knerlich, F., Bohn, M., Poser, W., Ruther, E., Kochen, M., Gefeller, O., Gleiter, C., Wessel, T. C., De Ryck, M., Itri, L., Prange, H., Cerami, A., Brines, M., Siren, A. L. Erythropoietin therapy for acute stroke is both safe and beneficial. *Mol. Med*. 2002;8:495-505.

[120] Zhang, F., Wang, S., Cao, G., Gao, Y., Chen, J. Signal transducers and activators of transcription 5 contributes to erythropoietin-mediated neuroprotection against hippocampal neuronal death after transient global cerebral ischemia. *Neurobiol. Dis*. 2007; 25:45-53.

[121] Ofir, R., Qing, W., Krup, M., Weinstein, Y. Identification of genes induced by interleukin-3 and erythropoietin via the Jak-Stat5 pathway using enhanced differential display-reverse southern. *J. Interferon Cytokine Res*. 1997;17:279-286.

[122] Morishita, E., Masuda, S., Nagao, M., Yasuda, Y., Sasaki, R. Erythropoietin receptor is expressed in rat hippocampal and cerebral cortical neurons, and erythropoietin prevents in vitro glutamate-induced neuronal death. *Neuroscience*. 1997;76:105-116.

[123] Erbayraktar, S., Yilmaz, O., Gokmen, N., Brines, M. Erythropoietin is a multifunctional tissue-protective cytokine. *Curr. Hematol. Rep*. 2003;2:465-470.

[124] Moon, C., Krawczyk, M., Paik, D., Coleman, T., Brines, M., Juhaszova, M., Sollott, S. J., Lakatta, E. G., Talan, M. I. Erythropoietin, modified to not stimulate red blood cell production, retains its cardioprotective properties. *J. Pharmacol. Exp. Ther*. 2006;316: 999-1005.

[125] Brines, M., Grasso, G., Fiordaliso, F., Sfacteria, A., Ghezzi, P., Fratelli, M., Latini, R., Xie, Q. W., Smart, J., Su-Rick, C. J., Pobre, E., Diaz, D., Gomez, D., Hand, C., Coleman, T., Cerami, A. Erythropoietin mediates tissue protection through an erythropoietin and common beta-subunit heteroreceptor. *Proc. Natl. Acad. Sci. US.* 2004;101: 14907-14912.

[126] Poggi, M., Sorrentino, F., Pascucci, C., Monti, S., Lauri, C., Bisogni, V., Toscano, V., Cianciulli, P. Malignancies in beta-thalassemia patients: first description of two cases of thyroid cancer and review of the literature. *Hemoglobin*. 2011;35:439-446.

[127] Karimi, M., Giti, R., Haghpanah, S., Azarkeivan, A., Hoofar, H., Eslami, M. Malignancies in patients with beta-thalassemia major and beta-thalassemia intermedia: a multicenter study in Iran. *Pediatr. Blood Cancer*. 2009;53:1064-1067.

[128] Borgna-Pignatti, C., Vergine, G., Lombardo, T., Cappellini, M. D., Cianciulli, P., Maggio, A., Renda, D., Lai, M. E., Mandas, A., Forni, G., Piga, A., Bisconte, M. G. Hepatocellular carcinoma in the thalassaemia syndromes. *Br. J. Haematol.* 2004;124: 114-117.

[129] Joosten, E., Meeuwissen, J., Vandewinckele, H., Hiele, M. Iron status and colorectal cancer in symptomatic elderly patients. *Am. J. Med.* 2008;121:1072-1077.

[130] Toyokuni, S. Role of iron in carcinogenesis: cancer as a ferrotoxic disease. *Cancer Sci.* 2009;100:9-16.

[131] Caro, J. J., Salas, M., Ward, A., Goss, G. Anemia as an independent prognostic factor for survival in patients with cancer: a systemic, quantitative review. *Cancer*. 2001;91: 2214-2221.

[132] Hirst, D. G. What is the importance of anaemia in radiotherapy? The value of animal studies. *Radiother. Oncol.* 1991;20 Suppl. 1:29-33.

[133] Harrison, L. B., Chadha, M., Hill, R. J., Hu, K., Shasha, D. Impact of tumor hypoxia and anemia on radiation therapy outcomes. *Oncologist*. 2002;7:492-508.

[134] Nordsmark, M., Overgaard, M., Overgaard, J. Pretreatment oxygenation predicts radiation response in advanced squamous cell carcinoma of the head and neck. *Radiother. Oncol.* 1996;41:31-39.

[135] Teicher, B. A., Holden, S. A., al-Achi, A., Herman, T. S. Classification of antineoplastic treatments by their differential toxicity toward putative oxygenated and hypoxic tumor subpopulations in vivo in the FSaIIC murine fibrosarcoma. *Cancer Res.* 1990;50: 3339-3344.

[136] Hockel, M., Schlenger, K., Hockel, S., Aral, B., Schaffer, U., Vaupel, P. Tumor hypoxia in pelvic recurrences of cervical cancer. *Int. J. Cancer*. 1998;79:365-369.

[137] Glaspy, J. The impact of epoetin alfa on quality of life during cancer chemotherapy: a fresh look at an old problem. *Semin. Hematol*. 1997;34:20-26.

[138] Bohlius, J., Langensiepen, S., Schwarzer, G., Seidenfeld, J., Piper, M., Bennett, C., Engert, A. Recombinant human erythropoietin and overall survival in cancer patients: results of a comprehensive meta-analysis. *J. Natl. Cancer Inst.* 2005;97:489-498.

[139] Ning, S., Hartley, C., Molineux, G., Knox, S. J. Darbepoietin alfa potentiates the efficacy of radiation therapy in mice with corrected or uncorrected anemia. *Cancer Res.* 2005;65:284-290.

[140] Thews, O., Kelleher, D. K., Vaupel, P. Erythropoietin restores the anemia-induced reduction in cyclophosphamide cytotoxicity in rat tumors. *Cancer Res.* 2001;61:1358-1361.

[141] Henke, M., Laszig, R., Rube, C., Schafer, U., Haase, K. D., Schilcher, B., Mose, S., Beer, K. T., Burger, U., Dougherty, C., Frommhold, H. Erythropoietin to treat head and neck cancer patients with anaemia undergoing radiotherapy: randomised, double-blind, placebo-controlled trial. *Lancet*. 2003;362:1255-1260.

[142] Leyland-Jones, B., Semiglazov, V., Pawlicki, M., Pienkowski, T., Tjulandin, S., Manikhas, G., Makhson, A., Roth, A., Dodwell, D., Baselga, J., Biakhov, M., Valuckas, K., Voznyi, E., Liu, X., Vercammen, E. Maintaining normal hemoglobin levels with epoetin alfa in mainly nonanemic patients with metastatic breast cancer receiving first-line chemotherapy: a survival study. *J. Clin. Oncol*. 2005;23:5960-5972.

[143] Hardee, M. E., Arcasoy, M. O., Blackwell, K. L., Kirkpatrick, J. P., Dewhirst, M. W. Erythropoietin biology in cancer. *Clin. Cancer Res*. 2006;12:332-339.

[144] Mittelman, M., Zeidman, A., Kanter, P., Katz, O., Oster, H., Rund, D., Neumann, D. Erythropoietin has an anti-myeloma effect - a hypothesis based on a clinical observation supported by animal studies. *Eur. J. Haematol*. 2004;72:155-165.

[145] Prutchi-Sagiv, S., Golishevsky, N., Oster, H. S., Katz, O., Cohen, A., Naparstek, E., Neumann, D., Mittelman, M. Erythropoietin treatment in advanced multiple myeloma is associated with improved immunological functions: could it be beneficial in early disease? *Br. J. Haematol*. 2006;135:660-672.

[146] Perron, N. R., Brumaghim, J. L. A review of the antioxidant mechanisms of polyphenol compounds related to iron binding. *Cell Biochem. Biophys*. 2009;53:75-100.

[147] Pari, L., Tewas, D., Eckel, J. Role of curcumin in health and disease. *Arch. Physiol. Biochem*. 2008;114:127-149.

[148] Jiao, Y., Wilkinson, Jt., Christine Pietsch, E., Buss, J. L., Wang, W., Planalp, R., Torti, F. M., Torti, S. V. Iron chelation in the biological activity of curcumin. *Free Radic. Biol. Med.* 2006;40:1152-1160.

[149] Ak, T., Gulcin, I. Antioxidant and radical scavenging properties of curcumin. *Chem. Biol. Interact*. 2008;174:27-37.

[150] Kalpravidh, R. W., Siritanaratkul, N., Insain, P., Charoensakdi, R., Panichkul, N., Hatairaktham, S., Srichairatanakool, S., Phisalaphong, C., Rachmilewitz, E., Fucharoen, S. Improvement in oxidative stress and antioxidant parameters in beta-thalassemia/Hb E patients treated with curcuminoids. *Clin. Biochem*. 2010;43:424-429.

[151] Srichairatanakool, S., Thephinlap, C., Phisalaphong, C., Porter, J. B., Fucharoen, S. Curcumin contributes to in vitro removal of non-transferrin bound iron by deferiprone and desferrioxamine in thalassemic plasma. *Med. Chem*. 2007;3:469-474.

[152] Aruoma, O. I., Hayashi, Y., Marotta, F., Mantello, P., Rachmilewitz, E., Montagnier, L. Applications and bioefficacy of the functional food supplement fermented papaya preparation. *Toxicology*. 2010;278:6-16.

[153] Amer, J., Goldfarb, A., Rachmilewitz, E. A., Fibach, E. Fermented papaya preparation as redox regulator in blood cells of beta-thalassemic mice and patients. *Phytother. Res*. 2008;22:820-828.

[154] Prus, E., Fibach, E. The antioxidant effect of fermented papaya preparation involves iron chelation. *J. Biol. Regul. Homeost. Agents*. 2012;26:203-210.

[155] Rimbach, G., Guo, Q., Akiyama, T., Matsugo, S., Moini, H., Virgili, F., Packer, L. Ferric nitrilotriacetate induced DNA and protein damage: inhibitory effect of a fermented papaya preparation. *Anticancer Res*. 2000;20:2907-2914.

[156] Fibach, E., Tan, E. S., Jamuar, S., Ng, I., Amer, J., Rachmilewitz, E. A. Amelioration of oxidative stress in red blood cells from patients with beta-thalassemia major and intermedia and E-beta-thalassemia following administration of a fermented papaya preparation. *Phytother. Res.* 2010;24:1334-1338.

In: Thalassemia
Editor: Makenzie Greene

ISBN: 978-1-63117-954-9

Chapter 11

Assessing Services for Haemoglobin Disorders: A Toolkit for Service Planning

Michael Angastiniotis*[*] *and Androulla Eleftheriou
Thalassaemia International Federation, Nicosia, Cyprus

Abstract

The thalassaemias are a group of hereditary disorders caused by over 300 mutations on the beta globin loci and - over 160 affecting the alpha globin genes, responsible for the production of haemoglobin. They are regarded as the commonest of the clinically serious single gene disorders affecting humans. The thalassaemia genes were endemic in areas where falciparum malaria was common, suggesting an epistatic relationship between these genes and resistance of carriers to malaria. The endemic areas of the globe include the Mediterranean basin, the Middle East, central Asia, the Indian subcontinent, southern China and South East Asia. Population migrations have now introduced the conditions to non-endemic areas such as Northern Europe and the Americas. This geographical distribution was referred to as the thalassaemia belt. Sickle cell disease covers much of the Middle East but mainly Africa and the countries which over the centuries have received populations of African origin.

It is estimated that there are over 200 million carriers of the thalassaemia genes and that almost 60000 babies are born annually affected by clinically significant thalassaemia syndromes. It is noted that most countries in the thalassaemia belt are low or middle income countries, burdened with many acute health problems and chronic, hereditary disorders are not high in their health agenda. Despite this it has been proven, especially in Mediterranean countries that these conditions are both treatable and preventable. Optimum lifelong care has resulted in survival to an age where patients can fulfil their lives, and have a good quality existence. In addition prevention programmes have limited new births of affected individuals and have saved resources for the benefit of patients.

Priority of patient support organisations is the provision of services which can favour the good outcomes that have been demonstrated in the relatively few countries which

[*] Corresponding author: Email: Michael.angastiniotis@thalassaemia.com.cy.

have introduced comprehensive and effective programmes for the thalassaemias in their health systems. Such planning and service development is however impossible without epidemiological information. The World Health Organisation has recognised the global problem and has issued resolutions urging governments to adopt both prevention and patient care policies. Political will, budgetary allocation and health planning require knowledge of the disease, knowledge of the carrier prevalence and birth incidence and importantly the number of patients and their location.

Such data are difficult to collect especially in large non- homogeneous populations and even more in locations where the diseases are rare and imported through migrations.

In this paper (chapter) we discuss the development of epidemiological tools, such as carrier screening, patient registers, cost effectiveness studies, outcome measures which will provide the information for service development. In addition we provide such epidemiological and service information as we have available with some mapping of available services and examples of outcome. The objective is to develop a toolkit for gathering useful information on existing services in order to diagnose deficiencies especially where patient care is concerned

Introduction

The thalassaemias are a group of hereditary disorders caused by over 300 mutations on the beta globin loci and over 160 affecting the alpha globin genes, responsible for the production of haemoglobin [1]. They are regarded as the commonest of the clinically serious single gene disorders affecting humans. The thalassaemia genes were endemic in areas where falciparum malaria was common, suggesting an epistatic relationship between these genes and resistance of carriers to malaria [2]. The endemic areas of the globe include the Mediterranean basin, the Middle East, central Asia, the Indian subcontinent, Southern China and South East Asia. Population migrations have now introduced the conditions to non-endemic areas such as Northern Europe and the Americas [3, 4]. This geographical distribution was referred to as the thalassaemia belt.

It is estimated that there are over 200 million carriers of the thalassaemia genes and that almost 60000 babies are born annually affected by clinically significant thalassaemia syndromes [5]. It is noted that most countries in the thalassaemia belt are low or middle income countries, burdened with many acute health problems and chronic, hereditary disorders are not high in their health agenda [6]. Despite this it has been proven, especially in Mediterranean countries that these conditions are both treatable and preventable. Optimum lifelong care has resulted in survival to an age where patients can fulfil their lives, and have a good quality existence. In addition prevention programmes have limited new births of affected individuals and have saved resources for the benefit of patients. Such achievements are not seen in all countries even those in which the thalassaemias are highly prevalent and in some locations children die even before diagnosis or in early childhood without proper treatment. This despite resolutions and directives to governments by the World Health Organisation which urge member states to design and implement national programmes for prevention and management of thalassaemia and other haemoglobinopathies [7].

Factors preventing the development of services are not only due to poor economic development but also the overall poor public health picture, reflected for example in high infant mortality. This general picture gives rise to other priorities for health authorities, such as infectious diseases and poor nutrition. Other factors however include the lack of epidemiological information concerning the contribution of hereditary diseases, the perception that these are 'small print' conditions and even ignorance of the conditions among health officials. Also there is a general perception among public health doctors that nothing can be done for congenital diseases. Nevertheless a child born with any birth defect, including a severe anaemia, is more vulnerable to infectious agents and the other environmental dangers that result from poor conditions and health services. The contribution of congenital disorders to overall childhood morbidity and mortality is often invisible to health statisticians.

The management of these conditions is lifelong and expensive. It requires planning involving many services and specialties in order to achieve the kind of outcomes that will enable survival and quality of life. It is for this reason that stakeholders other than health authorities often take the initiative to promote the development of services. These may be treating physicians, parents and surviving patients. NGOs have been created in most countries with members from these groups to act as advocates and even propose development plans for necessary services. In the field of haemoglobin disorders the Thalassaemia International Federation acts as an umbrella for national patient support groups, allowing them to benefit from international experience and the help of international experts in order to promote their concerns and help them on the road towards optimum care and prevention of these diseases.

As in all public health issues all stakeholders should work together for the best result to be achieved, so that collaboration with health authorities is of primary concern. Planning however requires knowledge of the current situation and which deficiencies need to be addressed. In this respect the Federation as an NGO supporting national groups, records and maintains data from each country which can be used in practical way. The databases, which are continuously under review, include:

- Epidemiological information – which includes carrier frequencies, birth incidence, patient numbers at regional level where possible
- Mapping of existing services
- Outcome indicators such as complication rates, age distribution, survival rates and quality of life indicators.

In this paper we present some of this information and the methodology used, in order to demonstrate the complexity of information that is required for service development.

Methodology

1. Epidemiological data
   A database has been created which derives information from published data, field visits and collaboration with local experts. This database includes: carrier rates of the clinically significant thalassaemias and haemoglobin variants: alpha and beta thalassaemia HbE, HbS and HbC. From these carrier rates and current demographic figures annual expected births of major syndromes (if no prevention measures are applied) are derived, which may be caused by homozygocity or double heterozygocity of these mutations. The number of patients known to be treated, is

also recorded. The accuracy of these data is frequently in doubt. However indicative figures are accepted and reviewed since the purpose is to approach the truth for service planning. Countries and TIF member organisations are urged to develop patient registries for more accurate and informative data.

2. Existing services are recorded in each country which will serve as indicators of the quality, as these affect the chances of survival. Such indicators include adequacy and safety of blood, the availability of the three approved iron chelating agents, whether out of pocket expenses are needed for any management modalities, whether there is sufficient monitoring for complications through multi-disciplinary care and especially if Cardiac Magnetic Resonance Imaging is available (T2*) which has been shown to reduce mortality by allowing early intervention if iron overload in the heart is detected at an early stage [8, 9].

   Results from a recent TIF survey on reference centres in various locations are reported in this paper. A questionnaire was sent to 220 centres treating haemoglobin disorders (these disorders and rare anaemias are usually treated in the same centre) in 38 countries and 147 (67%) responded but complete answers were provided by 143. The number of patients followed varied from 9 patients in a centre in Australia to 3950 in a centre in Egypt.
3. Outcome measures are the most important in evaluating quality of service but also the most difficult to information to collect. The basic information that is attempted to obtain is the age distribution of patients since this indicates not only the average age of survival and the oldest survivors but also indicates the effectiveness of prevention. Often even this information is not offered. Surveys periodically have provided figures on complications [10]. Survival rates are periodically published by countries or centres but cannot be accurately derived except where patient registries are kept. Likewise quality of life data are published by individual centres. Such data are noted and kept in the TIF archives and used in assessing country performance.

Results

The 143 centres serve a total of 50266 patients:

Beta thalassaemia major -23608

Beta thalassaemia intermedia – 5924

HbH Disease -2713

HbE/beta thalassaemia – 1968

Homozygous HbS – 10990

HbS/beta thalassaemia - 5063

Of the centres that have responded 36 catered for 500 to 4000 patients. This number of patients also brings a responsibility to provide more services and be centres of excellence. These large centres were located:

In Europe - 8

In the Americas - 5

In the Middle East – 21

In South East Asia - 2

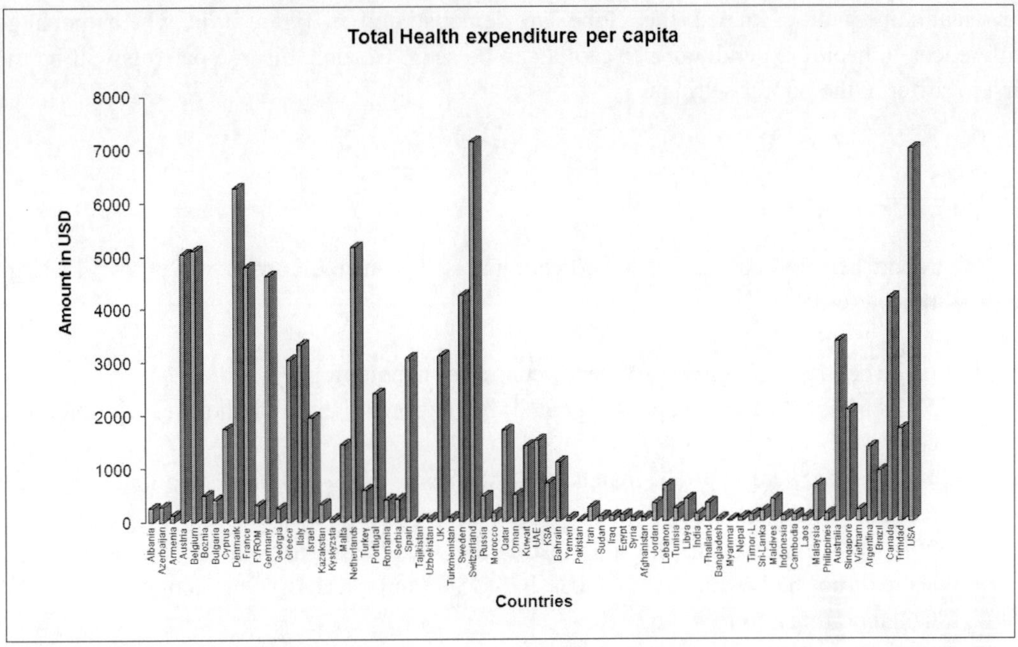

Chart 1. Showing the huge differences in health expenditure which inevitably affect service provision.

Epidemiology

Table 1 is derived from the TIF database. The expected thalassaemia births are similar to those estimated by Modell and Darlison in 2008 [5]. The thalassaemia patients known to clinics around the world is probably an underestimate but even so if around 55000 are expected to be born each year then treating only a maximum of 300000 shows that many are not known to services and may have perished at a very young age.

Table 1. The global epidemiology from the TIF database

WHO Region	B-thal carriers	Expected thal births	Sickle cell carriers	Expected SCD births	Known thal patients	Known SCD patients
Europe	11 million	1243	4.2 million	558	19183	29590
Middle East	32.6 million	9674	6.2 million	3716	120767	39164
South East Asia	140.2 million	41445	37.6 million	238730	155747	NA
West Pacific	23.8 million	5597	rare	rare	8740	NA
Americas	6.1 million	252	18 million	4791	1079	167500
Africa	rare	1500 estim	1-30%	244500 estim	4000	996711
Totals	214 million 3%of global population	59711	Approx 4% of global population	492295	309516	1232965

NB. 1. Annual births are calculated using the Hardy-Weinberg Rule

2. The number of carriers depends on figures being updated with new surveys

3. Known patients are those reported to TIF and do not represent the exact number of existing patients

Health inequalities across the globe are demonstrated in figure 1 in which the huge differences in health expenditure per capita can be seen. Chronic disease patients will be the first to suffer in the poorer settings.

Service Indicators

We report here indicators that have been analysed from the current survey of 147 large responding centres:

1. Is the centre a recognised reference centre for haemoglobin disorders?
   58 centres (40.5%) were designated by national health authorities as reference centres
   18 (12.6%) were self designated while the rest (46.9%) did not state that they were recognised as reference centres
   20 (14%) centres or the hospital hosting them had accreditation from an international accrediting body, mostly JACIE, JCI, ISO and AABB. One centre is a WHO Collaborating centre
2. Do centres keep a patient registry?
   107 (75%) keep a registry of patients attending the centre and in 81 of these (76%) this is partially or wholly computerised
   In 34 of the 107 centres (32%) the registry is part of a national patient registry
   Only 10/143 (7%) centres stated clearly that their registry was connected to electronic medical record for their haemoglobinopathy patients
3. Are any of the 3 approved iron chelating agents not available?
   14 centres did not respond to this question
   Deferiprone is not available in 21 centres: 9 centres in Iraq (indicating that this drug is not available in the country) but also in 4 Canadian centres, 2 Australian and 2 Romanian. Single centres in Greece, Egypt, Iran Malta and Qatar are also missing the drug
   Deferasirox is not available in 4 centres (in Greece, Indonesia, Iran and Iraq)
   Desferrioxamine is available in all the responding centres
   NB Despite this response TIF is aware that constant supply of these agents is problematic in many centres leading to inadequate treatment with adverse effects in the long term
4. *Magnetic resonance imaging to assess tissue iron*
   Of 143 centres 31 (21.5%) do not have Cardiac MRI (T2*). This includes most centres in some countries such as Iraq (where very large clinics are serving several thousands of patients)
   Liver iron measured by validated MRI technologies is not available in 83 (58%) of clinics. Even where available many patients need to pay for these services.
5. *Out of pocket expenses*
   - Completely free medical care is offered in 99 (69.2%) of centres
   - Partially free care is offered in 25 (17.5%) of centres
   - Exclusively out of pocket treatment is offered by 4 centres (2.8%)
   - 15 centres (10.5%) did not respond

6. *Provide leukodepleted blood*
   126 centres (88%) provide filtered blood
7. *Involved in research*
   108 (75.5%) centres responded that they are involved in research
   23 (16.1%) stated that they are not
   12 (8.4%) did not answer the question
8. *The staff/patient ratio* (See table 2 - investigated in the centres with more than 500 patients)

Outcome measures:

1. The average age of patients (see chart 2)
2. The age distribution curve (see chart 3). This indicator is the most informative and we use here the current curve for the Cyprus Thalassaemia Centres as an example. At present many centres could not provide such data because of the lack of a comprehensive register of patients

Discussion

The Thalassaemia International Federation has an interest in assessing the performance of the haematology centres which deal red cell disorders, which have the haemoglobin disorders as their main concern. This assessment is part of the assessment of the health care needs of multitransfused patients in various countries which will lead to efforts to improve both services and national plans through raising awareness and collaboration of all involved parties, including national support associations, the medical community and health authorities in order to affect necessary changes. Without information changes cannot come about so the preparation of a series of indicators to form a standard toolkit for assessment of services is an important step [11].

TIF is standardising a condition specific toolkit and some of the methods and preliminary list if indicators is presented in this paper. This is not a comprehensive list but includes some of the indicators which emerge from a recent survey of centres. The intention is to standardise and present in an electronic format a more complete questionnaire which may be used both by stakeholders both local and international.

Table 2. The centres catering for more than 500 patients Staff patient ratio

Region	Doctor patient ratio	Range	Nurse patient ratio	Range
Europe	1:145	1: 74-242	1:140	1: 43-285
Americas	1: 185	1: 85-245	1: 165	1: 72-350
Middle East	1: 270	1: 80-500	1: 150	1: 36-300
SE Asia	1:100		1: 60	1: 38- 80

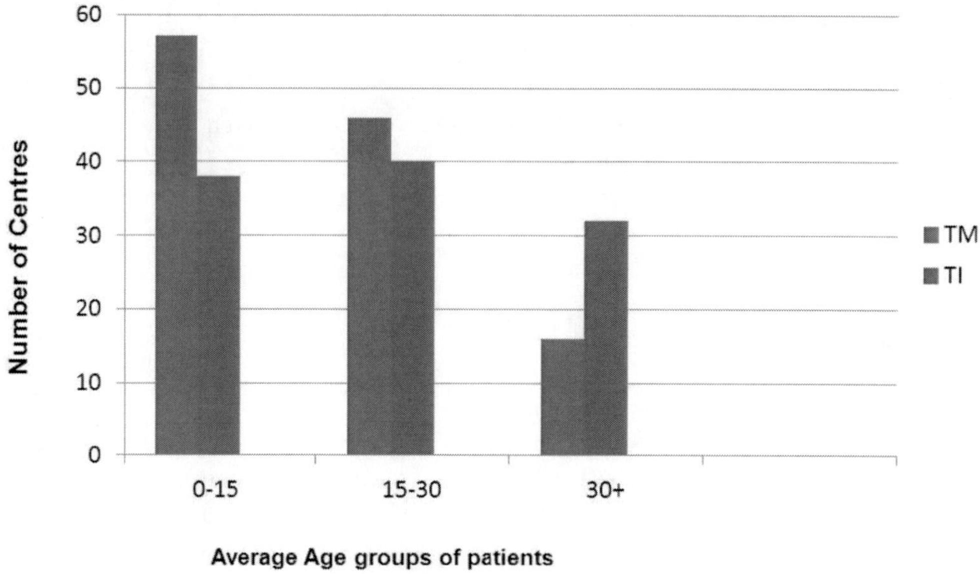

Comment: The majority of centres have very young patients with average ages in the 0-15 years category. This is both in thalassaemia major and intermedia, although there are more centres which have intermedia patients over 30 years. The differences between major and intermedia are to be expected and the over-representation of centres having 0-15y category patients, may be because more paediatric departments responded (this is not clearly seen from the departments listed).

Chart 2. The average age of patients in various centres comparing the average age of thalassaemia major and intermedia.

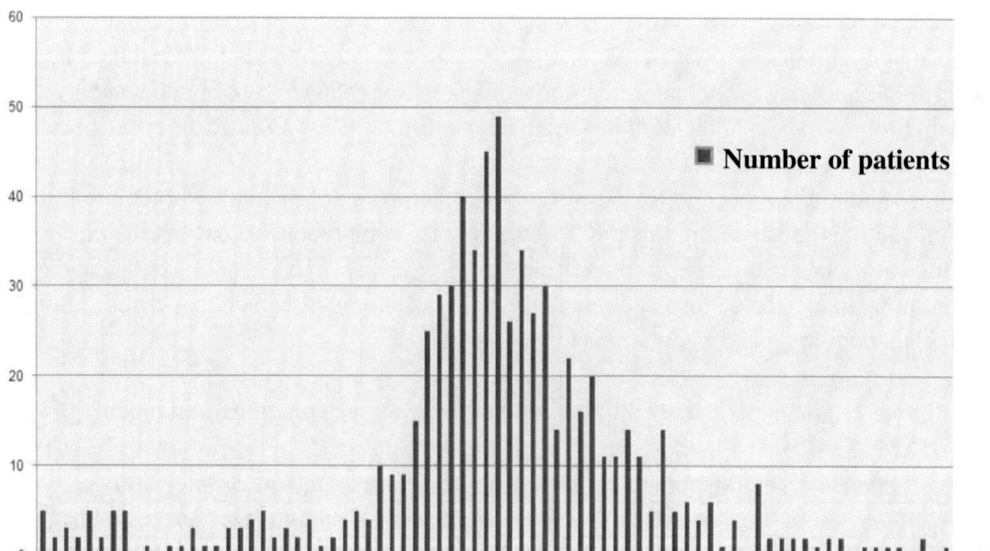

This chart indicates the reduced numbers in the younger age groups due to prevention. The falling numbers after the age of 50 is indicative of the higher mortality in patients who grew up with inadequate treatment regimes of a previous age. This chart includes thalassaemia intermedia as well as major.

Chart 3. Age distribution of beta-thalassaemia patients attending clinics in Cyprus in 2013.

Epidemiology is essential for policy making and the development of services. There are several databases in existence which concern red cell disorders [12] however few if any include service indicators which can be used for service development. Accurate population data of carrier rates are also essential and we agree with Piel et al. [12] that improving collaboration between different groups and integrating databases is now essential. However more patient oriented information needs to be added if the services available are to be understood. The methodology of gathering information needs to be improved and in this respect also collaboration of international experts is needed. In this respect the TIF toolkit is being tested and developed.

The indicators discussed in the survey reported here have revealed some major deficiencies in service provision even in centres which are regarded by health authorities as reference centres. One example is that 25 centres cannot provide al three chelating agents which may lead to inefficient iron chelation to patients; if to these are added another 14 centres which did not give an answer then a significant number of reference centres are providing inadequate treatment. This includes centres in Iran, Iraq and Egypt which serve over 500 patients each. Assessment of tissue iron measurements, which are important for early intervention to prevent serious life threatening complications, are also lacking in a significant number of centres. These important investigations often also suffer from poor accuracy of MRI quantification of iron due to lack of regular calibration and validation of the software.

The staff patient ratio is an important indicator but suffers from lack of studies to describe an optimum ration. A WHO advisory group many years ago suggested 1 physician per 50 patients and one nurse per 30 patients. These suggestions were never validated and are certainly difficult for services to provide, especially in large clinics. This is a subject that requires further studies.

In addition the fact that 30% of centres cannot provide completely free of charge services in a lifelong and potentially lethal disorder makes for inequalities in health service provision and potentially dangerous inadequacy in care.

The object of a standard tool is to identify and approach service deficiencies at local and county level so that with the help of all concerned corrective steps can be taken.

References

[1] Old, J; Angastiniotis, M; Eleftheriou, A; Galanello, R; Harteveld, CL; Petrou, M; Traeger-Synodinos, J. *Prevention of thalassaemias and other haemoglobin disorders*, Vol 1, Principles. TIF Publications no.18 2013

[2] Williams, TN; Weatherall, DJ. World distribution, population genetics and health burden of haemoglobinopathies. *Cold Spring Harb Prespect Med*, 2012, 2, a011692

[3] Modell, B; Darlison, M; Birgen, H; Cario, H; Faustino, P; Giordano, PC; Gulbis, B; Hopmeier, P, Lena-Russo, D; Romao, L; Theodorsson, E. Epidemiology of haemoglobin disorders in Europe: an overview. *Scand J Clin Investig*, 2007, 67, 39-70

[4] Angastiniotis, MA; Soteriades, ES; Vives-Corrons, JL; Eleftheriou, A. The impact of migrations on the health services of Europe: the example of haemoglobin disorders. An

Enerca enquiry. *Scientific World Journal*, 2013, 2013, 727905. doi: 10.1155/2013/727905. Epub 2013 Mar 18.

[5] Modell, B.; Darlison, M. Global epidemiology of haemoglobin disorders and derived service indicators. *Bull World Health Org*., 2008, 86(6), 704-712.

[6] Weatherall, DJ. Thalassemia as a global health problem; recent progress toward its control in the developing countries. *Ann NY Acad Sci*, 2010, 1202, 17-23

[7] WHO EB Resolution on thalassaemia and other haemoglobinopathies. EB118 R1 2006

[8] Modell, B; Khan, M; Darlison, M; Westwood, MA; Ingram, D; Pennell, DJ. Improved survival of thalassaemia major in the UK and relation to T2* cardiovascular magnetic resonance. *J Cardiovasc Magn Reson*, 2008, 10, 42

[9] Chouliaras, G; Berdoukas, V; Ladis, V; Kattamis, A; Chatziliami, A; Fragodimitri, C; Karabatsos, F; Youssef, J; Karagiorga-Lagana, M. Impact of magnetic resonance imaging on cardiac mortality in thalassaemia major. *J Magn Reson Imaging*, 2011, 34(1), 56-9

[10] De, Sanctis, V; Eleftheriou, A; Malaventura, C. Prevalence of endocrine complications and short stature in patients with thalassaemia major: a multicentre study by the Thalassaemia International Federation (TIF). *Pediatr Endocrinol Rev*., 2004, suppl 2, 249-55

[11] Nacul, LC; Stewart, A; Alberg, C; Chowdhuri, S; Darlison, MW; Grollman, C; Hall, A; Modell, B; Moorthie, S; Sagoo, GS; Burton, H. A toolkit to assess health needs for congenital disorders in low-and middle income countries: an instrument for public action. *J Pub Health (Oxf)*, 2013 May 10.

[12] Piel, FB; Howes, RE; Nyangiri, OA; Moyes, CL; Williams, TN; Weatherall, DJ; Hay, SI. Online biomedical resources for Malaria-related red cell disorders. *Hum Mutat*, 2013, 34(7), 937-44

In: Thalassemia
Editor: Makenzie Greene
ISBN: 978-1-63117-954-9

Chapter 12

Beta Thalasemia in Bahrain: An Overview

Shaikha Al Arrayed*
Genetic Department, Ministry of Health, Kingdom of Bahrain

Abstract

Genetic blood diseases are frequent in Bahrain as in all Middle Eastern countries. Previous neonatal screening study 1984-1985 showed that the incidence of sickle cell disease (SCD) was 2.1%, of sickle cell trait (SCT) 11%, while the carrier rate for beta Thalassaemia was 3%.

The total number of Bahraini patients with thalassemia is 88 patients, Non Bahraini is 21, Age group between 2-35 years.

A ten years study on the prevalence of β thalassemia among the students in Bahrain was performed. The aim of the program was to raise awareness among the youth. A total of 88,000 students were screened from 1999 to 2013. The mean prevalence of ß thalessemia trait and major were 3.5% and 0.035% respectively. The frequency of β thalassemia in Bahrain was found to be low to moderate, in comparison with the situation in many other gulf countries.

In another study we measure the public awareness level about Beta thalassemia in Bahrain, Conducted in 2006 to 2007. A questionnaire was distributed among 2000 persons from the general public. It showed that (65.1%) knew about beta thalassemia. A majority of (77.8) strongly agreed that premarital checking can prevent it. Females showed better knowledge than males.

The molecular characterization of B-thalassemia mutations among Bahrainis was studied by using a variety of polymerase chain reaction (PCR)-based procedures including reverse dot blot (RDB), denaturing gradient gel electrophoresis (DGGE) and DNA sequencing. Thirteen different β-thal mutations were identified. It showed that four mutations (Intervening Sequence I (IVSI)-3' end (-25 base pairs (bp)) deletion; Codon

* Corresponding author: Shaikha Al Arrayed, Chairperson of Genetic Department, Chairperson of Bahrain National Hereditary anemia Society, Genetic Department, Ministry of Health, Kingdom of Bahrain, POB 12, SMC hospital. Telephone: 00973-17284489, Fax: 00973-17284496, Tel: 00973 17689017, Fax: 00973-17689959 Email: ssarayed@batelco.com.bh, ssarrayed@gmail.com, web site www.bnhas.org.

(Cd) 39 (C→T) andIVSI-5 (G→C), account for ~80% of all β-thal alleles. and that IVSI-3' end (-25bp) deletion is the major β-thalassemic allele in Bahrain.

We have organized and directed the campaign to control genetic in the period between 1984-2013. The goals were to reduce the incidence, and to improve the standard of management for patients suffering from these diseases.

The prevention strategy depended on health education, screening and counseling. A comprehensive health education program has been launched, to increase public awareness of the diseases.

This program used the media, and targeted key opinion leaders in society and the community, in schools and other public places. Screening for haemoglobinopathies included sickle cell disease, thalassaemia, was undertaken on the following categories of the population: antenatal mothers, premarital couples, newborns, and school students, followed by counseling of families. The campaign was supported by both the policy makers and the community.

All these efforts continued for more than 25 years. It had tremendous effects in reducing the prevalence of Genetic Blood Diseases (GBD) among the newborns, in 1984 the incidence of SCD among newborn was 20 per thousand, now it is 4 per thousand with 75 % decline, while the number of affected newborn with beta thal is 0-2 per year.

During this campaign the Ethical legal and social issues were taken care of, such as: equity, informed consent, privacy, confidentiality and prevention of stigmatization and discrimination.

Treatment: available in Bahrain will be discussed, One of preventive measures is pnd prenatal diagnosis \ And pgd –preimplantation genetic diagnosis.

Introduction

The state of Bahrain is made up of an Archipelago of thirty-six islands, with an area of 694 square kilometers, located in the Arabian Gulf. The kingdom of Saudi Arabia is on the west and Qatar on the East. The estimated 2002 population was 627,123. The percentage of Bahraini is 62.4% and non-Bahraini 37.6%. Growth birth rate and population growth rates over the last five years have been stable. In 2002 the crude birth rate was 20.1 per 1000 population. The infant mortality rate has been reduced to 7/1000 live births in 2002. There has been a significant increase in life expectancy at birth. Children born today will on average live to 73.8 years. [1]

Falciparum malaria was endemic in Bahrain until 1970, and so the malaria associated genetic defects of red cells such as Sickle cell disease (SCD), thalassemia and glucose 6 phosphate dehydrogenase deficiency (G6PD) were expected to be common. These genetic diseases are passed from generation to generation through marriages between carriers. There is no real cure, and the management is supportive and symptomatic only. The preventive measures remain the best way of dealing with these diseases.

A new-born screening study conducted 1984-1985 in Bahrain revealed that 2.1% had sickle cell disease, 200 babies were born every year in Bahrain suffering from SCD, 11.2% were carriers for sickle cell disease, and 20% with G6PD deficiency [2]. The carrier status for Beta thalassemia was found to be 2-4% in a premarital counseling study. [3]

These statistics reflect the fact that a large number of children are suffering from these diseases. This affects individuals, families, and the society, both socially and economically.

The Cyprus Thalassemia Control Program has succeeded in reducing the incidence of B-thalassemia major in the country through measures such as health education, carrier screening, premarital counseling and prenatal diagnosis. This success has encouraged other countries to adopt same measures.[4-8]

In Bahrain, during the seventies patients attending the health services were treated symptomatically. Thalassaemia patients were under-treated and under-transfused. Many of them developed complications and dysmorphic features. Many families had 3-5 children with thalassaemia or sickle cell disease, and patients with sickle cell disease were treated as malingerer and subjected to neglect in emergency rooms and hospitals. They were often viewed as drug users since they often come for analgesics. At the beginning of the eighties, the service improved for these patients. The Ministry of Health started to organize services provided to them, through health centers, medical clinics and pediatric clinics. In 1984, the first genetic clinic was established, at Salmaniya medical complex. Premarital counseling started at the genetic clinic for families at risk. Information booklets were designed and distributed widely, Educational campaigns started in school and Clubs, to increase awareness among students and the public about these diseases.

In 1991 Bahrain Hereditary anemia society was formed with the aim of fighting these diseases, and raising the standard of care for the patients. 1992 the Minister of health formed a national committee for prevention of genetic disease in Bahrain. The committee put a plan aiming at preventing and eliminating these diseases. The committee advised to concentrate on screening and education.[9-12]. Screening all pregnant women started, and if the mother was found to be carrier the newborn was screened.

In 1993 the Premarital counseling services at health centers was organized by the genetic department and maternal and child health department. Training courses were given to all the primary health care physicians, and a form was designed to standardize the service through all health centers. The premarital counseling (PMC) become available on wide basis through all the health centers. Initially the acceptance was poor, but it gathers momentum gradually [3].

In 1998 student- screening project started. The aim of screening all students before they leave school was to raise awareness among the youth about hereditary anemia, and advice them to take the right decision to prevent these diseases in their future families. A card with blood result was given to each student with information booklet about the disease he carries.

This project is continuing for the 15th year, and it has tremendous effect on awareness, not only among the students, but also among the families. As the family ask to be tested if they knew that their son is carrier for certain disease. It also affects positively the attendance to premarital counseling.

All these efforts continued for more than 25 years. It had tremendous effects in reducing the prevalence of Genetic Blood Diseases (GBD) among the newborns, in 1984 the incidence of SCD among newborn was 20 per thousand, now it is 4 per thousand with 75% decline

During this campaign the Ethical legal and Social issues were taken care of, such as: equity, informed consent, privacy, confidentiality and prevention of stigmatization and discrimination.

Ref: Campaign to Control Genetic Blood Diseases in Bahrain, Community Genetic 2005:8: 52-55.

Beta Thalassemia Frequency in Bahrain: A Ten Years Study

Abstract

Hereditary blood disorders such as sickle-cell disease and thalassemia syndromes impose a significant burden on many countries. Their chronic nature makes them one of the leading causes of morbidity and mortality in these countries.1 Here we are reporting on a ten years study on the prevalence of β thalassemia among the students in Bahrain, from 1999 to 2008. Data was collected during the annual student screening program. The aim of the program was to raise awareness among the youth in Bahrain about hereditary anemia., and also to determine the prevalence of these disorders among Bahraini secondary school students.

Materials and Methods

The study plan was to screen all the students in the 11th grade (2nd Secondary class).

Awareness program and educational lectures were organized in school prior to sample collection. Informational booklets were distributed and permission from parents to test their children were obtained.

The blood samples were collected from the students by lab technicians and examined on the same day. Hemoglobin electrophoresis were carried out by using HPLC instrument.

Results

Thirty eight schools were visited per year, and a total of 60,000 students were screened from 1999 to 2008. The mean prevalence of ß thalessemia trait and major were 3.5% and 0.035% respectively.

Conclusion

The frequency of β thalassemia in Bahrain was found to be low to moderate, in comparison with the situation in many other gulf countries such as UAE, Qatar and Kuwait.. Sickle cell disease (SCD) is more common than β thalassemia in Bahrain. Preventive measures remain the best ways of dealing with these diseases.

Introduction

Genetic diseases are chronic in nature and require costly, lifelong care and management strategies. They causes significant health care and psychosocial burdens on the patient, the family, the health care system and the community as a whole. [1-5]

Epidemiological studies confirmed that the gene frequency of these diseases vary proportionately with malaria prevalence. These studies indicated that hemoglobinopathies and enzymopathies provide protection against malaria. The heterozygous suffer less frequently and less severely than normal individuals... [6, 7]

In general, Thalassemias are associated with, people of Asians and Mediterranean origin Maldives population shows the highest occurrence of 18% of carrier rate of Thalassemia, whereas the lowest prevalence are observed in North Europe (0.1%) and Africa (0.9%), especially northern Africa. The high occurrence are also observed in Latin America and Mediterranean countries like Greece, Italy, Portugal, Spain etc. The estimated occurrence of this disease shows 16% in Cyprus and 3-8% in Bangladesh, China, India, Malaysia and Pakistan. [8-11]

Incidence of beta in Arab and gulf countries states The frequency of this disease is high in Lebanon, Jordon, Iraq, Palestine, Egypt and other Arab countries. The carrier rate of β thalassemia of 3.6 – 4 %, 6.24% and 8 % were observed in Oman, Yemen. And UAE respectively. Nadkarni et al., 1991 and Al-Arrayed and Haites, 1995 have observed β thalassemia carrier rate of 2-4% in Bahrain population. [12-25]

The β thalassemia is characterised by a reduced production of β-globin chain (β+) or absent production of β-globin chain (β°). This result to an imbalanced α/non-α globin chain production. The molecular diagnosis is essential in the accurate diagnosis of these diseases as the inheritance of β-thalassemia might be masked by coinheritance of sickle cell gene and /or alpha thalasemia.

Thalassemia major patient shows severe anemia in the first year of life, and are unable to maintain the hemoglobin level around 5 gm/dl). Thus they need life long blood transfusion, which also causes iron overload. Hence, iron chelation treatment is necessary to prevent iron overload damage to the internal organs. Recent advances in iron chelation treatment help to solve this problem and leads to long life.

In general, the disease may affect the spleen (often enlarged), and causes heart failure.

In recent years, bone marrow transplant and stem cell transplant have shown success in some patients of thalassemia major. Successful transplant can eliminate the patients dependencies on transfusions.

Most of the β-thalassemia heterozygote carriers are clinically asymptomatic with distinctive hematological phenotype represent by hypochromic, microcytic anemia and characteristically raised levels of HbA2. The coinheritance of α-thalassemia will causes HbA2 into a normal/borderline level which will make the diagnosis of this condition difficult. [8-11]

Material and Method

The national project for prevention of hereditary blood diseases in Bahrain is a collaborative project between the Ministry of Health, Ministry of Education, and Bahrain Hereditary Anemia Society. The plan was to screen all the students in the 11th grade (2nd Secondary). This Included all Bahraini and non Bahraini students in the government, and also some private schools. Around 6000-7000 students were targeted annually for 10 years from 1999 to 2008.

The project duration was six months, which included planning, education sessions, blood collection, lab testing, data processing, distribution of cards, data analysis and reporting.

Permission for screening were obtained from parents,. Thirty eight schools were visited per year. Awareness program and educational lectures were organized in schools prior to sample collection. Informational booklets were distributed to all the students to create awareness about the program.

The blood samples were collected from the students by the lab technicians and examined on the same day. Hemoglobin electrophoresis were carried out by using HPLC instrument and G6PD deficiency were also tested.

The demographic information for each student and test result were recorded in a coded form.

Each student received a card with the result which can be used for his future life. The school also received the report about the prevalence of these diseases among their students.

Results

Total number of students screened during the ten years period was (60,000). The response rate of the parents to allow their children to have the test was 81-85% 96.5% of the students are normal for β thalassemia (i.e free of β thalassemia gene defect). Table 1 and figure 1 shows the prevelance of Beta thalassemia among these students

Beta Thalassemia Major

The Number of β thalassemia homozygous each year was 5, 0,3,2,3,1,1,1,0.2. Five cases with β thalassemia homozygous status, were detected in the first year.

The mean prevalence rate of β thalassemia homozygous, SD, SE was 0.03%, 0.029 and 0.00092 respectively. Significant difference was observed at 95% confidence (p=0.004). The lower and upper interval of difference was 0.0141 and 0.0559.

Prevalence of Beta Thal Trait

The number of carriers for beta thal during the years 1999-2008 was 164,212,187, 219,175,212,221,231,211 and 265 students respectively.

The observed mean, SD, SE of β thalassemia Trait were 3.5%, 0.614 and 0.194 respectively. The p value showed 0.000 at 95% of confidence. The lower and upper interval of difference were 3.09 and 3.97.

Hb A2 in β thalassemia trait ranged between 4% and 9%. Samples with lower figure of A2 (3.4-4) were suspected of having the gene and blood samples were directed for DNA studies to R/O heterozygosity.

Table 1. Prevalence of Beta Thalassemia among Students in Bahrain 1999-2008 Year

	1999	2000	2001	2002	2003	2004	2005	2006	2007	2008
Disease	**No and %**	**No and %**	**No and %**	**No and %**	**No and %**	**No and %**	**No and %**	**No and %**	**No and %**	**No and %**
β thal Disease	5 0.09%	0 0.00%	3 0.05%	2 0.03%	3 0.06%	1 0.02%	1 0.02%	1 0.02%	0 0.00%	3 0.06%
β tha l Trait	164 2.88%	212 3.72%	187 3%	219 3.72%	175 3.23%	212 3.40%	221 3.48%	231 3.64%	211 3.31%	265 5.05%
No of Student	**5685**	**5694**	**6244**	**5894**	**5418**	**6237**	**6358**	**6352**	**6376**	**5314**

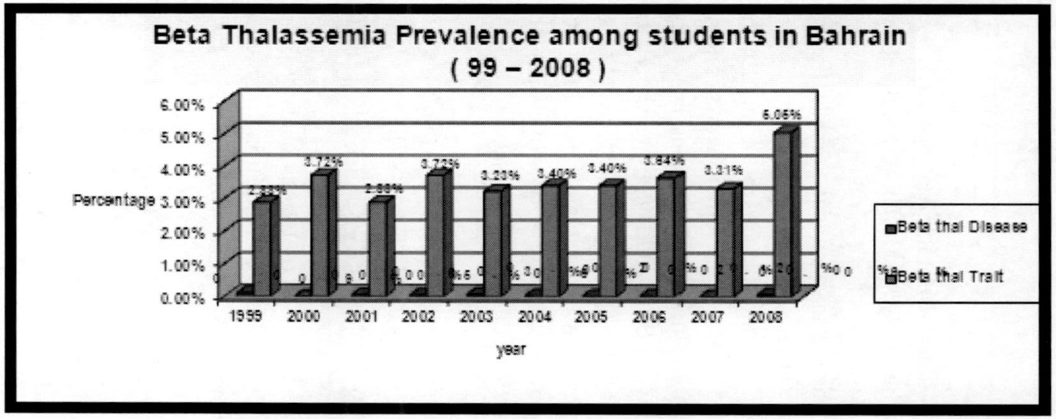

Figure 1. Beta Thalassaemia Prevalence (1999 – 2008).

Prevalence of Beta Thal by Region

According to the result of 1999, some regions were observed to have a higher rate of this disease like Hidd (5.4%), Sitra (5.3%), Riffa (3.3%) and Hamad town (3.35%). Other regions like Western region, Northern region, and Manama had only 2% of prevalence of this disease. Similar results were observed during the subsequent years also.

Discussion

The prevalence of β thalassemia in Bahrain was 3.5 % which was nearly the same figure obtained in the premarital study. [25]. The highest rate was found in Hidd 5.4% and Sitra 5.3%.

In the year 2008, there was a sudden increase in the frequency β thalassemia to 5%, which was not reported earlier. The cause of the rise of the carrier rate, and the future trend needs to be investigated. It could be due to the sudden increase in the population size from 700,000 to one million, or due to some other factors. The result of the study showed that there was a genetic heterogeneity in different regions in the state of Bahrain. The following was comparison between prevalence of sickle cell gene and beta thal gene among the regions.

The Western area had the highest prevalence rate of sickle cell disease (25%). It had the lowest prevalence rate of beta thalassemia (2%). In contrast with Al, Hidd region, had the highest prevalence rate of Beta thal (5.4%), while it has the lowest prevalence rate for sickle cell disease was 2.7%. Sitra region had the second highest rate for sickle cell disease (21%) and β thalassemia (5.3%). [24-28]

The malaria selection hypothesis could explain the higher rate of these diseases in Sitra and Hidd, as they are small islands surrounded by water. The higher frequency rate of β thalassemia in Riffa may be explained by the effect of migration from Hidd and Muharraq area (migration founder effect).

Internationally more than 500 mutations causing β-thalassemia have been characterized till date, the majority of which are non-deletional mutation. [3, 8-11] Previously, we studied the mutations causing the Beta Thal in Bahraini. A total of thirteen different β thalassemia mutations were identified. Four of which are considered to be of the (Mediterranean) type: Cd 39 (C—T), IVS1,1(G—A), IVS11,1 (G—A) and IVS1,110 (G—A); four are common in Indian sub continent: IVS1,5(G—C),Cd 8/9(+G), Cd 15(G—A)and Cd41/42(-CTTT); three mutations already described in the Kurdish people: Cd44(-C),nt-88(C—A) and nt-101 (C—T); one mutation already described in a Malay individual (Cd35(-C);and one mutation frequently encountered in the Middle East: IVS1,3' end (-25 bp) Four different mutations accounted for 80% of all β thalassemia alleles. These mutation are intervening sequence 1(IVS1)3'end (-25 bp)deletion; Codon (Cd) 39(C—T); IVS1,5(G—C); and IVS11,1(G—A). 26-27.

Sickle cell β thalassemia is found in few cases. It was expected that the clinical picture will vary according to level of HB A produced by the β thalassemia gene. They usually manifest milder form of the disease. [26-28]

Conclusion

The frequency of β thalassemia disease in Bahrain is not high, in contrast with the situation in many other gulf states such as UAE, Qatar and Kuwait.. Preventive measures such as health education, carrier screening and premarital counseling remain the best ways of dealing with these diseases. This can have significant financial saving, social benefits and health benefits.

Ref: Beta Thalassemia Frequency in Bahrain: A Ten Year Study, *Bahrain Medical Bulletin, Vol. 32, No. 2, June 1-5*

References

[1] WHO. (1999). Primary healthcare approaches for prevention and control of congenital and genetic disorders. Available at http://who.int/

[2] USPSTF. (US Preventive Services Task Force) (1996) Guide to Clinical Preventive Services. Screening for Hemoglobinopathies, 2nd edition. 43: p491. Available at http://www.ahcpr.gov/clinic/uspstf/uspshemo.htm.

[3] WHO. (2002). Genomics and World Health Report. Available at http://www.who.int/genomics/elsi/recommendations/en/

[4] WHO. (1983). Community control of hereditary anemia: memorandum from a WHO meeting. *Bulletin of the World Health Organization*, 61(1), 63-80.

[5] WHO. (1982). Hereditary anaemia: genetic basis, clinical features, diagnosis and treatment. *Bulletin of the World Health Organization*, 60(5), 643-60.

[6] Allison, A. C. (1954). Protection afforded by sickle-cell trait against subtertian malarial infection. *Brit. Med. J., I*, 290-294.

[7] Flint, J., Harding, R. M., Clegg, J. B. & Boyce, A. J. (1993). Why are some genetic diseases common? Distinguishing selection from other processes by molecular analysis of globin gene variants. *Hum. Genet. 91*, 91-117, PubMed ID: 8462981.

[8] The Thalassaemia Syndromes. (1981). Oxford: Blackwell (pub.) 1981. Oxford: Blackwefl Scientific Publications, Inc.

[9] Weatherall, D. J. & Clegg, J. B. (1995). The Thalassemia Syndromes. Weatherall, D. J.; Clegg, J. B.; Higgs, D. R.; Wood, W. G.: The hemoglobinopathies.In: Scriver, C.; Beaudet, A. L.; Sly, W. S.; Valle, D. (eds.): The Metabolic and Molecular Bases of Inherited Disease. (7th ed.) New York: McGraw-Hill. 3417-3484.

[10] Modell, B., Khan, M. & Darlison, M. (2000). Survival in beta-thalassaemia major in the UK: data from the UK Thalassaemia Register. *Lancet, 355*, 2051-2052. PubMed ID: 10885361.

[11] Flint, J., Harding, R., Boyce, A. C., et al. (1993). The Population Genetics of Hemoglobinopathies. In: Baillière's Clinical Hematology. London: *Baillière Tindall*, 215-62.

[12] Baysal, E. (2001). Hemoglobinopathies in the United Arab Emirates. *Hemoglobin*, *25*(2), 247-53.

[13] Miller, C. J., Dunn, E. V., Berg, B. & Abdouni, S. F. (2003). A hematological survey of preschool children of the United Arab Emirates. *Saudi Med J.*, *24*(6), 609-13.

[14] Makhoul, N. J., Wells, R. S., Kaspar, H., Shbaklo, H., Taher, A., Chakar, N. & Zalloua, P. A. (2005). Genetic heterogeneity of Beta thalassemia in Lebanon reflects historic and recent population migration. *Ann Hum Genet*, *69*(Pt 1), 55-66. 15.

[15] El-Kalla & Mathews, A. R. (1997). A Significant B -Thalassemia Heterogeneity in The United Arab Emirates. *Hemoglobin*, *21*,237-47.

[16] Al-Riyami, A. A., Suleiman, A. J., Afifi, M., Al-Lamki, Z. M. & Daar, S. (2001). A community-based study of common hereditary blood disorders in Oman. *East Mediterr Health J.*, *7*(6), 1004-11.

[17] Rajab, A. G., Patton, M. A. & Modell, B. (2000). Study of hemoglobinopathies in Oman through a national register. *Saudi Med J.*, *21*(12), 1168-72.

[18] Adekile, A. D., Gu, L. H., Baysal, E., et al. (1994). Molecular Characterization of a – Thalassemia Determinants, B -Thalassemia Alleles, and Bs Haplotypes among Kuwaiti Arabs. *Acta Haematologica*, *92*, 176-81.

[19] White, J. M., Byrne, M., Richards, R., Buchanan, T., Katsoulis, E. & Weerasingh, K. (1986). Red cell genetic abnormalities in Peninsular Arabs: sickle haemoglobin, G6PD deficiency, and alpha and beta thalassaemia. *J Med Genet.*, *23*(3), 245-51.

[20] El-Hazmi, M. A. F. & A1-Swailem, A. R. (1995).Warsy. Molecular Defects in Beta-Thalassemia in the population of Saudi Arabia. *Hum Hered*, *45*, 278-85.

[21] Hasounah, F. R., Sejeny, S. a. & Omer, J. A. (1995). Spectrum of B -Thalassemia Mutations in the Population of Saudi Arabia. *Hum Hered*, *45*, 231-4.

[22] El-Shanti, H. (2001). The impact of genetic disease on Jordanians: strategies towards prevention. *Journal of Biomedicine and Biotechnology, 1*, 45–47. p45.

[23] Nadkarni, K., Al Arrayed, S. S. & Bapat, J. (1991). Incidence of genetic disorders of haemoglobins in the hospital population of Bahrain. *Bahrain Medical Bulletin*, *13*(1), 19-23.

[24] Al-Arrayed, S. S., Hafadh, N. & Al Serafi, S. (1997). Premarital counseling: an experience from Bahrain. *Eastern Mediterranean Health Journal*, vol *3*, 3, 415-9.

[25] Bahrain Health Statistics report 2005-2007, http:// www.moh.gov.bh.

[26] Jassim, N. M., Al Arrayed, S. S., Al Mukhareq, H., Merghoub, T. & Krishmamoorthy, R. (2000). Spectrum of B Thalassemia In Bahrain, *bah Med Bull*, *22* (1), 8-12.

[27] Jassim, N., Merghoub, T., Pascadud, O., Al Mukhareq Ducrocoq, R. H. A., Labie, D., Elion, J., Krishmamoorthy, R., Al Arrayed, S. S., et al. B thalassemia in Bahrain. Annals New York Accademy of science.

[28] Jassim, N. & Al Arrayed, S. S. (2006) reported on the Molecular Basis of Benign form of Sickle Cell – B thalassemia Syndrome. *Bahrain Medical Bulletin*, *24*(4)168- 170.

Spectrum of B-Thalassaemia Mutations in Bahrain

Objectives: To study the molecular characterization of B-thalassemia mutations among Bahrainis.

Methods: We used a variety of polymerase chain reaction (PCR)-based procedures including reverse dot blot (RDB), denaturing gradient gel eiectrophoresis (DGGE) and DNA sequencing, to study the B-thai mutation In 87 Bahraini individuals from 51 unrelated Bahrainl families.

Results: Thirteen different β-thal mutations were identified. Four mutations (Intervening Sequence I (IVSI)-3' end (-25 base pairs (bp)) deletion; Codon (Cd) 39 (C→T) and IVSI-5 (G→C), account for ~80% of all β-thal alleles.

Conclusion: We conclude that IVSI-3' end (-25bp) deletion is the major β-thalassemic allele in Bahrain.

Recommendations: Based upon our findings, a preventive approach of β-thalassemia needs to be embloyed for the Bahraini people. This study can be used in implementing a cost effective strategy for screening and diagnosis of β-thal among Bahrainis.

Introduction

The hemoglobinopathies are the most common genetic disorders in Balirain, represented mainly By sickle cell disease (SCD) and thalassemias. Among thalassemias both α and β forms are identified. The βthalassemias are group of inherited anemias characterised by a reduced (β+) or absent (β°) production of β-globin chain from the affected allele2. This leads an imbalanced α/non-α globin chain production and subsequent accumulation of the α-chains which is the major pathophysiologic route in the β-thalassemia syndromes. The vast majority of mutations causing β-thalassemia are non-deletional forms of which more than 180 point mutations have been characterized to date3.

The incidence of β-thalassemia trait in Bahrain is as low as 2%2 but it is the most severe amongst other hemoglobinopathies. It is manifested clinically in homzygous state, with a life-long blood transfusion dependency phenotype2. On the other hand most of the β-thalassemia heterozygote states are clinically asymptomatic with a distinctive hematological phenotype repisented by hypochromic, microcytic red blood cells and characteristically raised levels of HbA2. Exceptions to ie latter include coinheritance of α-thalassemia which will render HbA2 into a normal/borderline level. Moreover, the inheritance of β-thalassemia might be masked by coinheritance of sickle cell gene. Thus, molecular diagnosis took an important place as a useful tool to overcome these diagnostic obstacles.

The techniques of denaturing gradient gel electrophoresis (DGGE) and reverse dot blot (RDB) technique as well as direct DNA sequencing were applied in this first study to uncover the molecular basis of β-thalassemia in Bahrain. Moreover, β-haplotypes (patterns of arrangements of the restriction fragment length polymorphisms (RFLPs) in the β-globin gene cluster), were investigated for the uncovered mutations in order to identify possible origin(s) of these mutations.

The aim of this study is to identify the β-thal mutations among Bahrainis..

Methods

Patients: Eighty seven native Bahraini individuals representing 51 unrelated families were studied. The patients were divided as follows: 33 clinically homozygote β-thalassemia. 17 S-β thal and 37 simple heterozygotesAll of these individuals are attendees of the genetic and pediatrics departments at Sa]rnaniya Medical Complex, Bahrain. The genetic study was done in the mo]ecular laboratories in Robert Debré Hopital in Paris, France.

Some of the individuals studied were having β-thal major. They were blood transfusion dependent. Others were heterozygous (carrier) for β-thal with elevated HbA2 microcytosis and hypochromia.

Blood Analysis: The whole blood samples were collected in EDTA-anticoagulated vacutainers and analysed in automatic cell counter. Hb electrophoresis and HPLC analysis were performed according to established methodologies2'4.

DNA Extraction: Genomic DNA was isolated from leucocytes by the phenol-chloroform extraction method as described by Dracopli et a15.

PCR-DGGE and Sequencing: The specific amplification of the different β-globin gene fragments with subsequent DGGE analysis were performed according to previously published procedures6. Sequencing protocol was performed according to the dideoxy termination method7'3 utilizing the Sequenase Version 2.0 DNA sequencing kit (US Biochemical, Cleveland, USA). The same PCR products and primers of DGGE were used for sequencing.

Reverse Dot Blot: The reverse dot blot technique was used for further searching of explored mutations as described in previous studies9.10, except for utilising hybridization and washing at temperature of 42°C instead of 45°C.

Haploype Analysis: It is defined by seven polymorphic sites in the β-globin gene cluster, was performed using a PCR-RFLP procedure as described11-3. The polymorphic restriction sites studied were Xmnl-5'Gy, HindIII-Gy, HindIII-Ay, HincII-YB, HincII-Ψβ', AvaII- B, and HincfI-3' B

Figure 2. Haplotype analysis of the major J3-rhal mutations in Bahrain. fi-globin gene cluster is indicated with the restriction enzymes used as follows: Hf I, Hinf I; Av H, Ava II; Hc I?, Hinc II; Hd HI, Hind HI and Xm I, Xmn I. The Positive sign indicate presence of the recognition site for the enzyme and hence cutting, while negative sign indicate absence of the recognition site and thus no cleavage.

Results

A total of 70 B~1 chromosomes were characterized in this study. The frequency of each mutation is presented in Table 1 along with previously published freqüency data from three neighboring countries. The IVSI3' end (-25 bp) deletion allele represents the first major mutation in Bahrain with a frequency of 36%, followed by Cd 39 (C-4T), a nonsense

Meditenanean type mutation, that accounts for 26% of the mutations. The third major mutation is P151-5 (G—~C) which was found at a frequency of 16%. Thus, four B~' alleles comprised —80% of all charaterized β-thai mutations. The remaining 20% of the β-thai alleles were distributed among 10 different less frequent or rare mutations.

Haplotype analysis of the major and most common β-thalassemia mutations in Bahrain revealed each of them to be in linkage disequilibrium with specific haplotype(s) (Figure 2). However, each single mutation has a common framework background (defined here by the presence or absence of the restriction sites for Ava II and Hinf I).

In addition to the above findings the following technical 'features are noteworthy:

1. DGGE profile of homozygous state for codon 44 (-C) was behaving like normal pattern without any alteration in the melting profile. Consequently this mutation was not possible to be discovered by ordinary DGGE analysis. However by premixing PCR product of the patient with a homologous normal PCR product succeeded by instant denaturation and annealing steps prior to DGGE analysis. it was possible to characterize the abnormality in DGGE fragment under study through the induction of heteroduplex formation.
   Heteroduplex analysis in DGGE. (a) Identical melt-big profiles for both normal BA allele and homozygote mutant of Cd 44 (-C) (BCd44). (b) Induction of heterodreplex formation by mixing normal and mutant allele.c prior to DGGE.
   Another observation is the very distinct DGGE profile of the 25 bp deletion allele of heterozygote individuals which failed to give any of the expected heteroduplexes and displayed merely as two hornoduplexes (Figure 4). This is due to the internal deletion in the mutant allele which prevents formation of encompassing the deleted region with subsequent agarose gel elecnophoresis.
2. DGGE analysis showing failure of hererozygote cases of the 25 bp Deletion to give heteroduplexes. Samples 1,2,3 and 6 are normal controls for Framework (FW): 1/2, 1/3, 1/3a and 3a/3a, respectively. Samples 4,5 and 7 are Del/del (homozygote sample for deletion). del/3a and del/I, respectively.
3. Sequencing gel of the 25bp deletion allele. 'A' Stands for adenin, 'G'. guanin; 'C'. cytosine and 'T',

Figure 5b. A simple diagnostic strategy of the 25 bp deletion Sample 1 and .5 normal alleles: 2. 3 and 6 heterozygotes and sample 4 is homozvgote for the 25 bp deletion allele.. M is molecular weight marker No. VIII (Boehringer Mannheim, Germany).

Discussion

Thirteen different β thal alleles have been discovered in the Bahraini population throughout this study. However, three mutations. IVS I-3 end (-25 bp) deletion; Cd 39 (C→T) and IVSI-5 (G→C). comprised —80% of all B'~ alleles: Further three mutations, IVSII,1 (G→A); Cd 44 (-C) and IVSI. I (G→A). found to be less frequent with a total frequency of 13%, though the remaining seven mutations are rare.

Table 1. Spectrum of β-thalassemia mutations in Bahrain and three neighbouring countries

	c/c (No. of Chromosomes)					
Mutation	Bahrain	Kuwait(14)	UAE131	(Saudi Arabw'161	Western Saudi Arabiatt~2	Original Description
IVSI.3' end (~25 bp)	36 (25)	7.3 (7)	9.5 (24)	12.9 (24)	7.3 (3)	Asian Indian
Cd 39 (C→T)	26(18)	7.3 (7)	.4 (10)	12.9 (24)		Mediterranean
IVSI.5(G→C)	16 (11)	18.7 (18)	54..5 (138)	12.9 (24)	22.5 (9)	Asian Indian
IVSII.I (G→A)	6 (4)	29 (28)	3.5 (9)	12.9 (24)	25 (10)	Mediterranean
Cd44(-C)	4(3)	1(1)	1.6(4)	-	-	Kurds
IVSI,I (G→A)	3 (2)	7.3 (7)	-	-	-	Mediterranefln
nt - 101 (C→T)	1(1)	-	0.4 (1)	-	-	Turkish
nt – 88 (C→A)	1(1)	-	-	-	-	Kurds
Cd 8/9(+G)	1(1)	3.1 (3)	5.9(15)	-	-	Asian Indian
Cd 15 (G→A)	1(1)	-	0.8 (2)	-	-	Asian Indian
IVSI,110 (G→A)	1(1)	-	2 (5)	26.9 (50)	(17.5 7)	Mediterranean
Cd35(-C)	1(1)	-	-	-	-	Malay
Cd 41/42 (-CTIT)	1(1)	-	-	-	-	Chinese
Other mutations	-	26 (25)	17.5 (44)	20.4 (35)	42.5 (17)	
Total chromosomes	70	96	253	186	40	

Our results revealed similarities in type of mutations with published spectrums of 3t~~ mutations from other neighbouring countries, and in particular for the first four mutations found in Bahrain. albeit their different frequencies (Table 1. This may reflect a genetic admixture among people of these countries.

However, the IVSI-3' end (-25 bp) deletion seems to be the outstanding feature of this region with the frequency in Bahrain being the highest ever reported. This mutation was originally described in an Asian Indian individual18. However, it was reported as a rare defect in the Indian subcontinent at a frequency of Q•4%8• Adding all these observations together, this study proposes a unicentric origin of this mutation somewhere around the Arabian Gulf including the island of Bahrain.

Moreover, haplotype analysis indicate that IVSI-3' end (-25 bp) deletion is in linkage disequilibrium with two different haplotypes, both haplotype I and IX19. However both of these haplotypes have a common framework background (Figure 2). This finding along with the observed higher frequency of the mutant allele that is in linkage disequilibrium with haplorype IX more than haplotype I may suggest emergence of this mutation being exclusively on haplotype IX with subsequent dispersion of the deletion toward haplotype I by recombination event in the presumed hot spot 5' of the β-globin gene20.

Haplotype analysis of Cd 39 (C→T), a typical Mediterranean mutation, may exclude the possibility of introduction of this mutation into Bahrain via Mediterranean people. The majority of Cd 39 (C→T) alleles in the Mediterranean basin are in linkage disequilibrium with haplotypes I and II21• However, this study found it to be in linkage disequilibrium with haplotype VII, that lied on a different framework background19. This observation has been previously described in the Kurdish people22. Nevertheless, the mentioned study showed all of the major haplotypes bearing Cd 39 (C→T) mutation (haplotypes I and II as well as haplotype VII) are sharing a common identical (ATTT)n tandem repeats and (At)x (T)y motif in the 5' highly polymorphic region of the β -globin gene[22]. Thus, they concluded the unlikliness of recurrent mutational event of this mutation on haplotype VII versus haplotype I and II.

Haplotype analysis of the third major mutation in Bahrain. IVSI-5 (G→C), revealed this mutation to be in linkage disequilibrium with haplotype I. This is identical to a previously reported haplotype analysis from the United Arab Emfrates[23] but in contrast to haplotype VII found in Asian Indian by Varawalla, et al.[24]. The possibility of introducing this mutation via the Indian subcontinent cannot be excluded, however this conclusion is based upon realising that Varawalla's study did not include all of the Indian ethnic groups such as the Baluchis ethnic group, for example. In this group (Pakistan) this mutation has been described previously with a very high frequency of 76.2%[8]. The Baluchis are living in the vicinity of the Arabian Gulf region. Hence the possible introduction of this mutation via Baluchistan. Haplotype analysis is needed to assess this possibility. Alternatively, the mutation might be originated in the Arabian Gulf region as was proposed previously[23] and introduced subsequently into the neighboring people by gene flow through population migration and genetic drift.

Regarding technical aspects of this study, the DGGE analysis despite being a powerful and potent technique to detect any nucleotide variation on the DNA level should be utilized with a caution. In particular with the suspected homozygote states. As it was noticed in the 11 case of Cd 44 (-C) (Figure 3a & 3b), the diagnosis may not be reached without the deliberately induced heteroduplex formation prior to DGGE

Conclusion

We conclude that IVSI-3' end (-2Sbp) deletion is the major β-thalassemic allele in Bahrain.

Ref: Spectrum of Beta thalassemia mutation in Bahrain, Bahrain Medical Bulletin, Vol. 22, No 1, March 2000. page 8-12.

References

[1] Nadkarni, K. V., Al-Arrayed, 5. & Bapat, J. P. (1991). Incidence of Genetic Disorders of Haemoglobins in the Hospital Population of Bahrain. *Bahrain Med Bull, 13*, 19-24.

[2] Weatherall, D. J. & Clegg, J. B. (1981). The Thalassemia Syndromes. Oxford: Blackwefl Scientific Publications, Inc.

[3] Huisman, T. H. j. & Carver, M. (1998). The B and a Thalassemia 3- Repository. *Hemoglobin*, *22*, 169-95.

[4] Wilson, J. B., Headlee, M. E. & Huisman, T. H. J. (1983). A New High-performance Liquid Chromatographic Procedure for the Separation and Quantitation of Various Hemoglobin 1Variants in Adults and Newborn Babies. *J Lab Clin Med*, *102*, 174-86.

[5] Dracopli, N. C., et al. (1998). Isolation of Genomic DNA from Mammalian cells. Appendix 3B. Vol.2. Current Protocol in Human Genetics: John Wi1e~' & Sons Inc.

[6] Ghanem, N., Girodon, E., Vidaud, M., et al. (1992). Comprehensive 6-G Scanning Method for Rapid Detection of B -Globin Gene Mutations and Polymorphisms. *Bum Mutation*, 229-39.

[7] Sanger, F., Nicklen, S. & Coulson, A. R. (1977). DNA Sequencing with Chain-terminating Inhibitors. *Proc Natl Acad Sci USA*, *74*, 5463-9.

[8] Ahmed, S., Petrou, M. & Saleem, M. (1996). Molecular Genetics of BThalassemia in Pakistan: Basis for Prenatal diagnosis. *Br J Haematol*, *94*, 476-82.

[9] Maggio, A., Giambona, S. P., Cai, 5., et al. (1993). Rapid and Simultaneous Typing of Hemoglobin 5, Hemoglobin C, and Seven Mediterranean B -Thalassemia Mutations by Covalent Reverse Dot-Blot Analysis: Application to Prenatal Diagnosis in Sicily. *Blood*, *81*, 239-42.

[10] Cai, S. P., Wall, J., Kan, Y. W., et al. (1994). Reverse dot Blot Probes for the Screening of B-Thalassemia Mutations in Asians and American Blacks. *Hum Mutation*, *3*, 59-63.

[11] Sutton, M., Bouhassira, E. E. & Nagel, R. (1989). Polymerase Chain Reaction Amplification Applied to the Determination of B- Like Globin Gene Cluster Haplotypes. *Am J Hematol*, *32*, 66-9.

[12] Semenza, G. L., Dowling, C. E. & Kazazian, H. H. (1989). Hinf I Polymorphism 3' to the Human B -Globin Gene Detected by the Polymerase Chain Reaction (PCR). *Nucleic Acids Res*, *17*, 2376.

[13] Sampietro, M., Them, S. L., Cornreras, M., et al. (1992). Variation of HbF and F cell number with the G? Xmn I (C 'T) polymorphism in normal individuals. *Blood*, *79*, 832-3.

[14] Adekile, A. D., Gu, L. H., Baysal, E., et al. (1994). Molecular Characterization of a - Thalassemia Determinants, B -Thalassemia Alleles, and Bs Haplotypes among Kuwaiti Arabs. *Acta Haematologica*, *92*, 176-81.

[15] El-Kalla, 5., Mathews, A. R. (1997). A Significant B -Thalassemia Heterogeneity in The United Arab Emirates. *Hemoglobin*, *21*, 237-47.

[16] El-Hazmi, M. A. F. & A1-Swailem, A. R. (1995). Wars~' AS. Molecular Defects in Beta-Thalassemia in the population of Saudi Arabia. *Hum Hered*, *45*, 278-85.

[17] Hasounah, F. R., Sejeny, S. a. & Omer, J. A. (1995). Spectrum of B -Thalassemia Mutations in the Population of Saudi Arabia. *Hum Hered*, *45*, 231-4.

[18] Orkin, S. H., Sexton, J. P., Goff, S. C., et al. (1983). Inactivation of an Acceptor RNA Splice Site by a Short Deletion in B -Thalassemia. *J Biol Chenz*, *12*, 7249-51.

[19] Orkin, S. H., Kazazian, H. H., Antonarakis, S. E., et al. (1982). Linkage of 13-Thalassemia Mutations and B-G]obin Gene Polymorphisms with DNA Polymorphisms in Human B-Globin Gene Cluster. *Nature*, *296*, 627-31.

[20] Smith, R. A., Ho, P. J., Clegg, J. B., et al. (1998). Recombination Breakpoints in the Human B -Globin Gene Cluster. *Blood*, *92*, 4415-21.

[21] Flint, J., Harding, R., Boyce, A. C., et al. (1993). The Population Genetics of Hemoglobinopathies. In: Baillière's Clinical Hematology. London: *Baillière Tindall*, 215-62.

[22] Rund, D., Cohen, T., Filon, D., et al. (1991). Evolution of a Genetic Disease in an Ethnic Isolate: B -Thalassemia in Jews of Kurdistan. *Proc Natl Acad Sci USA*, *88*, 310-4.

[23] De Leo, R., Deidda, G., Novelletto, A., et al. (1995). Analysis of B - Thalassemia Mutations in the Unitded Arab Emirates Provides Evidence for Recurrent Origin of the IVSI nt 5 (G-C) Mutation. *Hum Mutation*, *5*, 327-8.

[24] Varawalla, N. Y., Fitches, A. C. & Old, J. M. (1992). Analysis of B -Globin Gene Haplotypes in Asian Indians: Origin and Spread of B -Thalassemia on the Indian Subcontinent. *Hum Genet*, *90*, 443-9.

Borderline HbA_2 Is Associated with β Thalasemia Hetrozygosity

Objectives: The aim of this study is to determine the prevalence of β thalasemia hetrozygosity among healthy subjects with borderline HbA_2.

Methods: Data were collected from student screening program for hemoglobin-opathies in the Kingdom of Bahrain among years 2004 and 2005. A total of 12000 students were examined. The examinations include full blood count and HPLC chromatograms. A total of 140 students had borderline HbA_2 level (3.4 – 4.0 %) with normal HbA, HbF, and HbS. Direct DNA sequencing of β globin gene was done to uncover the hotspot of β thalasemia mutation. SPSS was used for data analysis.

Results: 25 % of the total sample of borderline HbA_2 was found to have β thalasemia mutation. The major types of this mutation were nt -101 (C-G) (65.7%) and nt -71 (C-T) (22.8%) and (11.5%) had other sub mutation.

Conclusion: Based on our findings, we recommend that all borderline HbA_2 (3.4 – 4.0 %) should undergo DNA examination for β thalasemia mutations.

Prenatal Diagnosis in Bahrain

Introduction: Prenatal diagnosis is testing for conditions in a fetus before it is born. The aim is to detect birth defects such as neural tube defects, Down syndrome, chromosome abnormalities, genetic diseases, such as sickle cell anemia, thalassemia, cystic fibrosis, Muscular dystrophy.

Common testing procedures include chorionic villi biopsy, amniocentesis, ultra sonography, and serum marker testing, followed by genetic screening.

In KSA, in 1990 ruling (Fatwa) allows termination of pregnancy in the first 120 days after conception if the fetus is shown beyond doubt to be affected with a severe malformation that is not amenable to treatment. The Islamic republic of Iran has same Fatwas for certain condition such as thalassemia.

This service is available in many Islamic and Arab countries such as Turkey, Iran, Pakistan Palestine, Jordan, Egypt, Syria, United Arab Emirates, Saudi Arabia, Tunisia, Iraq, and Gaza. It is available internationally in countries such as India, Malaysia, south East Asia, Canada, Europe, and USA etc.

In Bahrain the service started in 2002, in a private setting, where prenatal testing only is provided.

Material and method: Patients were referred to the private clinic from their obstetricians. Indications being at risk for chromosomal abnormalities such as advanced maternal age, or presence of abnormal ultrasound finding. The other Indications being at risk of getting affected babies with SCD or betathalassemis.

Prenatal testing is done early in pregnancy either by CVS at (11 weeks) or amniotic fluid testing at 14 weeks. Samples were sent to genetic laboratories where cytogenetic or molecular testing was performed. Result was available within 7-10 day.

This service is provided in many other hospitals and clinics in Bahrain now.

Results: Total number of patients who undergo PND during the last 10 years in our clinic was 150 patients. Fifty patients were for chromosomal testing and 100 patients for genetic blood diseases.

Number of affected fetuses was low. In the chromosome cases, it was 4 babies/50 =8%. Among blood disease it was 5 babies/100 = 5%.

Genetic counseling provided prior to testing and after getting the results

Conclusion: PND service aim is to ensure the well being of babies and mothers, it also aim is to give the parents and healthcare staff the chance to prepare medically, psychologically and socially for the delivery of a child with a health problem It allow couple to have further healthy babies. The affected babies' number in our series was low. Further action has to be decided by the couple themselves.

Concerning patient care, free treatments are available, and depend on the type and severity of the disorder. These include blood transfusions, iron chelation therapy, and folic acid supplements.

Transfusions of red blood cells are the main treatment for people who have moderate or severe thalassemias. (often every 2 to 4 weeks). Iron Chelation Therapy: Deferoxamine and Deferasirox exjade are available. Many patients were sent abroad for Blood and Marrow Stem Cell Transplant as it is not available in Bahrain

Ref: unpublished data

Public Awareness about Beta Thalassemia in Bahrain

Abstract

Objectives: To measure the public awareness level about Beta thalassemia in Bahrain.

Methods: A questionnaire was distributed among 2000 persons from the general public. It was conducted from December 2006 to February 2007. The participants got personally interviewed face to face either by a health professional or a trained interviewer.

Results: Most (65.1%) had heard of beta thalassemia and (40.5%) knew that both parents have to be carriers to have an affected child. A majority of 1547 (77.8) strongly agreed that premarital checking can prevent beta thalassemia. Females showed better knowledge than males and married persons seems to know more about beta thalassemia than unmarried ones.

Conclusion: Our study sample seems to have a fair knowledge about beta thalassemia. Implicating the need for improving their basic knowledge of the disease. Further stress on the importance of continuing the screening campaigns specially the student screening program, premarital counseling and newborn screening service is also urged.

Introduction

Genetic diseases, especially hereditary blood disorders such as thalassemia syndromes and sickle-cell disease impose a significant burden on many countries. Their chronic nature with no prospect of cure makes them one of the leading causes of morbidity and mortality.

Beta thalassemia is a genetic disorder caused by mutations in the HBB gene on chromosome 11 and is inherited in an autosomal recessive fashion. The defective gene results in the absence of normal hemobglobin synthesis (β^o) or a reduced amount of functional hemoglobin (β^+). Individuals affected by Beta thalassemia major (β^o) develop severe anemia necessitating life long blood transfusion. If untreated, it causes in addition to anemia, splenomegaly,, and severe bone deformities with death occurring before the age of twenty. Therefore, a life long treatment with blood transfusion and iron-overload chelating medications is necessary to maintain life. A cure is possible with bone marrow or stem cell transplantation.

The incidence of genetic blood diseases in Bahrain is considered high. Previous neonatal screening in 1984-1985 showed that the birth prevalence of sickle cell disease (SCD) was 2.1%, of sickle cell trait 11% and of glucose-6-phosphate dehydrogenase (G6PD) deficiency 25% [1]. Recent student screening study for beta thalassemia major showed a prevalence of 0.06%, and beta thalassemia trait 5% in 2008 [2].

As a result of the high incidence of hemoglopinopathies in Bahrain the first genetic clinic was established in 1984, which started several educational campaigns. It was followed by launching the Bahrain Hereditary Anemia Society in 1991. In 1992, a national committee for the prevention of genetic diseases in Bahrain was established and a screening program dedicated to all pregnant women began, followed by newborn testing if the mother was found to be a carrier. Premarital counseling (PMC) service was started in 1993 and expanded to include all health centers [3]. In 2004 It the Bahrain Government has passed a law by which requires that all couples, who are planning to marry, undergo free mandatory premarital counseling [3]. Meanwhile student-screening project has been running annually since 1998 [4]. In 2007 newborn screening program for blood diseases has been launched [5]. All these programs have been accompanied by educational campaigns which aimed at increasing public awareness about beta thalassemia among other common hereditary blood disorders. In Bahrain and as far as we know there is no previous study to measure the people awareness about beta thalassemia. In this research we aimed at measuring the public awareness level about beta thalassemia in Bahrain.

Methodology

This is a cross sectional study. A questionnaire was constructed to cover three of the commonest inherited blood diseases in Bahrain which are Beta thalassemia, SCD and G6PD reduced activity. The first part of the questionnaire was some demographic data including personal information such as age, sex, job, level of education and social status. Only the part covering beta thalassemia is presented in this paper. The questionnaire was distributed among 2000 persons from the general public including different categories of the general population such as school teachers, secondary school students and others (non-probability convenience sample). It was conducted from December 2006 to February 2007. The participants got personally interviewed face to face either by a health professional or a trained interviewer.

As the study didn't implicate any ethical violations, no ethical approval has been obtained.

The obtained data was coded and processed by using SPSS (15.0). Frequency tables were obtained and special statistical tests were calculated such as Mann-Whiteny U test (nonparametric tests algorithms) and Kruskal-Wallis One-Way Analysis of Variance (nonparametric tests algorithms).

Results

The response rate was almost 100%. 1,106 females (55%) and 894 (45%) were males. While 689 (34.5%) of the respondents fall in the age group of 10 to 19 years only 15 (0.8%) were above the age of 30 [Table 1].

Of the respondents 583 were professionals, 406 (20.5%) were students and 618 (31.3%) were unemployed. The level of education for the interviewers ranged between illiterate to postgraduate. There were 966 (48.8%) school students, 900 (45.5%) university graduates, and 92 (4.6%) postgraduates, while 22 (1.1%) respondents were illiterate. One thousand fifty (53%) were single and 932 (47%) were married.

The questionnaire was composed of multiple choice questions and open-ended questions. The part that tested the level of awareness of beta thalassemia was composed of 12 multiple choice questions. The first question asks if they have ever heard of beta thalassemia. A majority of 1297 (65.1%) answered yes, in contrast to the 500 (25.1%) who have not heard of it. Upon asking if they knew about their blood status in regards to being affected, healthy or a carrier of beta thalassemia, only 560 (28.1%) answered yes, while 1431 (71.8%) didn't know. See table 2. When we asked about the genetic basis for the disease 809(40.5%) knew that both parents have to be carriers for beta thalassemia to have an affected child, 445 (22.3%) answered (No) and 742 (37.2%) didn't know.

Table 1. Age distribution

Age	No.	Percent
10-19	689	34.8
20-29	627	31.7
30-39	376	19.0
40-49	213	10.8
50-59	61	3.1
>50	15	0.8
Total	1,981	100.0

Table 2.

	Yes	No	Don't know
Have you ever heard of beta thalassemia?	1297 (65.1)	500 (25.1)	196 (9.8)
Do you know about your blood status in regards to being affected, healthy or a carrier of beta thalassemia?	560 (28.1)	1038 (52.1)	393 (19.7)
Do both parents have to have beta thalassemia trait for a baby to be born with beta thalassemia?	809 (40.5)	445 (22.3)	742 (37.2)
If one parent have SCT and the other parent have Beta thalassemia, can they have a baby with sickle cell disease?	891 (44.7)	274 (13.7)	828 (41.5)
Is beta thalassemia related to food?	344 (17.3)	643 (32.2)	1007 (50.5)
Do you think that regular blood transfusion is the treatment of beta thalassemia?	670 (33.9)	304 (15.4)	1003 (50.7)
33. Can beta thalassemia be cured by:			
a. Bone marrow transplant	542 (27.3)	247 (12.4)	1196 (60.3)
b. Gene therapy	507 (25.5)	221 (11.1)	1257 (63.3)
c. Stem cell transplant	394 (19.9)	360 (13.3)	1330 (67.1)

We also intended to test public knowledge of the possible genetic interaction between sickle cell trait (SCT) and beta thalassemia trait. 891 (44.7) recognized the possibility of having a child affected with SCD, 274 (13.7) answered (No) and **828** (41.5%) didn't know.

Upon asking whether the disease is related to food, 344 (17.3%) wrongly answered (Yes), 643 (32.2%) correctly answered (No) and 1007 (50.5%) didn't know.

Six hundred and seventy (33.9%) knew that blood transfusion is the treatment of the disease, 304 (15.4%) answered (No) and 1003 (50.7%) didn't know.

The majority didn't know that beta thalassemia can be cured by bone marrow or stem cell transplant 1195 (60.2%) and 1329 (67%) respectively. A majority of 1547 (77.8) strongly agreed that premarital checking can prevent beta thalassemia, so do health education and premarital laws 1350 (68.1%) and 1418 (71.3%) respectively. Table 3.

Those who had previously heard of SCD correctly answered all the 12 questions related to beta thalassemia (100%) (P<0.05). When we tested the relationship between the level of knowledge and gender, the responses were significantly different for 5 questions (42%) (P<0.05). Four of them answered correctly by females. Females showed better knowledge of beta thalassemia in regards to the nature of the disease and the mode of inheritance. While males had shown a better knowledge of the negligible effect of food on this disease (P<0.05).\

Table 3.

31. Do you think that beta thalassemia is preventable by:	Strongly Agree	Agree	Neither agree nor disagree
A. Premarital checking	1547 (77.8)	309 (15.5)	133 (6.7)
B. Health education	1350 (68.1)	498 (25.1)	135 (6.8)
C. Laws	1418 (71.3)	397 (20)	174 (8.7)

University students gave more accurate answers than the rest of respondents, five out of the 12 questions were answered correctly (42 %) (P<0.05). When we tested the relationship between the respondents' occupation and their level of awareness, the results were significant in 6 items. Professionals seemed significantly more knowledgeable in answering four questions of the total 12 (33.3%) and students were significantly more knowledgeable in answering two questions (17%) (P<0.05).

Respondents aged 60 and above and those falling in the 40-49 years age group gave equally significant correct answers compared to the rest of age groups. Both gave correct five answers (42%) (P<0.05). Married individuals correctly answered 7 of the12 questions (58%), which was significantly better than the knowledge of single individuals (P<0.05).

Discussion

In general respondents showed a fair basic knowledge of beta thalassemia. Almost two third (65.1%) have heard of beta thalassemia compared to 93.4% who have heard of SCD in the same sample (SS). In an Italian study (Armeli, et al.), 85% of their respondents had heard of beta thalassemia compare to 19 % Among Italian-Americans and 21% of Other-Americans [6]. In our sample, the majority didn't know about their own status (71.8%). Our results are similar to the Italian study in which 70% of the participants were not tested for beta thalassemia [6]. Only 40.5% understood the basis of inheriting the disease. A higher percentage has been scored in (Armeli) study (67%) but a lower one was found among Americans of non Italian origin (39%) [6]. In contrast to a study done among university students in Turkey where the percentage of students who had accurate knowledge was 25% for thalassemia. But this percentage was raised to 86.2 % following an informative lecture [7]. However, 44.7% of our respondents recognized the possible interaction between sickle cell trait and beta thalassemia trait. About one third of them knew that this disease is not related to ingesting specific food items. Only 33.9% knew that regular blood transfusion is the mainstay treatment for beta thalassemia compared to 63% among Italians and 19% among Americans [6]. In a Turkish study, 6.3% of the eleventh grade students wrote that blood exchange was used to treat the disease [7]. Almost two third of our respondents didn't know about bone marrow or stem cell transplant as a curative modalities for the disease (60.2%) and (67%) respectively. While in the Turkish study 6.3% of the students knew that blood exchange was used [7]. As expected, the majority agreed with the importance of premarital checking, health education and laws to prevent or reduce the incidence of the disease. Interestingly, those who have good knowledge about the disease have also good knowledge about other common blood diseases such as SCD. In general females showed better knowledge than males and these results are consistent with the results we obtained for other hemoglobinopathies [8]. This can be explained by the fact that females receive a considerable amount of knowledge during their antenatal care. Therefore, we recommend more educational campaigns targeting male population.

The respondents' level of education has also an impact on the level of awareness. It was noticed that respondents at the university level are more aware of hereditary blood disease than postgraduate. This can be explained by the fact that this category had been a target for the annual student screening program which started 10 years ago in 1999. Most of these students have graduated from school by the time this questionnaire has been conducted. In contrast to the post graduates who didn't have the exposure because of the time factor. These results are congruent with our findings in testing the awareness of SCD [8] However, Adewuyi, found that undergraduates in Nigeria had markedly deficient knowledge regarding SCD while the undergraduates in our study had a good knowledge regarding beta thalassemia, SCD as well as G6PD deficiency [9] and [8]. Lane et al., also found that knowledge of SCD was closely related to educational level [10].

As expected, married people know better than single people. Married couples have gone through premarital testing and counseling by law. Therefore, they appear to be more knowledgeable about these diseases. Therefore we strongly recommend that student screening program, premarital counseling, and newborn screening service must be continued as these national programs have proved to have tremendous impact. We also recommend that essential information about common blood diseases, including beta thalassemia, be included in school curriculums. Informational programs should target the male population, educate the public through the different media such as TV broadcasts, life lectures, and seminars, emphasize on the nature of inheritance of the common blood diseases, emphasize preventive measures, emphasize the differences between a carrier of an inherited blood disease and an affected individual.

Even though our study might have some limitations such as the sampling method, whom some might argue against. In this type of sampling a potential bias might be unknowable and the relationship between the target population and the survey sample might be immeasurable. Nevertheless, our justification is the large number of our sample.

Conclusion

In view of the relatively low incidence of beta thalassemia in Bahrain, our people seem to have a fair knowledge about the disease. These results show a substantial room for improving the basic knowledge of beta thalassemia among our population. We recommend further studies to test patients' awareness and attitude toward their illness. We further stress on the importance of continuing the screening campaigns specially the student screening program, premarital counseling and newborn screening service as these national programs proved to have tremendous impact in raising the awareness of beta thalassemia among the other common hemoglobinopathies in Bahrain.

Ref: Public awareness of G6PD in Bahrain, *Bahrain* Medical Bulletin **v33, no3, September 2011, page 147-149.**

References: Public Awareness about Beta thalassemia in Bahrain. Amani Al Hajeri, MD, CABFM, IBFM, MSc MG*,Shaikha Al Arrayed, MBCHB. DHCG. DHCM PhD**.

[1] Al Arrayed, S. (2005). Campaign to Control Genetic Blood Diseases in Bahrain. *Community Genetics*, *8*, 52-55.

[2] Al Arrayed, S. (2010). Beta Thalassemia Frequency in Bahrain: A Ten Year Study. Bahrain Medical Bulletin, *32* (2), 65-67.

[3] Al Arrayed, S. & Al Hajeri, A. (2005). Premarital genetic counseling: A new law in the Kingdom of Bahrain, *Journal of Health, Social and Environmental Issues*, *6* (2), 31-34.

[4] Al-Arrayed, S., Hafadh, N., Amin, S., Al-Mukhareq, H. & Sanad, H. (2003 May). Student screening for inherited blood disorders in Bahrain. *East Mediterr Health J.*, *9*(3), 344-52

[5] Al Arrayed, S., Hamza, A., Sultan, B., Shome, D. & Bapat, J. (2007). Neonatal Screening for Genetic Blood Diseases. *Bahrain Medical Bulletin*, *29* (3), 88-90.

[6] Armeli, C., Robbins, S. J. & Eunpu, D. (2005). Comparing knowledge of beta-thalassemia in samples of Italians, Italian-Americans, and non-Italian-Americans. *J Genet Couns*, *14*(5), 365-76.

[7] Gülleroğlu, S. K., Sarper, N. & Gökalp, A. S. (2007). Public education for the prevention of hemoglobinopathies: a study targeting Kocaeli University students. *Turk J Hematol*, *24*, 164–70.

[8] Al Arrayed, S. & Al Hajeri, A. (2010). Public awareness of sickle cell disease in Bahrain. *Annals of Saudi Medicine*, *30*(4), 284-288.

[9] Adewuyi, J. O. (2000). Knowledge of and attitudes to sickle cell disease and sickle carrier screening among new graduates of Nigerian tertiary educational institutions. *Niger Postgrad Med J*, *7*, 120-3.

[10] Lane, J. C. & Scott, R. B. (1969). Awareness of sickle cell anemia among negroes of Richmond, Va. *Public Health Rep.*, *84*(11), 949–953.

In: Thalassemia
Editor: Makenzie Greene
ISBN: 978-1-63117-954-9

Chapter 13

Dental and Orofacial Changes in Thalassemia Major: An Overview

Faiez N. Hattab, B.D.S., Ph.D., Odont. Dr.
Amman, Jordan

Abstract

Background. Thalassemia is one of the most common genetic disorders worldwide and presents public health and social challenges in areas of high incidence. The manifestations of the condition are modulated by several genetic, racial, and environmental factors. The homozygous type of β-thalassemia (thalassemia major, TM) is associated with most severe signs and symptoms.

Subjects and methods. A total of 54 TM patients aged 5.5 to 18.3 years and healthy controls (when appropriate) were examined for dental caries, oral hygiene, periodontal status, orofacial features, tooth size and dental arch dimensions, dental development, and physical pattern.

Results. The caries prevalence in TM patients was significantly higher ($P<0.001$) than the control group. Among cases, 61.1% had poor oral hygiene. Supra- and subgingival calculus was found in 32.5% of TM patients versus 21.8% in the controls. Only 7.8% of TM patients showed no sign of gingivitis versus 25.2% in the controls. The mean periodontal pocket depth in the patients was 2.7 ±1.4 mm versus 2.3 ± 1.2 mm in the controls. Clinical orofacial features of TM were: frontal bossing (61.1%), saddle nose (59.2%), dental and jaw pain (40.7%), maxillary protrusion (24.1%), "chipmunk" like face (16.7%) and malocclusion. Radiographical examination showed the followings: thickened frontal bone (67%), thinned mandibular cortex (65%), and maxillary sinus hypoplasia (42%). More than one-third of the patients exhibited enlarged marrow spaces with course trabeculation producing "chicken-wire" appearance of the alveolar bone, thin lamina dura, faint inferior alveolar canal and widened dipolic spaces. All means of tooth size and dental arches dimensions were reduced relative to the controls, with 20 of the 24 and 14 of the 16 measurements, respectively were statistically significant ($P<0.05$ to $P<0.001$). Growth retardation was present in 75.9% of the thalassemic patients, worsened after the age of 10 years. Mean body mass index was 16.5 ± 2.2 kg/m^2.

Conclusion. TM produces a variety of signs, symptoms and complications including high risk dental caries, periodontal diseases and oral infection as well as dental and orofacial changes. These changes should be taken into account when planning treatment with emphasis to maintain preventive program.

Introduction

Thalassemia is one of the most common genetic disorders worldwide and presents major public health and social challenges in areas of high incidence. The frequency of this disorder varies considerably with geographic locations and racial groups. Thalassemia refers to a group of inherited hemolytic anemia disorders that involve defects in the synthesis of hemoglobin α- or β-polypeptide chains.

It leads to decreased hemoglobin production and hypochromic microcytic anemia associated with erythrocyte dysplasia and destruction. Homozygous β-thalassemia (also known as thalassemia major, Cooley's anemia, or Mediterranean anemia) is associated with the most severe signs and symptoms.

Thalassemia major (TM) is a life-threatening condition that commonly manifests during early infancy, after which progressive pallor, severe anemia, and failure to thrive are common. Children with TM often develop feeding problems, recurrent fever, bleeding tendencies (especially epistaxis), susceptibility to infection, pathologic fractures of long bones and vertebrae, endocrine abnormalities, splenomegaly, lack of sexual maturation, and growth retardation (Lukens, 1993; Weatheral and Clegg, 2001). Hemoglobin level may be as low as 3 to 5 g/dL when a child with TM becomes symptomatic (Modell, 1976).

Skeletal and craniofacial deformities are the common manifestation of TM. They result primarily from hypertrophy and expansion of the erythroid marrow due to ineffective erythropoiesis. A close relationship between bone metabolism and erythropoietic activity has been documented as thalassemic patients show osteopenia with increased bone resorption, decreased mineralization, and decreased bone-forming sites (Lukens, 1993).

The aim of this review is to provide description of TM manifestations including: dental caries, oral hygiene and periodontal status, orofacial and craniofacial features, tooth crown size and dental arch dimensions, dental development, and physical growth. Discussion and practical recommendation is addressed.

Overview of Evidence

Dental Caries

The sample consisted of 54 Jordanian patients with TM, 31 males and 23 females aged 5.5 to 18.3 years, with the mean age (± SD) of 11.6 ± 3.2 years. The sample was divided into four subgroups according to age. The caries prevalence in TM patients was significantly higher ($P<0.001$) than the healthy control group, with an overall mean DMFT for 12-18 year olds was 6.26 compared to 4.84 for the control group.

The mean dmft/DMFT for the primary / permanent teeth and their individual components for each age group are presented in Table 1. The major contributors to dmft and DMFT were decayed teeth, accounting for 95.2% of total dmft and 92.7% of total DMFT (Hattab et al., 2001).

Kaplan et al. (1964) studied caries prevalence among 50 TM patients resident in Philadelphia. They found that thalassemic patients had caries activity 15.7% higher than the normal population. In a study on 21 Greeks with TM, it was found that TM patients had caries experience almost twice as high as that in control group. They exhibited a lower concentration of salivary immunoglobulin A (Siamopoulou-Mavridou et al., 1992). In addition, TM patients shown to have reduced salivary flow rate (Hattab et al., 2001) and higher levels of salivary *Strepotococcus mutans* compared with healthy subjects (Luglie et al., 2002).

Table 1. Caries experience in primary teeth (dmft) and permanent teeth (DMFT) and the mean values of decayed (d/D), missing (m/M), and filled (f/F) teeth in each age group of the thalassemic patients standard deviations of dmft/DMFT score in paranthesis

	Primary teeth	Permanent teeth
Age group	6-7 8-9	12-14 15-18
Decayed	6.59 4.29	6.09 5.33
Missing	0.25 0.18	0.26 0.35
Filled	0.08 0.25	0.22 0.27
Total dmft/DMFT	6.92 4.72	6.57 5.95
(±SD)	(4.54) (3.86)	(4.28) (3.74)

Hattab FN et al. (Int Dent J, 2001).

Oral Hygiene and Periodontal Status

The oral hygiene and periodontal status was assessed using plane mouth mirror, sickle explorer, and periodontal probe with William's marking. Plaque deposits were evaluated at four surfaces of six indexed teeth. The amount of accumulated plaque was graded according to the criteria of plaque index (P1.I) (Silness and Löe, 1964). Both supra- and subgingival calculus was recorded. Gingivitis was assessed using the criteria of gingival index (GI) (Löe and Silness, 1963). Periodontal condition was assessed by measuring the distance from the free gingival margin to the bottom of the gingival crevice (probing pocket depth, PPD). Results showed that 61.1% had poor oral hygiene (plaque score $\geq$ 2.0); that is moderate to accumulation of soft deposits within the gingival pocket. Thin plaque film (score 1) was found in 33.4% of the patients. Only 5.5% of the patients showed no visible plaque deposits. Supra- and subgingival calculus was found in 32.5% of thalassemic patients versus 21.8% in the controls The mean P1.I and GI scores in the thalassemic and control groups are presented in Table 2 (Hattab, 2012).

Thalassemic patients showed a tendency of higher P1.I and GI scores than the control groups, but the differences were statistically not significant. In both thalassemic and control groups, GI was significantly higher in older ages than the younger ones ($P<0.025$). The GI showed that 49.2% of the thalassemic patients had mild gingivitis (no bleeding on probing; score 0.1-1.0), 34.7% moderate gingivitis (bleeding on probing; score 1.1-2.0), 8.3% severe gingivitis (spontaneous bleeding; score 2.1-3.0). Only 7.8% showed no sign of gingivitis versus 25.2% in the controls. Of the thalassemic patients, 16.7% had gingival sulcus depth of 3 mm, 6.1% had pocket depth of 4-5 mm, and 1.9% exhibited pocket depth of $\geq$ 6 mm. The mean PPD in thalassemic patients was 2.7 ±1.4 mm versus 2.3 ± 1.2 mm in the controls (Hattab, 2012).

Table 2. Oral hygiene status and periodontal condition of thalassemic patients and unaffected control group measured by plaque index (P1.I) and gingival index (GI)

Age group	Thalassemic group	Control group
Years	(Mean ± SD)	(Mean ± SD)
	P1.I GI	P1.I GI
6-11 (n=23)	1.54 ± 0.44 1.30 ± 0.49	1.43 ± 0.63 1.24 ± 0.40
12-18 (n=31)	1.74 ± 0.57 1.56 ± 0.69	1.67 ± 0.68 1.48 ± 0.61

Hattab FN. (J Clin Pediatr Dent, 2012).

Clinical Orofacial Features

Frequencies of orofacial features of TM patients evaluated clinically and photographically are shown in Table 3 (Hattab, 2012).

More than half of the patients exhibited frontal bossing, saddle nose and to less extent maxillary protrusion; giving in severe cases a distinctive "chipmunk" like appearance. Observations indicate that the facial disfigurement increased with age and duration of symptoms in uncontrolled cases. Of the 54 patients examined, 33% had almost normal appearance (grade 0), 26% (grade 1), 24% (grade 2), and 16.7% (grade 3) (Figure 1). A study on Greek TM patients (mean age 10 ± 4 years) showed that 32% had normal appearance, 23% had mild maxillary overgrowth, and 14% displayed "rodent like facies" (Logothetis et al., 1971). Dental abnormalities in TM are shown in Figure 2.

Radiographic Craniofacial Features

Panoramic and lateral cephalometric radiographs were taken to evaluate dental, mandibular and craniofacial abnormalities in TM group. The findings are presented in Table 4 and depicted in Figure 3. The majority of the patients had thickened frontal bone and thinned inferior border (cortex) of the mandible.

Table 3. Prevalence of clinical orofacial complications in 54 thalassemic patients aged between 5.5 and 18.3 years

Manifestations	Number	Percentage
Frontal bossing	33	61.1
Saddle nose	32	59.2
Lip incompetence	28	51.8
Discolored teeth	24	44.4
Dental and jaw pain	22	40.7
Pallor oral mucosa	21	38.9
Headache	16	29.6
Increased overjet	14	25.9
Maxillary protrusion	13	24.1
"Chipmunk" facies	9	16.7

Manifestations	Number	Percentage
Nasal airway problem	9	16.7
Lower lip paresthesia	7	13
Parotid gland enlargement	3	5.6

Hattab FN. (J Clin Pediatr Dent, 2012).

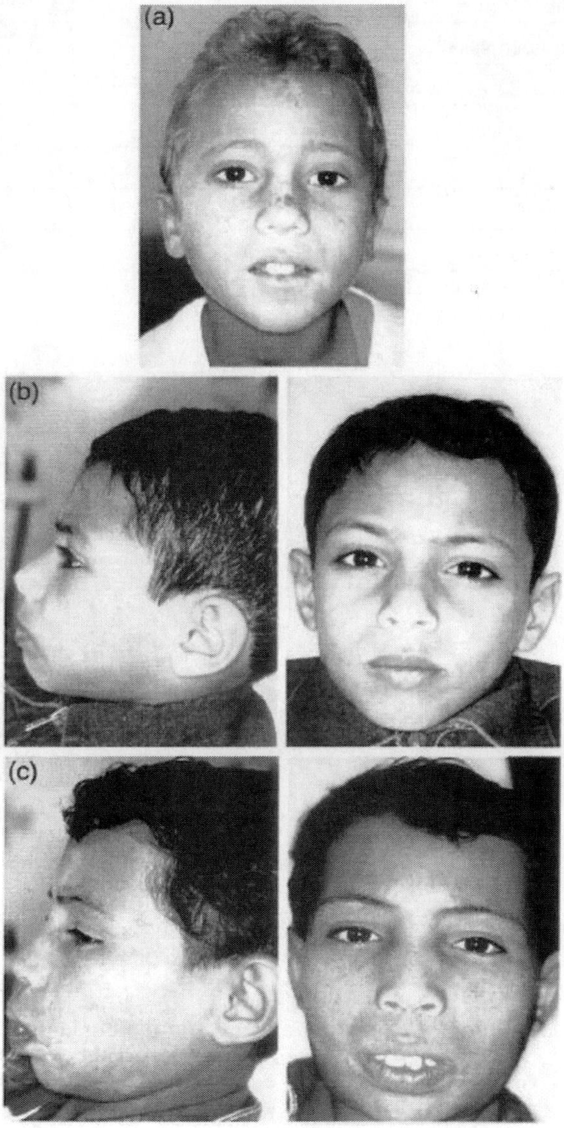

Figure 1. Grades of cephalofacial deformities in TM children. (a) Slight depression of the nose, puffiness of the eyelids with no maxillary overgrowth (grade 1). (b) Mild maxillary overgrowth and slight bulging of the frontal and cheek bones (grade 2). (c) Gross maxillary overgrowth (protrusive premaxilla), prominent frontal and malar bones, distinct saddle nose, drifting of the maxillary anterior teeth, and lip incompetence "chipmunk" faces (grade 3).

Table 4. Panoramic (n= 48) and lateral cephalometric (n= 33) radiographs showing the prevalence of oro-maxillofacial abnormalities in thalassemic group

Manifestations		Number		Percentage
Thickened frontal bone*		22		66.7
Thinned mandibular cortex**		31		64.6
Maxillary sinus hypoplasia*		14		42.4
Faint lamina dura**		19		39.6
Enlarged marrow spaces**		18		37.5
Widened dipolic spaces*		12		36.4
Spiky short roots**		16		33.3
"Hair-on-end" calvarium*		2		6.1

* Lateral radiographs, ** Panoramic radiographs.
Hattab FN. (J Clin Pediatr Dent, 2012).

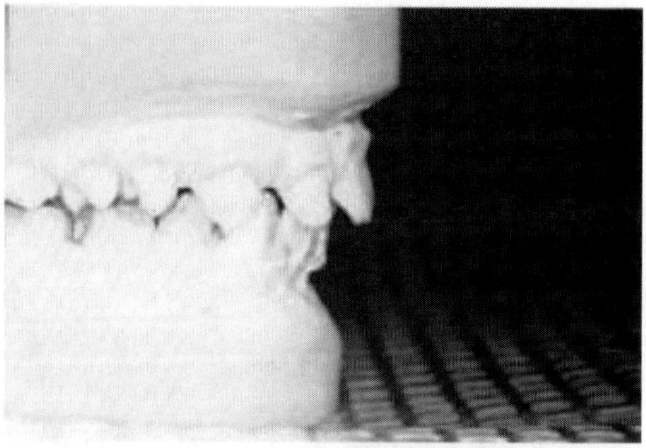

Figure 2. Dental cast showing maxillary protrusion, increased overjet, flaring of the maxillary anterior teeth, spacing of teeth, and malocclusion (Hattab FN. J Clin Pediatr Dent, 2012).

More than one-third of the patients exhibited enlarged marrow spaces with course trabeculation producing “chicken-wire” appearance of the alveolar bone, delayed pneumatization of the maxillary sinus, thin lamina dura, faint inferior alveolar canal and widened dipolic spaces (Hattab, 2012). In a study on 16 thalassemic cases, Poyton and Darvey (1968) reported that 88% of the cases had thickening of calvarium, faint lamina dura, and thin mandibular cortex.

The high frequency of abnormalities recorded in their study could be due to the limited number of cases. In a more recent study on 60 Thai thalassemic patients, Wisetsin (1990) showed that 73.3% had thin mandibular cortex, 63.3% had thickening of frontal bone, 8.3% had “hair-on-end” calvarium, and 5% showed absence of maxillary sinus. Cephalometric measurements showed that typical TM patients had a Class II skeletal pattern, short cranial base length, short mandible, increased anterior and reduced posterior vertical dimensions (Abu Alhaija et al., 2002; Amini et al., 2007).

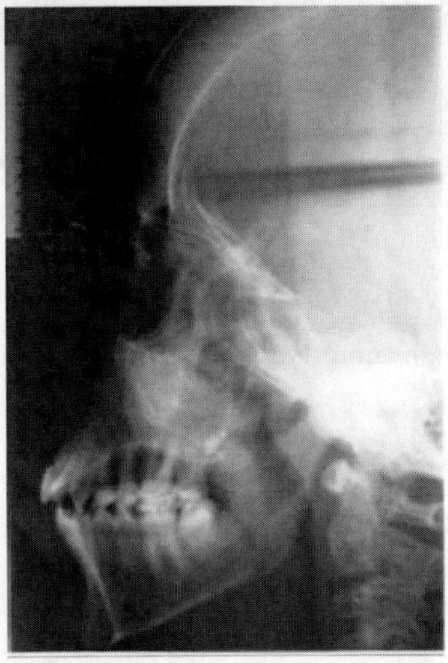

Figure 3. Cephalometric radiograph of a 15-year-old boy with TM disclosing thickened frontal bone, thinned inferior border of the mandible, and prominent premaxilla causing drifting of maxillary anterior teeth and increased overjet. Note partially obliterated maxillary sinus and widened dipolic spaces in the frontal bone (Hattab FN. J Clin Pediatr Dent, 2012).

Radiographic Measurements of Mandibular Dimensions

The linear and angular measurements of the mandible in the thalassemic and control groups were obtained from tracing the panoramic radiographs. The mean ramus length (62.5 ± 4.8 mm) and width (32.8 ± 2.6 mm) in thalassemic patients were reduced by 3.2 and 1.8 mm; respectively, compared with the control group. The differences were statistically significant ($P<0.001$). The mean intercondylar distance in thalassemic group (195.4 ± 11.7 mm) was reduced by 6.9 mm. Interestingly, the gonial angle was significantly larger in thalassemic than that in controls (Hattab, 2012).

Tooth Crown Size and Tooth Size Discrepancy

Measurement of the mesiodistal crown diameters (MD) was carried out using fine tips electronic digital sliding caliper reading to 0.1 mm. Results showed that all means for MD of thalassemic males and females were smaller than their controls, with 20 of the 24 comparisons being statistically significant (ranged from $P<0.05$ to $P<0.001$). In both thalassemic and control groups, males exhibited significantly larger MD than females in most instances (Hattab et al., 2000; Hattab, 2013a).

The tooth size ratio between maxillary and mandibular teeth was calculated as described by Bolton (1958):

$$\text{Anterior ratio} = \frac{\text{Sum of MD of mandibular six anterior teeth (33 to 43)}}{\text{Sum of MD of maxillary six anterior teeth (13 to 23)}} \times 100$$

$$\text{Overall ratio} = \frac{\text{Sum of MD of mandibular 12 teeth (36 to 46)}}{\text{Sum of MD of maxillary 12 teeth (16 to 26)}} \times 100$$

There was no statistically significant differences in the anterior and overall tooth size ratios between thalassemic and control groups. The mean anterior ratio was 79.5% and overall ratio 92.4%.

Dental Arches Dimensions

Measurements of arch dimensions were made on the dental casts (Figure 4). The segmental arch lengths in the maxilla and mandible of thalassemic group were reduced by an average of 2.59 and 2.55 mm respectively, compared with the control group. The mean maxillary and mandibular arch depths (lengths) were shorter by 3.21 and 2.63 mm respectively, relative to the controls ($P<0.001$). All arch widths in thalassemic patients were significantly reduced by an average ranged from 1.33 to 1.90 mm in the maxilla and 1.37 to 1.77 mm in the mandible (Hattab and Yassin, 2011).

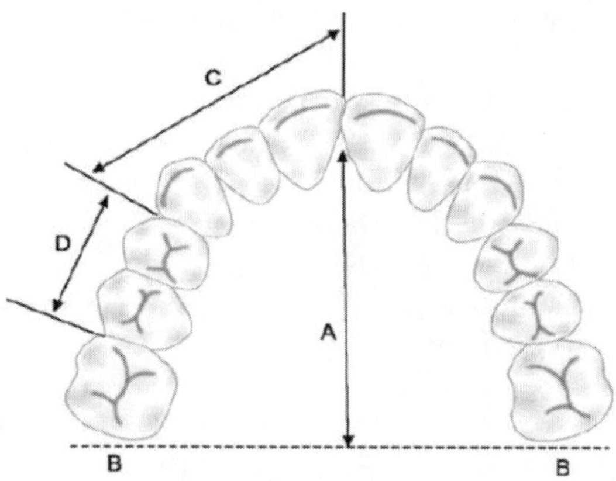

Figure 4. Dental arch measurements: (A) arch depth; (B) arch perimeter; (C) anterior arch length; (D) posterior arch length (Hattab FN, Yassin OM. J Contemp Dent Pract. 2011).

Physical Growth and Dental Development

Growth retardation (<10th percentile for height and weight) was present in 75.9% of the thalassemic patients. Height less than the 3rd percentile were noted in 41.9% of males and 34.8% of females. The data show that growth retardation was worse in patients older than 10 years: 45.4% of patients aged 6-10 years had heights less than the third percentile versus 68.7% of patients older than 10 years. The body mass index (BMI) of thalassemic patients was 16.5 ± 2.2 kg/m^2. BMI was less than the 10th percentile in 21.6% of participants younger than 10 years versus 37.2% of those older than10 years (Hattab, 2013b).

The development of the dentition is an integral part of craniofacial growth. Dental development or maturity, expressed as dental age (DA), is considered one of the most reliable indictors of chronological age (CA). Panoramic radiographs of thalassemic patients were taken and the dental development of the seven left mandibular teeth was assessed applying the method of Demirjian et al., (1973). Results revealed a delay in dental development in 79.5%; with mean delay 1.12 years in males and 0.81 in females. Dental development in thalassemic patients was significantly delayed relative to their CA (average = 0.97 years, $P<0.001$). Dental development was more advanced in females had in males. The association between DA and CA was stronger than that between DA and body growth ($r = 0.87$ vs. 0.58) (Hattab, 2013b).

Discussion and Practical Recommendations

Primary management of patients with TM can be considered under four headings: transfusion therapy, iron chelation agents, splenectomy, and bone marrow transplantation. The goals of transfusion include correction of anemia, suppression of erythropoiesis, retard the development of splenomegaly, and inhibition of increased gut absorption of iron (Modell, 1976; Lukens, 1993). Iron overloading (hemosiderosis) from high gut absorption and from repeated transfusions eventually leads to cardiomyopathy, liver and pancreas dysfunction. Iron deposition in the parotid glands can result in painful facial swelling but is rare (Goldfarb et al., 1983; Hattab, 2012). Iron deposits have also been found in the gingivae (Caliskan et al., 2011). Deposition of bilirubin; a degraded product of hemoglobin, during the formation of hard dental tissues been found to cause yellow discoloration of teeth (Hattab et al., 1999).

Infections are major complications and a main cause of morbidity in patients with TM which should be taken into account when providing dental care. Patients who have undergone a splenectomy are at higher risk of massive infection following bacteremia (Wang et al., 2003). In such cases antibiotic prophylaxis similar to that used for the prevention of bacterial endocarditis should be prescribed prior to invasive procedure. All splenectomized children under five years of age should be treated with prophylaxis antibiotics; oral penicillin125 mg twice daily for children under two years, and 250 mg twice daily for children two years and over (Terezhalmy, 1984). Multiple immune abnormalities (Vento et al., 2006), defective neutrophils and macrophage chemotaxis (Khan et al., 1984; Wiener, 2003) and increased the oral *Candida albicans* colonization (Van Dis and Langlais, 1984) have been noted in the thalassemic patients. Children should receive immunization with pneumococcal vaccine and influenza vaccination after six months of age, and meningococcal vaccination after 2 years of age. Because thalassemic patients are at increased risk of viral hepatitis, appropriate precautions should be taken by the dental team when these patients are to be treated.

TM patients suffer from chronic anemia manifested by loss of appetite, fatigue, lethargy, and headache. Dental care should be adapted to their tolerance of the planned procedure on the day of treatment. As in other hemolytic disorder, TM patients are susceptible to folate deficiency. Affected subjects should avoid foods that contain iron such as infant cereal, liver, oysters, pork, beef, beans, peas, and spinach. Foods that inhibit iron absorption are coffee, tea, chocolate, and soy products. Because osteoporosis is common in thalassemia, patients must obtain plenty of calcium with vitamin D. Dairy products are a good sources of calcium and they reduce iron absorption.

The evidence presented indicates that patients with TM are at risk for dental caries and periodontal disease. This could primarily be related to local factors including poor oral hygiene, improper dietary habits, reduced salivary flow rate, malocclusion, lack of dental awareness, and neglected dental care. In addition, periodontitis may be aggravated by systemic factors including lowered resistance to infection, nutritional deficiencies, and chronic anemia. Therefore, patients should be maintained on a preventive program with regular follow-up. Oral hygiene instructions, diet counselling, and preventive measures including prophylaxis, fluoride application, and fissure sealant should be emphasized to minimize the need for extensive dental procedures.

Reduction in tooth size and dental arches in thalassemic patients have an impact on the occlusal relationships. An appropriate maxillary to mandibular tooth size ratio is important for the achievement of proper interdigitation, overjet, and overbite during the final stages of orthodontic treatment. Discrepancy between tooth size and arch length result in dental crowding being the most common cause of malocclusion. Correction of forward drifted maxillary anterior teeth and increased overjet should be undertaken to improve esthetic, reduce susceptibility to trauma, avoid gingival inflammation, and improve functional ability. It is recommended that orthodontic treatment be initiated as early as possible concentrating on preventive and interceptive approaches.

The cause of growth retardation in children with TM is multifactorial and includes chronic anemia and hypoxia, iron overload, low somatomedin activity, endocrinopathies, low socioeconomic status, and racial factors (Lukens, 1993; Gulati et al., 2000; Weatheral and Clegg, 2001). A review of the literature reveals some inconsistency regarding the age at which growth retardation occurs in children with TM. Some reports found that slowing of growth was more evident as puberty approached (Borgna-Pignatti et al., 1985; Kattamis et al., 1990), while others noted a tendency for retarded growth at age 8-10 years (Yesilipek et al., 1993). Recent study of Indian children with TM showed marked growth retardation in height and weight after age 11 years in boys and after age 9 years in girls (Saxena, 2003). Our data on Jordanian patients shows that growth retardation worsened after the age of 10 years (Hattab, 2013b). Lapatsanis et al. (1978) noted that half of TM children aged 5-7 years had bone retardation (> 6 months), whereas after this age bone retardation was found in almost two-thirds of the cases. Saxena (2003) found that bone age retardation in TM increased with age and that it started much earlier than height and weight retardation.

Physical growth patterns of individuals with TM have been studied in a number of populations. Borgna-Pignatti et al. (1985) reported that, among 250 Italian adolescents with TM, 62% of males and 35% of females had short stature. Kattamis et al. (1990) found that 21.7% of males and 13% of females had growth retardation among a group of 405 Greeks with TM; the highest incidence of growth retardation was among those aged 15-20 years. A study of 68 Chinese children with TM in Hong Kong showed that 75% of girls and 62% of boys older than 12 years were below the third percentile of height (Kwan et al., 1995). The considerable variation in the prevalence of growth retardation among TM patients must be interpreted in the light of anemia severity, timing and frequency of blood transfusion, age at initiation of iron chelation therapy, bone marrow transplantation, and socioeconomic background. In addition, thalassemia is a disease in which manifestations are modulated by several genetic, racial, and environmental factors.

There was a significant delay in dental development among TM participants. Further, there was a significant correlation between the extent of this delay and CA, but not between dental maturity and physical development (Hattab, 2013b). This is in accordance with the findings that dental development is less influenced than somatic development by environmental factors (Garn et al., 1965; Demirjian et al., 1985; Cardoso, 2007). In parallel with the general growth retardation; a significant delay in the dental development, reduction in tooth crown size and dental arches dimensions was evident.

Most patients with TM can be treated normally, using local anaesthetic supplemented if necessary with inhalation sedation (Duggal et al., 1996). Because of the possibility of impairing local circulation, short procedure can be performed using anaesthetic without vasoconstrictor. However, if the procedure requires long, profound anaesthesia, 2% Lidocaine with 1/100,000 epinephrine is the anaesthetic of choice. Nitrous oxide can be safely used as far as the concentration of oxygen is greater than 50%, the flow rate is high, and the patient is able to ventilate adequately. General anaesthesia is hazardous in this group of patients because of anemia hypoxia. Psychological adjustment should be considered to improve the quality of life, enabling patients to live normal life.

Conclusion

Thalassemia major is a lifelong condition requiring ongoing medical and dental treatment. It produces a variety of signs, symptoms and complications including high risk dental caries, periodontal diseases and oral infection as well as dental and orofacial changes.

Pediatric dentists and orthodontists must be mindful of these changes when planning treatment. Emphasis should be given to maintain preventive program, with consideration to improve appearance and function in patients with malocclusion and facial deformities. Regular nutritional assessments should be done, with specific attention to iron-containing foods, calcium, vitamin D, and diabetes. The psychosocial needs of thalassemic patients should be prioritized in ongoing treatment.

References

Abu Alhaija ESJ, Hattab FN, al-Omari MA. Cephalometric measurements and facial deformities in subjects with β-thalassemia major. *Eur J Orthod.* 2002;24:9–19.

Amini F, Jafari A, Eslamian L, et al. A cephalometric study on craniofacial morphology of Iranian children with beta thalassemia major. *Orthod Craniofac Res.* 2007;10:36-44.

Borgna-Pignatti C, De Stefano P, Zonta L, et al. Growth and sexual maturation in thalassemia major. *J Pediatr.* 1985;106:150-155.

Bolton WA. Disharmony in tooth size and its relation to analysis and treatment of malocclusion. *Angle Orthod.* 1958;28:113-130.

Calişkan U, Tonguç MO, Ciriş M, et al. The investigation of gingival iron accumulation in thalassemia major patients. *Pediatr Hematol Oncol.* 2011;33:98-102.

Cardoso HFV. Environmental effects on skeletal versus dental development: using a documented subadult skeletal sample to test a basic assumption in human osteological research. *Am J Phys Anthropol.* 2007;132:223-233.

Demirjian A, Goldstein H, Tanner JM (1973) A new system of dental age assessment. *Hum Biol.* 45, 211-227.

Demirjian A, Buschang PH, Tanguay R, et al. Interrelationships among measures of somatic, skeletal, dental and sexual maturity. *Am J Orthod.* 1985;88:433-438.

Duggal MS, Bedi R, Kinsey SE, et al. The dental management of children with sickle cell disease and β-thalassaemia: a review. *Int J Paediatr Dent.* 1996;6:227-234.

Garn SM, Lewis AB, Blizzard RM. Endocrine factors in dental development. *J Dent Res.* 1965;44:243-258.

Goldfarb A, Nitzan DW, Marmary Y. Changes in the parotid salivary gland of beta-thalassemia patients due to hemosiderin deposits. *Int J Oral Surg.* 1983;12:115-119.

Gulati R, Bhatia V, Agarwal SS. Early onset of endocrine abnormalities in β-thalassemia major in developing country. *J Pediatr Endocrinol Metab.* 2000;13:651-656.

Hattab FN, Qudeimat MA, Al-Rimawi HS. Dental discoloration: an overview. *J Esthet Dent.* 1999;11:291-310.

Hattab FN, Abu-Alhaija ESJ, Yassin OM. Tooth crown size of the permanent dentition in subjects with thalassemia major. *Dent Anthlop.* 2000;14:7-13.

Hattab FN, Hazza'a AM, Yassin OM, et al. Caries risk in patients with thalassemia major. *Int Dent J.* 2001;51:35–38.

Hattab FN, Yassin OM. Dental arch dimensions in subjects with β-thalassemia major. *J Contemp Dent Pract.* 2011;12:429-433.

Hattab FN. Periodontal condition and orofacial changes in patients with thalassemia major: a clinical and radiographic overview. *J Clin Pediatr Dent.* 2012; 36:301-308.

Hattab FN. Mesiodistal crown diameters and tooth size discrepancy of permanent dentition in thalassemic patients. *J Clin Exp Dent.* 2013a;5:239-244.

Hattab FN. Patterns of physical growth and dental development in Jordanians children and adolescents with thalassemia major. *J Oral Sci.* 2013b;55:71-77.

Kaplan RI, Werther R, Castano FA. Dental and oral findings in Cooley's anemia: a study of fifty cases. *Ann NY Acad Sci.* 1964;119:664–666.

Kattamis C, Liakopoulou T, Kattamis A. Growth and development in children with thalassemia major. *Acta Paediatr Scand Suppl.*1990;366:111-117.

Khan AJ, Lee C-K, Wolff JA, et al. Defects of neutrophil chemotaxis and random migration in thalassemia major. *Pediatrics.* 1977;60:349-351.

Kwan EY, Lee AC, Li AM, et al. A cross-sectional study of growth, puberty and endocrine function in patients with thalassaemia major in Hong Kong. *J Paediatr Child Health.* 1995;31:83-87.

Logothetis J, Economidou J, Constantoulakis M, et al. Cephalofacial deformities in thalassemia major (Cooley's anemia). *Am J Dis Child.* 1971;121:300-306.

Löe H, Silness J. Periodontal disease in pregnancy. Part I. Prevalence and severity. *Acta Odontol Scand.* 1963;21:533-551.

Luglie PF, Campus G, Deiola C, et al. Oral condition, chemistry of saliva, and salivary levels of streptococcus mutans in thalassemic patients. *Clin Oral Investig.* 2002; 6:223-226.

Lukens JN. *The thalassemia and related disorders: quantitative disorders of hemoglobin synthesis*. In Lee GR, Bithell TC, Foster J, Athens JW, Lukens JN, editors. Wintrobe's Clinical Hematology, 9th ed. Philadelphia: Lea &Febiger, 1102-1133, 1993.

Modell B. Management of thalassemia major. *Br Med Bull*. 1976;32:270-276.

Poyton HG, Davey KW. Thalassemia: Changes visible in radiographs used in dentistry. *Oral Surg Oral Med Oral Pathol*. 1968;25:564-576.

Saxena A. Growth retardation in thalassemia major patients. *Int J Hum Genet*. 2003;3: 237-246.

Siamopoulou-Mavridou A, Mavridis A, Galanakis E, et al. Flow rate and chemistry of parotid saliva related to dental caries and gingivitis in patients with thalassemia major. *Int J Pediatr Dent*. 1992;2:93-97.

Silness J, Löe H. Periodontal disease in pregnancy. Part II. Correlation between oral hygiene and periodontal condition. *Acta Odontol Scand*.1964; 22:121-135.

Terezhalmy GT, Hall ET. The asplenic patients: a consideration for antimicrobial prophylaxis. *Oral Surg Oral Med Oral Pathol*. 1984;57:114-117.

Van Dis ML, Langlais RP. The thalassemias: Oral manifestations and complications. *Oral Surg Oral Med Oral Pathol*. 1986;62:229-233.

Vento S, Cainelli F, Cesario F. Infections and thalassemia. *Lancet Infect Dis*. 2006; 6: 226-233.

Wang SC, Lin KH, Chern JPS, et al. Severe bacterial infection in transfusion-dependent patients with thalassemia major. *Clin Infect Dis*. 2003;37:984-988.

Weatheral JD, Clegg JB. The Thalassemia Syndrome, 4th ed. Oxford: *Blackwell Scientific*; 2001.

Wiener E. Impaired phagocyte antibacterial effector functions in β-thalassemia: A likely factor in the increased susceptibility to bacterial infections. *Hematology*. 2003;8:35-40.

Yesilipek MA, Bircan I, Oygur N, et al. Growth and sexual maturation in children with thalassemia. *Haematologica*. 1993;78:30-33.

Index

A

B

C

D

E

F

H

I

J

K

L

M

N

O

P

Q

R

S

T

U

V